Late-Life Depression and Anxiety

Late-Life Depression and Anxiety

Edited by

Art Walaszek, M.D.

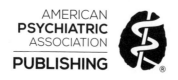

AMERICAN
PSYCHIATRIC
ASSOCIATION
PUBLISHING

If you wish to buy 50 or more copies of the same title, please go to www.appi.org/specialdiscounts for more information.

Copyright © 2022 American Psychiatric Association Publishing

ALL RIGHTS RESERVED

First Edition

Manufactured in the United States of America on acid-free paper
26 25 24 23 22   5 4 3 2 1

American Psychiatric Association Publishing
800 Maine Avenue SW, Suite 900
Washington, DC 20024-2812
www.appi.org

Library of Congress Cataloging-in-Publication Data
Names: Walaszek, Art, 1972– editor. | American Psychiatric Association Publishing, issuing body.
Title: Late-life depression and anxiety / edited by Art Walaszek.
Description: First edition. | Washington, DC : American Psychiatric Association Publishing, [2022] | Includes bibliographical references and index.
Identifiers: LCCN 2021053640 (print) | LCCN 2021053641 (ebook) | ISBN 9781615373475 (paperback ; alk. paper) | ISBN 9781615374410 (ebook)
Subjects: MESH: Depression | Aged | Anxiety Disorders | Geriatric Assessment—methods
Classification: LCC RC537.5 (print) | LCC RC537.5 (ebook) | NLM WM 171.5 | DDC 618.97/68527—dc23/eng/20220106
LC record available at https://lccn.loc.gov/2021053640
LC ebook record available at https://lccn.loc.gov/2021053641

British Library Cataloguing in Publication Data
A CIP record is available from the British Library.

CONTENTS

Contributors

Eileen Ahearn, M.D., Ph.D.
Clinical Adjunct Professor of Psychiatry, University of Wisconsin School of Medicine and Public Health, Madison, Wisconsin

Anna Borisovskaya, M.D.
Psychiatrist, SeattleNTC, Seattle, Washington

Lisa L. Boyle, M.D., M.P.H.
Adjunct Clinical Professor of Psychiatry, University of Wisconsin School of Medicine and Public Health, Madison, Wisconsin

William Bryson, M.D., Ph.D.
Acting Assistant Professor, Department of Psychiatry and Behavioral Sciences, University of Washington; Veterans Affairs Puget Sound Healthcare System, Seattle, Washington

Elizabeth Chmelik, M.D.
Clinical Assistant Professor, Department of Psychiatry and Behavioral Sciences, University of Washington; Veterans Affairs Puget Sound Healthcare System, Seattle, Washington

Samantha May, M.D.
Psychiatry Resident, Department of Psychiatry, Samaritan Health Services, Corvallis, Oregon

Marcella Pascualy, M.D.
Associate Professor, Department of Psychiatry and Behavioral Sciences, University of Washington; Veterans Affairs Puget Sound Healthcare System, Seattle, Washington

Rebecca M. Radue, M.D.
Geriatric Psychiatrist, William S. Middleton Memorial Veterans Hospital, Madison, Wisconsin

Courtney Roberts, M.D.
Psychiatry Resident, Department of Psychiatry, UCLA–Olive View Medical Center, Los Angeles, California

Matthew Schreiber, M.D.
Acting Assistant Professor, Department of Psychiatry and Behavioral Sciences, University of Washington; Veterans Affairs Puget Sound Healthcare System, Seattle, Washington

Art Walaszek, M.D.
Professor of Psychiatry, University of Wisconsin School of Medicine and Public Health, Madison, Wisconsin

Lucy Y. Wang, M.D.
Assistant Professor, Department of Psychiatry and Behavioral Sciences, University of Washington School of Medicine, Seattle, Washington

DISCLOSURES

The following contributor to this book has indicated a financial interest in or other affiliation with a commercial supporter, a manufacturer of a commercial product, a provider of a commercial service, a nongovernmental organization, and/or a government agency, as listed below:

Art Walaszek, M.D.   *Grant support:* National Institute on Aging, U.S. Administration on Community Living, UW Wisconsin Partnership Program. *Honoraria:* Advocate Lutheran General Hospital, United Way/Pharmacy Society of Wisconsin Investigator. *Not compensated:* Eisai Network Companies.

The following contributors have indicated that they have no financial interests or other affiliations that represent or could appear to represent a competing interferes with their contributions to this book:

Eileen Ahearn, M.D., Ph.D.; Anna Borisovskaya, M.D.; Lisa L. Boyle, M.D., M.P.H.; William Bryson, M.D., Ph.D.; Elizabeth Chmelik, M.D.; Samantha May, M.D.; Marcella Pascualy, M.D.; Rebecca M. Radue, M.D.; Matthew Schreiber, M.D.; Lucy Y. Wang, M.D.

Preface

We all want to age well. What this mean varies from person to person, so here's my list: to have loving and respectful relationships with my family and friends; to live with meaning and purpose and in a way that is consistent with my values; to be emotionally, cognitively, and physically healthy; to be able to make choices that benefit my community, my family, and myself; and to be resilient in the face of the inevitable stressors of aging.

Depression and anxiety disorders threaten our ability to age successfully. Whereas sadness, grief, and worry are core parts of being a human, depression and anxiety disorders are not inevitable. But they are emotionally painful, physically uncomfortable, disabling, and potentially fatal. Suicide is a significant global health problem, especially among older adults, and depression contributes mightily to the risk of suicide.

Thankfully, we can identify people with late-life depression and anxiety, we can diagnose them accurately, and we can offer treatment that works. In other words, people suffering from these conditions can find relief, maintain their independence, and lower their risk of dying from suicide.

My coauthors and I wrote this book to provide health care professionals with evidence-based, pragmatic, and clear recommendations regarding the care of people with late-life depression and anxiety. Although we certainly wanted to be scholarly, we wrote in a conversational tone—as if we were all in a room together discussing how best to assess and help our patients. We believe that anyone involved in the care of older adults—primary care physicians, geriatricians, psychiatrists, neurologists, residents and fellows, medical students, psychologists, advanced practice providers, social workers, and nurses—will find this book useful.

The book begins with an overview of late-life depression (Chapter 1) and late-life anxiety (Chapter 2), including their public health impact, epidemiology, clinical presentation, and course, as well as consequences, complications, and comorbidities. We move on to the assessment of the depressed or anxious older adult in Chapter 3 and guide the reader from interviewing a patient to making the diagnosis. Given how important it is to assess and reduce the risk of suicide among older adults, we have devoted Chapter 4 to the topic. In Chapter 5, we try to answer the question "How can we best help our patients suffering from late-life depression or anxiety?" In other words, we review the evidence base and present recommendations regarding psychotherapy, medications, electroconvulsive therapy, complementary and alternative medicine, and other approaches. We close with the crucial topic of ensuring that health care professionals provide culturally sensitive care to racial/ethnic, sexual, and other minority elders (Chapter 6); we have also tried to weave this consideration into the narrative throughout the book. In each chapter, we list key points to provide readers with a quick summary of the content; provide online and other resources for patients, family members, and clinicians; and include plenty of figures to help illustrate the material.

We hope that our readers will find *Late-Life Depression and Anxiety* to be readable and helpful. And we hope that older adults who are suffering from depression or anxiety will benefit—and will age well.

Art Walaszek, M.D.
Madison, Wisconsin
April 2021

Acknowledgments

Eileen Ahearn: Many thanks to Dr. Art Walaszek for organizing and guiding this project. I am thankful for my wonderful colleagues at the William S. Middleton Memorial Veterans Hospital, including Dr. Lisa Boyle and Dr. Rebecca Radue. It is a privilege to work with them and to serve our aging veteran population.

Lisa Boyle: I would like to thank all of the wonderful mentors, residents, fellows, interprofessional team members, and patients I have learned from and been fortunate to work with over the past 20 years of my career at the University of Wisconsin, University of Michigan, University of Rochester, and the William S. Middleton Memorial Veterans Hospital. Specifically, my deepest gratitude for all the support over the years from Drs. Molly Carnes, Steve Barczi, Timothy Howell, Barbara Kamholz, Susan Maixner, Helen Kales, David Knesper, Michael Jibson, Jeffrey Lyness, Yeates Conwell, Carol Podgorski, Deborah King, Anton Porsteinsson, Paul Katz, Annie Medina-Walpole, P.J. Chen, E.J. Santos, Tom Caprio, Eileen Ahearn, Rebecca Radue, and Art Walaszek, and also to Teresa Swader and Daniel Goldman. I would like to acknowledge my family, who have supported me through all the highs and lows of my training and career as a physician and psychiatrist: my mother, Tzu-Yueh, who has been my biggest cheerleader; my dad, Daniel; my brother, Dan, and sister-in-law, Jennifer, and their three girls; and the bright lights in my life, my children, Lucille and Lloyd. I could never do any of this without all of your love and support and can never thank you enough for your patience and inspiration.

Anna Borisovskaya: My colleagues and I are grateful for the support of the University of Washington Department of Psychiatry and Behavioral Sciences, as well as the Veterans Administration Medical Center in Seattle, Washington. Geriatric Psychiatry faculty from both institutions were instrumental in encouraging our dedication to scholarship.

Rebecca Radue: Special thanks to my many mentors in geriatric psychiatry, including Lisa Boyle, Lynn Verger, Tim Howell, and especially to Art Walaszek for his mentorship and the opportunity to collaborate here. I also must thank my dear friend Rebecca Nierengarten for her advice and edits as I wrote, and my wife, Ashley, for supporting me through all my endeavors.

Lucy Wang: I would like to acknowledge my many mentors in geriatric psychiatry, some of whom include Elaine Peskind, Murray Raskind, Marcella Pascualy, and Debby Tsuang. I also consider it a privilege to work at the VA Puget Sound Health Care System, which has supported my clinical practice focused on older adults and sparked my interest in learning more about suicide risk reduction strategies in this important population.

Art Walaszek: Thank you to my wonderful co-authors—Eileen, Lisa, Rebecca, Lucy, and Anna and her colleagues at the University of Washington—for their commitment to this project, even as a pandemic raged. I learned a tremendous amount from reading and editing their chapters, which will benefit my patients and hopefully many other patients. I very much appreciate their patience with me and their collaborative spirit. I hope we can work together again.

I have been graced with many mentors and colleagues at the University of Wisconsin, both in Psychiatry and in Geriatrics, who have been instrumental in my writing about how best to relieve the suffering of older adults who have problems with mood, behavior, and cognition.

Thank you to Erika Parker, Laura Roberts, and John McDuffie at American Psychiatric Association Publishing for their continued support and their remarkable patience.

And my deepest gratitude to my always supportive family: Suzanne, Maddy, Lucy, Dewey, and even Percy.

CHAPTER 1

Introduction to Late-Life Depression

Art Walaszek, M.D.

PRÉCIS

Depression is not a normal part of aging. But depression is common among older adults, and it is distressing, disabling, and sometimes fatal. Older adults with depression follow one of these clinical courses: earlier onset of major depressive disorder or bipolar disorder, with recurrence or chronicity into older adulthood; subclinical depression or anxiety through early adulthood or midlife, worsening into clinical depression in late life; or late-life onset of depression that is either a risk factor for or harbinger of dementia. A number of biological, psychosocial, cultural, and spiritual factors contribute to the development of late-life depression. Depression can manifest differently in older adults, including more somatic concerns, subtle psychotic symptoms (such as delusional guilt), and greater cognitive impairment—in fact, there is a strong two-way relationship between depression and dementia. Many older adults with depressive symptoms do not meet criteria for major depressive disorder but can still have significant dysfunction and worse outcomes. Whereas bereavement and grief are universal experiences, depression is pathological and can be clinically distinguished from grief. Late-life depression is associated with a number of negative outcomes, including suicide, increased all-cause and cardiovascular mortality, onset of or exacerbation of various medical conditions (e.g., stroke), disability, and caregiver burden. Comorbidities are common and include anxiety, dementia, substance use disorders, personality disorders, sleep disorders, and frailty. Thus, it is critical that clinicians assess for and address depression and associated conditions in older adults.

Public Health Impact of Late-Life Depression

The concept of depression dates back to Hippocrates, who defined melancholia, an ancient incarnation of depression, as "when fright or despondency lasts for a long time" (Scholtz 1941). Thomas Burton, a seventeenth-century cataloger of the disease and a sufferer himself, metaphorically linked melancholy and aging, referring to the former as "a kind of dotage" (Burton 2001, p. 169). Although Emil Kraepelin's major diagnostic contribution to modern psychiatry was distinguishing *manic-depressive insanity* (bipolar disorder or recurrent major depressive disorder in the parlance of the *Diagnostic and Statistical Manual of Mental Disorders, 5th Edition* [DSM-5]; American Psychiatric Association 2013) from *dementia praecox* (schizophrenia), he also introduced *involutional melancholia*, that is, depression that arises later in life (Hirshbein 2009). Kraepelin described people suffering from involutional melancholia as having been free of psychiatric illness until involution—that is, menopause in women or a comparable age in men. American psychiatrists included involutional melancholia in their first diagnostic manual in 1918 and continued to diagnose patients with this condition well into the twentieth century, strongly linking aging with depression (Hirshbein 2009). Although DSM-5 does not include involutional melancholia, the false public perception that aging inevitably leads to depression remains pervasive.

Aging and depression are not synonymous. In fact, the prevalence of major depressive disorder (MDD) is lower in late life (roughly 65 years and older) than during midlife (Byers et al. 2010). Psychological well-being, resilience to adversity, an arc toward wisdom, and continued capacity for gratifying relationships are the norm in older adults.

When MDD does occur, it can be distressing, disabling, and even deadly for older adults. Late-life depression (LLD) has been associated with loss of quality of life, functional decline, increased mortality from comorbid medical conditions, and suicide (Fiske et al. 2009). (From here on, I use the term LLD when referring to depression in older adults in general and MDD when referring to the specific DSM diagnosis of major depressive disorder; people with LLD meet DSM criteria for MDD.) Depressed older adults, compared with older adults who are not depressed, are more likely to visit primary care, be hospitalized, and seek help within the home (e.g., nursing care, meals on wheels) (Luppa et al. 2012a). Depression in older adults is also associated with higher medical costs as compared with older adults without depression, including increased cost of outpatient care, inpatient care, emergency care, and medications (König et al. 2019). Severity also matters: health care costs, including the cost of informal caregiving for depressed elders, are higher in those with severe depression compared with those with mild depression (Luppa et al. 2012a). LLD contributes to and complicates other geriatric syndromes, including dementia, stroke, cardiac disease, falls, chronic pain, and frailty—in fact, LLD is one of the core geriatric syndromes affecting the quality of life and functioning of older adults and their caregivers. The number of older adults worldwide is projected to increase from 962 million in 2017 to 2.08 billion in 2050; therefore, clinicians should expect to see more cases of LLD over time (United Nations, Department of Economic and Social Affairs, Population Division 2017).

Older adults are more likely to seek mental health care from a primary care provider than from a mental health specialist (Fiske et al. 2009), but primary care providers have limited time to discuss mental health issues (median time of 2 minutes; Tai-Searle et al. 2007) and might easily miss the diagnosis. Further, older adults with depression may present with somatic symptoms such as fatigue, headache, or gastrointestinal distress, delaying the recognition of underlying LLD (Niles and O'Donovan 2019). Despite a number of public health and clinical interventions to promote the detection of LLD (e.g., U.S. Preventive Services Task Force recommendations for screening for depression), many elders with depression remain undiagnosed or undertreated (Rhee et al. 2018).

Ethnic and sexual minority elders face even more challenges. Compared with white older adults, ethnic minority elders are less likely to have their depression recognized, be prescribed antidepressants, or receive specialty mental health care and are more likely to have poorer outcomes (Mansour et al. 2020). Lesbian, gay, bisexual, transgender, and queer (LGBTQ+) elders may have experienced discrimination and threats to their safety for most of their lives, possibly preventing them from receiving appropriate mental health care (Yarns et al. 2016). We cover these topics in greater detail in Chapter 3, "Assessment of Late-Life Depression and Anxiety," and Chapter 6, "Comprehensive Cultural Assessment of the Older Adult With Depression and Anxiety."

Etiology of Depression

Understanding the clinical types of depression in late life is important for predicting clinical course and for choosing appropriate treatment. Clinical subtypes of depression in this older population include the following:

1. Major depressive disorder that arises in adolescence or early adulthood, likely has significant genetic and developmental roots, and then either recurs repeatedly as the person ages or becomes a chronic condition
2. Bipolar disorder that arises in early adulthood, likely has significant genetic and other biological causes, and then persists into late life, perhaps with more frequent mood episodes over time
3. Subclinical depression or anxiety that is present throughout early adulthood and midlife but is not disabling or even necessarily distressing but then emerges as clinically significant depression as the person ages
4. Major depressive disorder that arises in late life in a person with no prior psychopathology and either puts that person at high risk of developing a neurocognitive disorder or represents the prodrome of a neurocognitive disorder
5. Depression that arises after the onset of a neurodegenerative disorder (Alzheimer's disease, Parkinson disease) or cerebrovascular disease, likely due to dysfunction of neural circuitry involved in emotion regulation compounded by psychological distress, and whose symptoms overlap with those of the syndrome of apathy

We might label the latter two subtypes as *late-onset depression*, a neuropsychiatric condition that is likely etiologically distinct from the first three presentations. Bearing in mind these manifold manifestations of LLD, we present multiple models of how depression can arise in older adults (for a synthesis, see Figures 1–1, 1–2, and 1–3).

NEUROBIOLOGY

LLD may arise from disruption of the neural circuitry involved in emotion regulation, especially frontal-executive and corticolimbic circuits (Rashidi-Ranjbar et al. 2020). Various networks are thought to be involved in emotion regulation, including the default mode network, an executive control network, and a network involved in reward and reinforcement (Kupfer et al. 2012). These networks include parts of the prefrontal cortex (e.g., the dorsolateral prefrontal cortex), hippocampus,

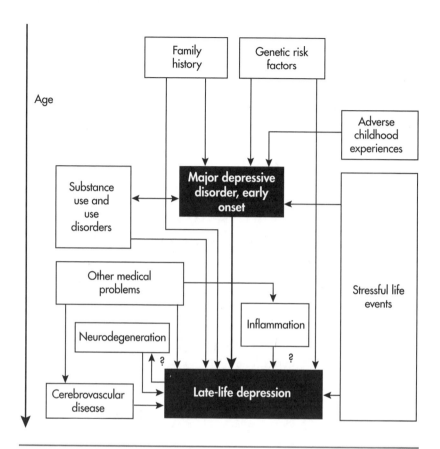

Figure 1–1.   Life course of late-life depression.

In general, late-life depression follows one of two courses: early onset and late onset. Family history, genetic factors, and adverse childhood events are more common in early-onset depression. Neurodegenerative disease, cerebrovascular disease, and other medical problems are more prominent contributors to late-onset depression.

Source.   Adapted from Kupfer et al. 2012 and Alexopoulos 2019.

amygdala, posterior cingulate cortex, and white matter tracts connecting these and other structures (see Figure 1–3). Anhedonia may arise from abnormalities in the reward network, executive dysfunction may arise from abnormalities in the executive control network, and rumination may arise from abnormalities in the default mode network.

Cerebrovascular disease, especially ischemic changes in white matter, is a primary cause of this disruption of neural circuitry (Alexopoulos 2019). Location of disease in white matter and extent of white matter disease have been associated with LLD, especially late-onset depression. Persons with LLD have been found to have decreased resting ce-

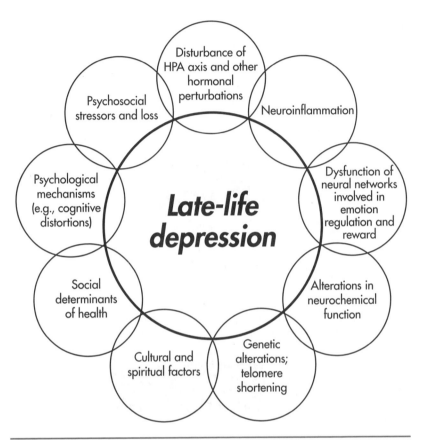

Figure 1–2.   Mechanisms of late-life depression.

Various proposed mechanisms likely interact with each other to give rise to late-life depression.
Abbreviation. HPA=hypothalamic-pituitary-adrenal.
Source.   Adapted from Kupfer et al. 2012 and Alexopoulos 2019.

rebral blood flow in the frontal lobes. Vascular risk factors in midlife, including hypertension and diabetes, are also risk factors for LLD. This strong link between cerebrovascular disease and depression has led to the construct of *vascular depression*, discussed in greater detail in the subsection "Vascular Depression."

The high rate of depression in persons with Alzheimer's disease and Parkinson's disease suggests that neurodegeneration affects not only cognition but also emotional functioning. Several Alzheimer's disease biomarkers (e.g., burden of amyloid plaques in the frontal cortex and hippocampus) have been associated with depression in older adults with and without dementia (Alexopoulos 2019). Depression, especially

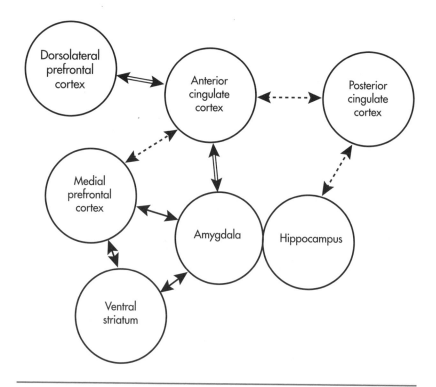

Figure 1–3.   Neural networks involved in late-life depression.
Simplified model of the neural networks thought to be involved in depression, including the reward network (solid lines), executive control network (double lines), and the default mode network (dotted lines). See text for further discussion.
Source.   Adapted from Kupfer et al. 2012 and Alexopoulos 2019.

late-onset depression, may be a risk factor for dementia and for progression from mild cognitive impairment to dementia, suggesting a two-way relationship between dementia and depression; we discuss this in greater detail below.

Peripheral inflammatory markers have been associated with LLD, suggesting a pathway from aging to peripheral inflammation to central nervous system inflammation to depression (Martínez-Cengotitabengoa et al. 2016; Miller et al. 2013). For example, a large longitudinal study measured an inflammatory marker, C-reactive protein (CRP), in midlife, 7 years later, and another 14 years later, at which time depressive symptoms were also assessed; elevated CRP at two or more time points was associated with LLD (Sonsin-Diaz et al. 2020). This link raises the possibility of anti-inflammatory approaches to preventing or treating depression.

LLD has low to moderate heritability (14%–55%), suggesting a modest role for genetic factors (Tsang et al. 2017). Elders with early-onset depression are more likely to have a family history of depression than do those with late-onset depression (Gallagher et al. 2010). However, most genetic studies of LLD have not distinguished between early-onset and late-onset depression, making it hard to figure out how much of the genetic contribution to LLD is mediated by depression earlier in life. Carriers of the e4 allele of the *APOE* gene, an allele associated with increased risk of Alzheimer's disease, may also be at slightly increased risk of LLD (Tsang et al. 2017). Cognitively intact elders with depression who are *APOE* ε4 carriers may be at higher risk for cognitive decline (Morin et al. 2019). Note that most subjects in the *APOE* studies have been non-Hispanic white people, limiting generalizability. Polymorphisms involving genes encoding neurotrophins such as brain-derived neurotrophic factor (BDNF) have also been associated with LLD (Miao et al. 2019; Tsang et al. 2017). In younger populations, carrying the S allele of *SLCA64* (which results in less transcription of serotonin transporter) moderates the relationship between stressful life events and depression; the same polymorphism confers a slightly increased risk of LLD (Tsang et al. 2017). Depression has been associated with telomere shortening, a marker of cellular aging (Ridout et al. 2016).

Dysfunction of the hypothalamic-pituitary-adrenal (HPA) axis is a hallmark of depression in younger adults. Older adults with depression can have either hypocortisolemia or hypercortisolemia, with the latter possibly associated with smaller hippocampal volumes (Bremmer et al. 2007; Geerlings and Gerritsen 2017). Women who undergo menopause later (i.e., have greater exposure to estrogen) have a lower risk of subsequently developing depression, even among women with a history of premenopausal depression (Georgakis et al. 2016). Estrogen has antidepressant and neuroprotective properties, although perhaps only during the perimenopausal period because estrogen has not been found to be effective for depression in women after menopause (Georgakis et al. 2016). The literature on the relationship between low testosterone and depression in older men is mixed (Walther et al. 2019).

Aside from neurodegenerative disorders, stroke, hypertension, and diabetes, other medical conditions have been associated with LLD. These conditions include coronary artery disease (including myocardial infarction), chronic pain, arthritis, hearing loss, vision loss, sleep apnea, cancer, thyroid disease, hyperhomocysteinemia, and vitamin B_{12} deficiency (Aziz and Steffens 2013; Kerner and Roose 2016). This list becomes especially pertinent when we seek to identify reversible causes of depression in our patients, which we cover in Chapter 3. A number of medications have been associated with LLD, including steroids, β-blockers, benzodiazepines, opioids, and antiparkinsonian agents (Aziz and Steffens 2013). (Note that some of these medications can also cause euphoria or mania, in particular steroids and antiparkinsonian agents.) Excessive use of alcohol, benzodiazepine use disorder, and opioid use disorder have been associated with LLD (Wu and Blazer 2014).

PSYCHOSOCIAL, PSYCHOLOGICAL, AND PERSONALITY FACTORS

For a comprehensive review, readers are referred to incisive articles by Areán and Reynolds (2005) and Laird et al. (2019). Table 1–1 summarizes the findings from these reviews. In general, older adults experience a number of stressful life events, most notably the deaths of a partner and other loved ones, which in turn may result in loss of social supports and loneliness. Some stressors may be somewhat unique to aging, such as the loss of driving privileges due to physical or cognitive decline, which has been associated with a doubling of the risk of depression (Chihuri et al. 2016). The stressors do not have to be recent: older adults who had experienced one or more adverse childhood experiences (ACEs), especially those with low perceived social support, are at higher risk of LLD (Cheong et al. 2017). Older women, ethnic and racial minority elders, and sexual minority elders may continue to face sexism, racism, homophobia, and transphobia as they age. Increased living expenses while on a fixed income, neighborhood crime, food insecurity, and problems with access to and affordability of medical care may contribute to depression. Like younger adults, older adults may have a number of maladaptive personality traits and coping strategies that precipitate or perpetuate depression. Conversely, resilience may be protective (Laird et al. 2019).

In my practice, I have found older adults' despair about a perceived loss of meaning and purpose to be an especially powerful and difficult-to-address component of LLD. For a more in-depth review of the role of meaning and purpose in psychological well-being, cognition, and survival, I recommend reading the section "Capacity Assessment" in Chapter 6.

It is helpful to understand how the psychology of LLD informs evidence-based psychotherapy (Kiosses et al. 2011). For example, the recognition that grief, loneliness, role transitions (e.g., retirement, becoming a caregiver), interpersonal skills deficits, and interpersonal conflicts can contribute to depression forms the basis of interpersonal

---

Table 1–1.   Psychosocial and psychological contributors to late-life depression

---

Stressful life events

- Interpersonal loss and bereavement
- Social isolation and decreased emotional support
- Medical illness and associated burden and disability
- Trauma, including interpersonal violence and fear of violence
- Role transitions (e.g., retirement)
- History of adverse childhood experiences

Socioeconomic factors

- Low income, difficulty affording medications, poor access to medical care
- Problems with transportation (e.g., following loss of driving privileges)
- Racism, sexism, homophobia, transphobia
- Stigma regarding mental illness and ageism

Personality factors

- Passive coping style (e.g., avoidance)
- Harm-avoidant or behaviorally inhibited temperament
- Insecure attachment
- Low extroversion, high neuroticism, low conscientiousness

Beliefs and values

- Low self-esteem
- Internalized mental illness stigma
- Negative stereotypes about aging
- Loss of sense of meaning and purpose

Source.   Adapted from Areán and Reynolds 2005; Cheong et al. 2017; Laird et al. 2019.

---

psychotherapy. Cognitive-behavioral therapy seeks to address negative dysfunctional thoughts, distorted perceptions and beliefs, and the withdrawal or inactivity that accompany depression. Because cognitive impairment and executive dysfunction can accompany depression in older adults, problem-solving therapy focuses on "teaching patients skills for improving their ability to deal with specific everyday problems and life crises…. Patients identify problems, brainstorm different ways to solve their problems, create action plans, and evaluate their effectiveness in implementing the best possible solution" (Kiosses et al. 2011).

CULTURAL AND SPIRITUAL FACTORS

We devote Chapter 6 to a comprehensive review of cultural and spiritual factors in the care of older adults with depression and anxiety. Here we discuss the roles of culture and spirituality in contributing to LLD. Please note that I use the ethnic/racial terminology used in the original papers.

Culture refers to "a set of shared symbols, beliefs and customs that shapes individual and/or group behavior" (Dilworth-Anderson and Gibson 2002). Culture influences how people define a mental health problem, how they perceive the cause of the problem, how they cope with the problem, and whether and how they seek help for the problem (Aggarwal 2010). A tool such as the DSM-5 Cultural Formulation Interview, discussed in Chapter 6, can help the clinician better understand the role of culture in an elder with depression.

Culture may affect how depression manifests in older adults. For example, Black African, Caribbean, and South Asian elders in the United Kingdom are less likely to report guilt, hopelessness, and suicidal ideation than are White British elders. This could reflect a different presentation of LLD (fewer affective, more somatic symptoms) or lower acceptability of reporting such symptoms (Mansour et al. 2020).

The experience of being an ethnic minority or immigrant may contribute to developing LLD. Being an older adult who immigrated may be protective against depression (e.g., because of the *healthy migrant effect*, the hypothesis that the immigration process selects for more psychologically resilient people) or a risk factor (e.g., because of loss of power or status within the new culture) (Mansour et al. 2020; Sadavoy et al. 2004). Among immigrants to Western nations, intergenerational conflict over traditional versus Western-based values may serve as a stressor contributing to depression (Sadavoy et al. 2004). For example, Asian elders may feel disappointment in their adult children with respect to *filial piety*, "the spirit and principle of being considerate and respectful toward one's parents and older family members": Asian older adults' satisfaction with their children's filial piety is correlated with lower level of depression (Wu et al. 2018, p.370). Latinx elders may have expectations regarding *familismo*, the "intergenerational obligation, respect, and the duty to care for aging parents" (Wu et al. 2018, p.376).

Language barriers and challenges navigating social and medical systems may contribute to social isolation, in turn a risk factor for LLD (Sadavoy et al. 2004). Elders of various cultural backgrounds may view depression as a personal or familial matter not requiring a medical intervention (Flores-Flores et al. 2020; Ward et al. 2014). Ethnic minority elders may face challenges with respect to accessing linguistically and culturally appropriate services and are less likely to receive appropriate treatment, including antidepressants and psychotherapy (Mansour et al. 2020; Sadavoy et al. 2004). African American and other ethnic minority elders in the United States experience psychological distress as a result of racism, discrimination, prejudice, and poverty (Conner et al. 2010). African American elders are less likely to seek treatment for depression than are white elders because of mistrust of the health care system, stigma about mental illness, and alternative methods of coping (e.g., religious practices) (Conner et al. 2010). Depressed Black elders are 61% less likely to receive any depression treatment than are non-Hispanic white elders (Vyas et al. 2020).

In general, religion and spirituality have been associated with reduced risk of depression. There is some evidence that religious practices (such as attendance at religious services and prayer) are more protective against LLD than are religious beliefs alone (Laird et al. 2019). Spirituality may be especially important with respect to addressing LLD. For example, older African Americans may be more likely to turn to religious counsel (e.g., clergy) and may wish to incorporate religious practices into treatment of depression (Pickett et al. 2013).

We cover social determinants of health in Chapter 6.

Epidemiology of Depression

The prevalence of depression in older adults is around 5%–10%. Estimates across epidemiological studies vary, depending on how depression is defined (namely, using DSM-5 criteria [categorical] vs. using a rating scale with a cutoff score [dimensional]), on the population studied (e.g., some samples include older adults residing in nursing homes), and on which measure of prevalence is used (lifetime, 12-month, or point prevalence). Older adults with depressive symptoms may suffer from MDD (discussed in the following paragraphs) or from subsyndromal depression (sometimes also referred to as *minor depression*, discussed further in the subsection "Persistent Depressive Disorder (Dysthymia)").

In general, the prevalence of MDD is lower among older adults than among younger adults and seems to decrease with age among older adults, although not all studies agree on the latter point. It is not clear why rates of depression are lower in older adults than younger adults. Possible explanations include cohort effects (i.e., current older adults had lower rates of depression as younger adults than do current younger adults), survivor effect (i.e., middle-age people with mood disorders are less likely to live into late life or are less likely to be ascertained because they become institutionalized), and methodological issues (e.g., older adults may have more difficulty recalling symptoms or may be less likely to report them) (Byers et al. 2010). The prevalence of MDD and depressive symptoms has uniformly been found to be higher among older women than older men. Relative rates of depression among ethnic minority elders have varied from study to study.

The National Comorbidity Survey Replication (NCS-R) examined the rates of depression among community-dwelling Americans 60 years and older. The *lifetime prevalence* of DSM-IV-defined MDD and dysthymia were 10.6% and 1.3%, respectively—lower than rates found in 18- to 59-year-old subjects (American Psychiatric Association 1994; Kessler et al. 2005). As would be expected, using 12-month prevalence yields lower rates than using lifetime prevalence. The *12-month prevalence* of MDD in the NCS-R declined with age: ages 55–64, 6.2%; ages 65–74, 3.1%; ages 75–84, 1.1%; ages 85 and older, 1.8% (Byers et al. 2010). Older women had higher 12-month prevalence of mood disorders (including MDD, dysthymia, and bipolar disorder) than did older men (6.4% vs. 3.0%) (Byers et al. 2010). Comorbidity was common, with a 12-month prevalence of both a mood and an anxiety disorder of 3%.

The worldwide numbers are somewhat different, with higher rates of depression reported. A meta-analysis of 24 epidemiological studies from around the world estimated that the pooled *point prevalence* of MDD in adults 75 and older is 7.2% (95% CI, 4.4–10.6%), with higher rates for women than men; the lowest rates were in North America (Luppa et al. 2012b). When depression was defined dimensionally (i.e., using rating scales rather than diagnostic criteria), the pooled point prevalence was higher: 17.1% (95% CI, 9.7–26.1%). Note that this meta-analysis included studies of older adults residing in nursing homes, which may help explain the higher prevalence than in NCS-R, which included only community-dwelling older adults. See below for further discussion of depression among nursing home residents.

With respect to relationship status, the NCS-R data set yielded statistically significant differences in 12-month prevalence of mood disorder by marital status: divorced/separated/widowed, 6.6%; never married, 6.2%; married/cohabiting, 3.9% (Byers et al. 2010). Although the NCS-R study did not reveal significant differences in prevalence by years of education, other studies have found that lower educational attainment increases the risk of LLD (as will be discussed in greater detail in Chapter 6, section "Social Determinants of Late-Life Depression and Anxiety").

Comparisons of rates of depression among older adults from various ethnic/racial groups have yielded conflicting results. Some studies have not found significant differences in prevalence of depression among ethnic/racial groups, whereas others have. For a detailed review of this literature, see Chapter 6, section "Ethnic and Racial Minority Elders."

Clinicians should note that the prevalence of LLD is higher in clinical populations (e.g., in primary care or inpatient settings) than the numbers in other studies (e.g., Luppa et al. 2012b). Also, although most older adults reside in the community, others live in nursing homes and long-term care facilities, where the prevalence is also higher. In a meta-analysis of 32 studies conducted in nursing homes around the world, the prevalence of MDD in nursing home residents without dementia was found to be 18.9% (95% CI 14.8–23.8%) (Fornaro et al. 2020). An older meta-analysis that did not exclude residents with dementia found the prevalence of MDD to be 10% and prevalence of depressive symptoms to be 29% (Seitz et al. 2010). The prevalence of depression is especially high in persons with certain diagnoses (e.g., 42% in those with dementia due to Alzheimer's disease; Zhao et al. 2016).

Rates of depression among LGBTQ+ elders are astonishingly high. At any given time, approximately 31% of LGB elders and 48% of transgender elders meet criteria for depression (Yarns et al. 2016).

As the population ages, the numbers of older adults experiencing homelessness and older adults who are incarcerated have been increasing. The prevalence of depression is 38.3% among homeless older adults and 25% among incarcerated older adults (Barry et al. 2017; Kaplan et al. 2019).

Clinical Presentation

As discussed in the section "Public Health Impact of Late-Life Depression," the diagnosis of *major depressive disorder* (MDD) replaced *involutional melancholia*, regardless of the age of the patient. However, involutional melancholia included many symptoms that we recognize as present in LLD, especially when severe: apprehension and anxiety; confusion and other cognitive symptoms; delusions; and somatic symptoms such as headache, chest pain, and vertigo (Hirshbein 2009). Thus, MDD, as defined in DSM-5 (Box 1–1), paints only part of the picture of LLD. In this section, we review the many ways that depression manifests in older adults.

Box 1–1.   DSM-5 Diagnostic Criteria for Major Depressive
Disorder

A. Five (or more) of the following symptoms have been present during the
same 2-week period and represent a change from previous functioning;
at least one of the symptoms is either (1) depressed mood or (2) loss of
interest or pleasure.
Note: Do not include symptoms that are clearly attributable to another
medical condition.
1. Depressed mood most of the day, nearly every day, as indicated by
either subjective report (e.g., feels sad, empty, hopeless) or observation made by others (e.g., appears tearful). (Note: In children and adolescents, can be irritable mood.)
2. Markedly diminished interest or pleasure in all, or almost all, activities
most of the day, nearly every day (as indicated by either subjective
account or observation).
3. Significant weight loss when not dieting or weight gain (e.g., a
change of more than 5% of body weight in a month), or decrease or
increase in appetite nearly every day. (Note: In children, consider failure
to make expected weight gain.)
4. Insomnia or hypersomnia nearly every day.
5. Psychomotor agitation or retardation nearly every day (observable
by others, not merely subjective feelings of restlessness or being
slowed down).
6. Fatigue or loss of energy nearly every day.
7. Feelings of worthlessness or excessive or inappropriate guilt (which
may be delusional) nearly every day (not merely self-reproach or
guilt about being sick).
8. Diminished ability to think or concentrate, or indecisiveness, nearly
every day (either by subjective account or as observed by others).
9. Recurrent thoughts of death (not just fear of dying), recurrent suicidal
ideation without a specific plan, or a suicide attempt or a specific plan
for committing suicide.
B. The symptoms cause clinically significant distress or impairment in social,
occupational, or other important areas of functioning.
C. The episode is not attributable to the physiological effects of a substance or another medical condition.
Note: Criteria A–C represent a major depressive episode.
Note: Responses to a significant loss (e.g., bereavement, financial ruin, losses
from a natural disaster, a serious medical illness or disability) may include the
feelings of intense sadness, rumination about the loss, insomnia, poor appetite, and weight loss noted in Criterion A, which may resemble a depressive
episode. Although such symptoms may be understandable or considered appropriate to the loss, the presence of a major depressive episode in addition
to the normal response to a significant loss should also be carefully consid-

ered. This decision inevitably requires the exercise of clinical judgment based on the individual's history and the cultural norms for the expression of distress in the context of loss.[1]

D. The occurrence of the major depressive episode is not better explained by schizoaffective disorder, schizophrenia, schizophreniform disorder, delusional disorder, or other specified and unspecified schizophrenia spectrum and other psychotic disorders.

E. There has never been a manic episode or a hypomanic episode.
   Note: This exclusion does not apply if all of the manic-like or hypomanic-like episodes are substance-induced or are attributable to the physiological effects of another medical condition.

Coding and Recording Procedures

The diagnostic code for major depressive disorder is based on whether this is a single or recurrent episode, current severity, presence of psychotic features, and remission status. Current severity and psychotic features are only indicated if full criteria are currently met for a major depressive episode. Remission specifiers are only indicated if the full criteria are not currently met for a major depressive episode. Codes are as follows:

Severity/course specifier	Single episode	Recurrent episode*
Mild (DSM-5 p. 188)	296.21 (F32.0)	296.31 (F33.0)
Moderate (DSM-5 p. 188)	296.22 (F32.1)	296.32 (F33.1)
Severe (DSM-5 p. 188)	296.23 (F32.2)	296.33 (F33.2)

---

[1]In distinguishing grief from a major depressive episode (MDE), it is useful to consider that in grief the predominant affect is feelings of emptiness and loss, while in an MDE it is persistent depressed mood and the inability to anticipate happiness or pleasure. The dysphoria in grief is likely to decrease in intensity over days to weeks and occurs in waves, the so-called pangs of grief. These waves tend to be associated with thoughts or reminders of the deceased. The depressed mood of an MDE is more persistent and not tied to specific thoughts or preoccupations. The pain of grief may be accompanied by positive emotions and humor that are uncharacteristic of the pervasive unhappiness and misery characteristic of an MDE. The thought content associated with grief generally features a preoccupation with thoughts and memories of the deceased, rather than the self-critical or pessimistic ruminations seen in an MDE. In grief, self-esteem is generally preserved, whereas in an MDE feelings of worthlessness and self-loathing are common. If self-derogatory ideation is present in grief, it typically involves perceived failings vis-à-vis the deceased (e.g., not visiting frequently enough, not telling the deceased how much he or she was loved). If a bereaved individual thinks about death and dying, such thoughts are generally focused on the deceased and possibly about "joining" the deceased, whereas in an MDE such thoughts are focused on ending one's own life because of feeling worthless, undeserving of life, or unable to cope with the pain of depression.

Severity/course specifier	Single episode	Recurrent episode*
With psychotic features** (DSM-5 p. 186)	296.24 (F32.3)	296.34 (F33.3)
In partial remission (DSM-5 p. 188)	296.25 (F32.4)	296.35 (F33.41)
In full remission (DSM-5 p. 188)	296.26 (F32.5)	296.36 (F33.42)
Unspecified	296.20 (F32.9)	296.30 (F33.9)

*For an episode to be considered recurrent, there must be an interval of at least 2 consecutive months between separate episodes in which criteria are not met for a major depressive episode. The definitions of specifiers are found on the indicated pages.
**If psychotic features are present, code the "with psychotic features" specifier irrespective of episode severity.

In recording the name of a diagnosis, terms should be listed in the following order: major depressive disorder, single or recurrent episode, severity/psychotic/remission specifiers, followed by as many of the following specifiers without codes that apply to the current episode.

Specify:
   With anxious distress (DSM-5 p. 184)
   With mixed features (DSM-5 pp. 184–185)
   With melancholic features (DSM-5 p. 185)
   With atypical features (DSM-5 pp. 185–186)
   With mood-congruent psychotic features (DSM-5 p. 186)
   With mood-incongruent psychotic features (DSM-5 p. 186)
   With catatonia (DSM-5 p. 186). **Coding note:** Use additional code 293.89 (F06.1).
   With peripartum onset (DSM-5 pp. 186–187)
   With seasonal pattern (recurrent episode only) (DSM-5 pp. 187–188)

Source. Reprinted from American Psychiatric Association: *Diagnostic and Statistical Manual of Mental Disorders*, 5th Edition, Arlington, VA, American Psychiatric Association, 2013. Copyright © 2013 American Psychiatric Association. Used with permission.

TYPICAL PRESENTATIONS

We begin by asking, what is depression? LLD is a sustained *affective*, *cognitive*, and *behavioral* syndrome that results in individuals having less ability to care for themselves and to engage in interpersonal relationships. The affective component of LLD has a negative valence that is experienced as discomfort or suffering; the predominant emotion is sadness, sometimes anxiety. People with depression also experience less positive affect, can lose pleasure and enjoyment in activities (i.e., anhedonia), and may not feel content or satisfied. The duration, intensity, and dysfunction of LLD distinguish it from the normal human emotion of sadness.

A person experiencing depression tends to have thoughts, beliefs, or cognitions that are inaccurate or incomplete:

- the belief that one is or not deserving of love
- the belief that one has done something wrong (regret or guilt); when severe, this belief can take on delusional intensity and can be complicated by hallucinations
- the belief that one is helpless or incapable of effective action
- hopelessness and the associated belief that life is not worth living (i.e., suicidal ideation)

Especially in older adults, depression is associated with cognitive impairment, including inattention, memory loss, and indecision.

The behaviors of depression include disturbances of core bodily functions: sleeping too much or too little; eating too much or too little; being withdrawn and inactive or being restless and purposelessly active; and somatization (e.g., nausea, headache, back pain). Depression increases the risk of suicidal behavior. Rarely, depression can result in catatonia.

The symptoms of depression result in distress, worse quality of life, and/or functional impairment. In older adults, we think about functioning in terms of instrumental activities of daily living (ADLs) and personal (or basic) ADLs (Katz 1983). Instrumental ADLs are higher-order functions described by the mnemonic SHAFT (University of Ottawa 2011):

- **S**=shopping for groceries, clothes, and other household items
- **H**=housekeeping
- **A**=accounting (i.e., managing one's finances, including paying bills)
- **F**=food preparation
- **T**=transportation—not necessarily driving, but more broadly the ability to get around, whether by cab or bus or by driving oneself

Use the mnemonic DEATH to recall the list of basic or personal ADLs (University of Ottawa 2011):

- **D**=dressing oneself
- **E**=eating (i.e., feeding oneself)
- **A**=ambulating
- **T**=toileting
- **H**=hygiene

LLD is a predictor of the onset of disability (the inability to carry out ADLs; Mendes de Leon and Rajan 2014), discussed below in the subsection "Disability."

Older adults have a somewhat different pattern of depression symptoms than do younger adults. Older adults are more likely to endorse somatic symptoms (sleep disturbance, fatigue, psychomotor agitation or retardation) and less likely to endorse worthlessness or guilt and suicidal ideation than are younger adults; most but not all studies have found older adults more likely to report cognitive symptoms (poor concentration or memory) (Balsis and Cully 2008; Fiske et al. 2009). The prevalence of specific symptoms from the National Epidemiologic Survey on Alcoholism and Related Conditions (NESARC) study is presented in Table 1–2; this study included 1,808 community-dwelling older adults in the United States who had endorsed either low mood or anhedonia. Older adults with early-onset depression may be more likely to experience guilt and worthlessness than those with late-onset depression, although not all studies are consistent with respect to symptomatic differences between the two groups (Gallagher et al. 2010). There may be racial and ethnic differences in the symptoms of LLD, such as higher rates of rates of sadness, dysphoria, and psychomotor symptoms among Black and Hispanic elders (Vyas et al. 2020).

Table 1–2.   Prevalence of specific symptoms in depressed older adults

Symptom	Prevalence
Low mood	92%
Anhedonia	68%
Weight or appetite change	58%
Sleep change	65%
Psychomotor agitation or retardation	33%
Fatigue	50%
Worthlessness or guilt	38%
Diminished concentration	51%
Thoughts of death or suicidal thoughts	31%

Source.   National Epidemiologic Survey on Alcoholism and Related Conditions (adapted from Balsis and Cully 2008).

LLD tends to be episodic, with a remitting-relapsing course, although it can become chronic. Grief is especially common in older adults and shares many characteristics with LLD, except that a loss or other severe stressor does not necessarily precede an episode of depression and grief is usually not associated with significant dysfunction.

(We spend more time on distinguishing grief from depression in the subsection "Depression and Grief").

PSYCHOTIC DEPRESSION

Psychotic depression is a particularly severe form of LLD that is defined by the presence of delusions and/or hallucinations. The psychotic features are thought to be mood-congruent if their content includes "personal inadequacy, guilt, disease, death, nihilism, or deserved punishment" (American Psychiatric Association 2013, p. 186). Psychotic depression in older adults has been associated with frontal and temporal lobe atrophy, impairments in executive function and psychomotor speed, greater depression severity, poorer treatment response, and generally worse outcomes than in nonpsychotic depression (Gournellis et al. 2014).

Delusions are the hallmark of psychotic depression. The most common types of delusions are paranoia, somatic delusions, delusions of guilt, and the belief that one ought to be punished; somatic delusions are more common in older adults with depression than younger adults with depression (Gournellis et al. 2014). One-third of patients with psychotic depression have hallucinations, usually auditory (Gournellis et al. 2014). Psychotic depression is distinguished from schizophrenia and other psychotic disorders by the psychotic symptoms being present only when the patient is depressed. Clinicians should have a high index of suspicion for psychotic depression because treatment is different from that for nonpsychotic depression, including combining antidepressant and antipsychotic medication and earlier consideration of electroconvulsive therapy (for further discussion, see section "Pharmacological Interventions" in Chapter 5, "Management of Late-Life Depression and Anxiety"). A case example of psychotic depression is presented next.

CASE EXAMPLE 1: "I LOST MY MIND"

Mrs. Williams is a 72-year-old widowed, retired social worker with a history of MDD who presents with 3 months of withdrawing from activities, weight loss, low energy, and poor sleep. Her only prior episode of depression occurred 3 years ago, soon after her husband's death, and resolved following treatment with sertraline and interpersonal psychotherapy. Recent medical evaluation (electrolytes, creatinine, hepatic enzymes, complete blood count, thyroid-stimulating hormone, vitamin B_{12} level, erythrocyte sedimentation rate) was negative. Sertraline was resumed 2 months ago and titrated to 150 mg/day, without benefit—in fact, her depression has only worsened. Alarmed by her deterioration, her daughters urge her to seek a second opinion regarding her depression.

Today, Mrs. Williams's chief complaint is "I lost my mind." The clinician reassures her that she has not lost her mind but is instead suffering from a treatable mental health condition. However, she insists that she has lost her mind, so the clinician asks her to clarify. Mrs. Williams states that she no longer has a brain, and she requests an MRI to demonstrate this.

Mrs. Williams recounts more of her history: About 3 months ago, she felt a tingling sensation in her scalp. She found herself ruminating about it, could not concentrate on other tasks, and started falling behind on housework. She lay in bed at night, unable to fall asleep, worrying that she might die in the middle of the night. She lost interest in her hobbies, and she started canceling activities with her daughters and with her friends. She wondered if perhaps she had done something wrong— not eaten the right food, for example—and that was why her scalp tingled. She became terrified that she might eat the wrong food and started eating less; she has lost 25 pounds in 3 months. Eventually, she determined that the tingling in her scalp was due to her brain going missing, although she cannot explain how this might have happened. Once in a while, at night, she hears a voice whispering to her that she has lost her mind. She does not want to go on living like this, but at the same time she is afraid of dying and does not want to harm herself—"The Lord would send me straight to hell if I did that." She does not endorse any religious, paranoid, or other delusions; other than the auditory hallucination of whispering and the possible tactile hallucination of scalp tingling, she does not endorse hallucinations. Mrs. Williams does not endorse any current or past manic symptoms, and there is no evidence of a substance use disorder. Bedside cognitive testing is slightly abnormal, with impairment in short-term memory.

The clinician diagnoses Mrs. Williams with MDD, recurrent, severe, with psychotic features, that is, psychotic depression. The clinician recommends psychiatric hospitalization and asks her to consider a course of electroconvulsive therapy.

CATATONIA

Catatonia is present in 18%–40% of patients admitted to a geriatric psychiatry inpatient unit, affecting about half of inpatient elders with depression in one study; depression was the most common cause (43%) of catatonia in this sample (Cuevas-Esteban et al. 2017). Catatonia is a severe behavioral syndrome whose features commonly include immobility and mutism but may also include agitation, catalepsy, waxy flexibility, negativism, posturing, mannerisms, stereotypies, grimacing, echolalia, and echopraxia (American Psychiatric Association 2013; Taylor and Fink 2003). Recognizing catatonia is critical because in older adults delayed treatment can result in adverse outcomes such as pneumonia, pulmonary embolus, physical restraint, misdiagnosis of dementia, and death (Swartz and Galang 2001).

BIPOLAR DEPRESSION

A full discussion of bipolar disorder is beyond the scope of this book; we provide only a brief review here. *Bipolar I disorder* includes episodes of mania, usually depression, and sometimes mixed states (features of both mania and depression). *Bipolar II disorder* is characterized by hypo-manic and depressive episodes, with the latter being far more distressing and impairing. A medication (typically an antidepressant) or other substance may precipitate a manic episode with or without mixed features (in DSM-5 terms, *substance/medication-induced bipolar disorder*), or a manic episode could be due to another medical condition (formerly known as *secondary mania* but now referred to as *bipolar and related disorder due to another medical condition*).

The estimated prevalence of bipolar disorder among older adults is 0.5%–1.0%; it accounts for 6% of outpatient geriatric psychiatry visits and 8%–10% of inpatient geriatric psychiatry admissions (Sajatovic et al. 2015). As with MDD, people with bipolar disorder generally fall into two groups: those with early-onset bipolar disorder who have aged into older adulthood and those with onset after age 50 years (making up about 5%–10% of older adults with bipolar disorder) (Sajatovic et al. 2015). Early-onset illness tends to be associated with family history of mood disorders, more depressive and mixed episodes, and substance use, whereas late onset is associated with more cognitive impairment and medical comorbidity (Chen et al. 2017). The female-to-male ratio in bipolar disorder in older adults is about 2:1, compared with 1:1 in younger adults (Chen et al. 2017).

There are conflicting data regarding risk of recurrence of mood episodes in older adults with bipolar disorder. In one study following people with bipolar disorder and MDD up to 40 years after hospitalization, the risk of recurrence of bipolar disorder was twice as high as for MDD (0.4 vs. 0.2 episodes per year), with no change in frequency of episodes up to about age 70 (Angst et al. 2003). It is possible that antidepressants are less likely to "flip" an older adult with bipolar disorder into a manic or mixed episode compared with a younger adult (Chen et al. 2017). Older adults with bipolar disorder often have medical comorbidities (including metabolic syndrome, diabetes, hypertension, and cardiovascular disease) and, in one study, had life expectancy 10 years shorter than that of the general population (Sajatovic et al. 2015). Cognitive impairment is common (even when patients are euthymic), and bipolar disorder is a risk factor for the development of dementia (Ahearn et al. 2020).

The clinical presentation of bipolar disorder in older adults is similar to that in younger adults, except that hypersexuality, psychosis, anxiety, and suicide may be less common in older adults, although the latter is likely due to a survivor effect (Chen et al. 2017; Sajatovic et al. 2015). Misdiagnosis is common, and clinicians should maintain an index of suspicion of bipolarity in older adults who present with depression. Careful clinical history and family history are important. The onset of mania in late life raises the possibility of an organic disorder and necessitates a full medical workup that includes neuroimaging.

DEPRESSION IN DEMENTIA

Sadness is common among people with dementia, especially when they are aware of loss of cognition—in other words, an experience akin to grief. The functional impairment of dementia may itself contribute to feeling helpless, worthless, or hopeless. The pathophysiological changes that accompany the major causes of dementia—hippocampal degeneration in Alzheimer's disease, dopaminergic dysfunction in Parkinson's disease, and disruption of white matter tracts connecting the frontal lobes with the rest of the brain in vascular dementia—can also lead to depression. Figure 1–4 illustrates the relationship between dementia and depression; it should be noted that depression itself can contribute to cognitive impairment and may represent a reversible component of dementia.

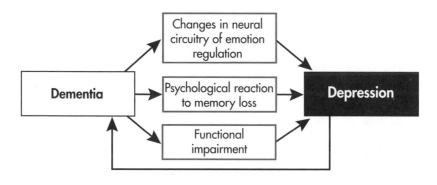

Figure 1–4.   Dementia as a cause of depression.
Dementia can lead to depression through the pathophysiological changes of Alzheimer's disease and other causes of dementia; through grief, that is, a psychological reaction to memory loss; or through functional impairment leading to feelings of worthlessness and helplessness. Depression in turn may exacerbate the cognitive impairment of dementia.

Depression is the second most common behavioral and psychological symptom of dementia (BPSD) overall (prevalence of 42%) and is the most common BPSD in mild dementia (25%) (Okura et al. 2010; Zhao et al. 2016). In 2002, a group of late-life depression and Alzheimer's disease researchers proposed criteria for depression in Alzheimer's disease (Olin et al. 2002). The prevalence of each criterion has been reported (Verkaik et al. 2009), and the criteria have been used in clinical trials of depression in Alzheimer's disease (e.g., Munro et al. 2012). The criteria are as follows:

1. Clinically significant depressed mood (e.g., depressed, sad, hopeless, discouraged, tearful) (point prevalence of 90%)
2. Decreased positive affect or pleasure in response to social contacts and usual activities (i.e., a variant of the anhedonia typically seen in MDD) (59%)
3. Social isolation or withdrawal (presumably due to decreased ability to cope with social situations, as opposed to loss of pleasure) (55%)
4. Disruption in appetite (45%)
5. Disruption in sleep (19%)
6. Psychomotor changes (differing from the agitation or apathy commonly seen in dementia itself) (42%)
7. Irritability (note that this is not one of the DSM-5 criteria for major depressive disorder, but it is quite common in depression of Alzheimer's disease) (64%)
8. Fatigue or loss of energy (61%)
9. Feelings of worthlessness, hopelessness, or excessive or inappropriate guilt (64%)
10. Recurrent thoughts of death, suicidal ideation, suicide plan, or suicide attempt (33%)

For a diagnosis of depression of Alzheimer's disease, a patient must have at least three of the above criteria, at least one of which must be the first or second criterion. A patient who had MDD well before the onset of Alzheimer's disease may be considered to have recurrent MDD rather than depression of Alzheimer's disease (Olin et al. 2002).

Distinguishing between depression and apathy (the most common BPSD) can be challenging; the following tips may be helpful: Guilt, worthless, and hopelessness are typically not present in patients with apathy (Walaszek 2019). Whereas patients with depression can be quite distressed, those with apathy may not be particularly bothered by their apathy; in fact, the family members of patients with apathy may be more frustrated with or distressed by the apathy than are the patients themselves (Walaszek 2019).

VASCULAR DEPRESSION

The observation of a strong relationship between cerebrovascular disease and LLD has led to the concept of vascular depression. People with vascular depression typically experience onset in late life, although exacerbation of early-onset depression is also possible (Alexopoulos 2019). The most common symptoms include psychomotor retardation, anhedonia, executive dysfunction, and poor insight into depression; guilt and family history of depression are less frequent than in patients with typical LLD (Alexopoulos 2019). The neurological signs associated with vascular depression vary and depend on the location and severity of ischemic changes—for example, patients with left temporal lobe stroke may have aphasia in addition to depression (Alexopoulos 2019).

A closely related concept is that of depression executive dysfunction syndrome. Disruption of frontal-subcortical networks leads to impairments in verbal fluency, inhibition, problem-solving, cognitive flexibility, working memory, and/or planning, in addition to anhedonia, psychomotor retardation, suspiciousness, and lack of insight (Alexopoulos 2019). My sense is that vascular depression and especially executive dysfunction syndrome represent syndromes that are actually closer to apathy (with respect to pathophysiology, presentation, and clinical course) than to what we would classically consider melancholic depression.

Why is this clinically relevant? When evaluating someone with late-onset depression, you should consider the possibility of underlying cerebrovascular disease, especially if the patient has not responded to antidepressants or psychotherapy. The prognosis of such patients is poorer, and other treatment options (e.g., psychostimulants, behavioral activation) may be more effective.

PERSISTENT DEPRESSIVE DISORDER (DYSTHYMIA)

Historically, *dysthymia* (or *dysthymic disorder*) represented a chronic syndrome of less intense depressive symptoms than seen with MDD. In DSM-5, *persistent depressive disorder* includes both dysthymia and chronic MDD. In addition to depressed mood, people with persistent depressive disorder experience at least two of the following: poor appetite or overeating, insomnia or hypersomnia, low energy or fatigue, low self-esteem, poor concentration or difficulty making decisions, or hopelessness (American Psychiatric Association 2013). Symptoms are present for at least 2 years, and no depression-free period lasts more than 2 months at a time. The symptoms cause clinically significant distress or functional impairment.

Most older adults with dysthymic disorder have onset of symptoms in late life (Devanand 2014). Family history of mood disorders is relatively uncommon, whereas bereavement, loss of social support, neuro-degenerative disease, and/or cerebrovascular disease are prevalent (Devanand 2014).

MINOR DEPRESSION

Although the prevalence of DSM-diagnosable MDD is lower in older adults than in younger adults, depressive symptomatology is actually fairly common in older adults and can be associated with dysfunction and poorer quality of life. This observation has led to the interrelated constructs of *minor depression*, *subsyndromal depression*, and *subthreshold depression*—which may be two to three times more prevalent than major depression in older adults (Meeks et al. 2011). We will consider these together under the label of minor depression, the most commonly used term. In DSM parlance, this would be considered *other specified depressive disorder*, specifically, a depressive episode with insufficient (fewer than five) MDD symptoms.

About 8%–10% of older adults with minor depression convert to MDD each year; having minor depression roughly doubles (incidence rate ratio of 1.95) the risk of developing MDD (Lee et al. 2019; Meeks et al. 2011). Minor depression has been associated prospectively with suicidal ideation and behavior, increased cognitive impairment (including dementia), worse physical health, increased risk of disability, and increased health care utilization (Lee et al. 2019). Elders with minor depression have outcomes that are intermediate in severity compared with nondepressed elders and those meeting criteria for MDD (Meeks et al. 2011). Clinicians should be alert to minor depression as a marker for increased risk of development of MDD and other adverse outcomes.

DEPRESSION AND GRIEF

Bereavement, the loss of a loved one, is a universal experience. Grief is a normal emotional response to bereavement. The clinician caring for older adults faces two challenges: to not pathologize grief, while at the same time to not dismiss psychopathology as a normal part of aging. Acute grief can be quite distressing, is associated with physiological changes (e.g., sleep disturbance, increased cortisol, increased heart rate or blood pressure), and may increase the risk of myocardial infarction or Takotsubo cardiomyopathy (Shear 2015). Clinicians note that intense emotions of acute grief gradually wane, yet the patient's sense of loss and of missing the loved one often persists. Adapting to the loss is the norm (Simon et al. 2020).

Pathological sequelae of bereavement include MDD, PTSD, and complicated grief. DSM-5 makes a significant point of describing how the manifestations of grief differ from the symptoms of MDD; I refer the reader to the notes to the DSM-5 criteria for MDD, which are summarized in Table 1–3. Bereavement is a severe stressful life event that can contribute to the development of a major depressive episode; grief is normal, but major depression is not.

Table 1–3. Distinguishing grief from depression

	Grief	Depression
Predominant emotions	Emptiness and loss	Depressed mood and anhedonia
Time course of emotions	Dysphoria decreases in intensity over days to weeks and occurs in *pangs* (waves) associated with thoughts or reminders of the deceased	Persistent; not tied to specific thoughts or preoccupations
Associated emotions	Positive emotions and humor may be present	Pervasive misery may be present
Thought content	Preoccupation with thoughts and memories of the deceased	Hopeless and pessimistic rumination
Cognitions about self	Self-esteem is preserved; if present, self-derogatory ideation refers to perceived failings with respect to the deceased	Worthlessness, self-loathing, self-critical thoughts
Thoughts of death	Focused on the deceased, including the possibility of "joining" the deceased	Suicidal ideation associated with feeling worthless, undeserving of life, or unable to cope with pain of depression
Hallucinations and delusions	Benign auditory or visual hallucination of the deceased or sensing the deceased's presence	Paranoia, somatic delusions, delusions of guilt, or the belief that one ought to be punished; marker of psychotic depression

Source. American Psychiatric Association 2013.

PTSD can arise following the death of a loved one in a traumatic way (e.g., a motor vehicle accident) and may include guilt focused on the traumatic event or its aftermath and nightmares related to the traumatic event (Shear 2015). Detailed discussion of PTSD is beyond the scope of this chapter.

Complicated grief is a severe form of acute grief that lasts longer than expected (usually at least 6 months) given the person's cultural and religious background and results in functional impairment (Shear 2015). It is estimated that complicated grief occurs in 10%–11% of adults bereaved by natural causes, with higher rates when the loved one died as a result of an accident, suicide, homicide, or disaster (Simon et al. 2020). Yearning and longing are core symptoms and are frequent and intense (Shear 2015). People with complicated grief may excessively avoid reminders of the loss and may angrily or guiltily ruminate about the circumstances or consequences of the death (Shear 2015). As of DSM-5-TR (American Psychiatric Association 2022), prolonged grief disorder is listed as a psychiatric diagnosis (Box 1–2). It is characterized by a maladaptive grief reaction that has persisted for at least 12 months after the death of a person who was close to the bereaved person. The core symptoms include intense yearning or longing for the deceased person and/ or preoccupation with thoughts or memories of the deceased person. The International Classification of Diseases, 11th Revision (ICD-11) also includes prolonged grief disorder (Simon et al. 2020).

Box 1–2.   DSM-5 Diagnostic Criteria for Prolonged Grief Disorder

---

A. The death, at least 12 months ago, of a person who was close to the bereaved individual (for children and adolescents, at least 6 months ago).

B. Since the death, the development of a persistent grief response characterized by one or both of the following symptoms, which have been present most days to a clinically significant degree. In addition, the symptom(s) has occurred nearly every day for at least the last month:

  1. Intense yearning/longing for the deceased person.
  2. Preoccupation with thoughts or memories of the deceased person (in children and adolescents, preoccupation may focus on the circumstances of the death).

C. Since the death, at least three of the following symptoms have been present most days to a clinically significant degree. In addition, the symptoms have occurred nearly every day for at least the last month:

  1. Identity disruption (e.g., feeling as though part of oneself has died) since the death.
  2. Marked sense of disbelief about the death.
  3. Avoidance of reminders that the person is dead (in children and adolescents, may be characterized by efforts to avoid reminders).

4. Intense emotional pain (e.g., anger, bitterness, sorrow) related to the death.

5. Difficulty reintegrating into one's relationships and activities after the death (e.g., problems engaging with friends, pursuing interests, or planning for the future).

6. Emotional numbness (absence or marked reduction of emotional experience) as a result of the death.

7. Feeling that life is meaningless as a result of the death.

8. Intense loneliness as a result of the death.

D. The disturbance causes clinically significant distress or impairment in social, occupational, or other important areas of functioning.

E. The duration and severity of the bereavement reaction clearly exceed expected social, cultural, or religious norms for the individual's culture and context.

F. The symptoms are not better explained by another mental disorder, such as major depressive disorder or posttraumatic stress disorder, and are not attributable to the physiological effects of a substance (e.g., medication, alcohol) or another medical condition.

Source. Reprinted from American Psychiatric Association: *Diagnostic and Statistical Manual of Mental Disorders,* 5th Edition, Text Revision. Washington, DC, American Psychiatric Association, 2022. Copyright © 2022 American Psychiatric Association. Used with permission.

Clinical Course

MDD tends to have a remitting-relapsing course, whereas dysthymic disorder is more chronic; a small subset of older adults may develop a steadily worsening course. Older adults with depression may experience a worse course than do younger adults with depression, including persistence of diagnosis of MDD or dysthymia, greater chronicity of symptoms, delayed time to remission, and worsening depression severity over time (Schaakxs et al. 2018). Many risk factors for worse trajectories of depression in older adults have been identified, including female gender; Black or Hispanic race/ethnicity; past psychiatric history of depression and/or anxiety; presence, number, and severity of medical conditions (e.g., ischemic heart disease, stroke, hypertension, diabetes mellitus, obesity, breast cancer); tobacco use; certain personality traits (e.g., avoidance coping, psychological inflexibility); lower educational level; severity of functional impairment; lack of social supports; and stressful life events (Musliner et al. 2016). Limitations in mobility (i.e., ability to do heavy housework, walk half a mile, and climb stairs) and adverse childhood experiences (in women) have also been associated with worse trajectories of LLD (Carrière et al. 2017). Interestingly, cognitive impairment has not been consistently identified as a predictor of a worse course of depression (Musliner et al. 2016).

In a primary care sample of older adults with MDD or dysthymia that had partially or fully remitted, 40% had recurrence of clinically significant depressive symptoms within a year (Katon et al. 2006). Predictors of relapse included severity of baseline depression and number of residual depressive symptoms at remission; for example, subjects with four residual symptoms had a 54% relapse rate versus 36% for those with only one residual symptom (Katon et al. 2006). The clinical implication is that a goal of treating depression in older adults should be complete remission of symptoms. In fact, persistence of depressive symptoms has been associated with a number of negative health outcomes, including increased mortality and increased risk of dementia, as discussed in the following section.

Consequences and Complications

A classic aphorism in geriatric psychiatry is that untreated depression in older adults can lead to a downward spiral of disability and worsening depression that culminates in death. In this section, we cover some of the consequences of LLD.

SUICIDE

Suicide is the topic of Chapter 4, "Suicide Risk Reduction in Older Adults," and we very briefly summarize the chapter here. Age is a powerful predictor of suicide risk, with men 75 years old and older at the highest risk of dying from suicide (Figure 1–5) (Centers for Disease Control and Prevention 2020). Older adults are more likely than younger adults to choose lethal means (notably firearms) and are less likely to survive suicide attempts. Depression is the most common psychiatric diagnosis associated with suicide in older adults, although a significant proportion of older adults who die from suicide do not have a history of MDD. Interestingly, the risk of suicide does not appear to be higher in patients with dementia compared with elders without dementia, although the time immediately after the diagnosis of dementia is a period of higher risk of suicide (Seyfried et al. 2011). An essential part of the evaluation of any older adult with depression is conducting a suicide risk assessment, which is discussed in greater detail in Chapter 4.

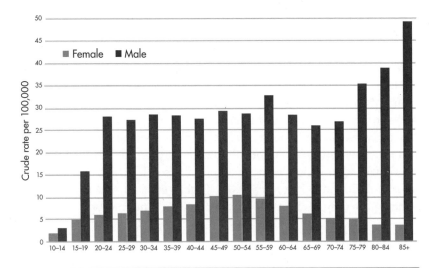

Figure 1–5. Suicide across the life span: crude rate of suicide by age per 100,000 people in the United States in 2019.

Women experience a midlife peak in suicide rate, with a decline afterward. Men experience peaks in midlife and again as older adults. Men die by suicide more frequently than women at all ages.

Source. Centers for Disease Control and Prevention: WISQARS—Web-Based Injury Statistics Query and Reporting System. Atlanta, GA, Centers for Disease Control and Prevention, July 1, 2020. Available at: www.cdc.gov/injury/wisqars/index.html. Accessed April 11, 2021.

MORBIDITY AND OTHER CAUSES OF DEATH

Older adults with depression are at heightened risk of dying from causes other than suicide. LLD is associated with a 34% increase in all-cause mortality and 31% increased cardiovascular mortality; for late-onset depression, the increases are 51% and 40%, respectively (Wei et al. 2019). In one cohort of 4,000 older adults with depression in the United Kingdom (mean age of 77 years), nearly 55% of subjects died within 3.5 years; predictors of mortality included older age, male gender, specific symptoms (cognitive impairment, apathy, lack of appetite), older age at diagnosis of depression, physical illness, impairments of ADLs, and (only in new-onset depression) depression severity (Cai et al. 2020). Another large cohort study of older adults, this time in Brazil, also found that LLD predicted mortality, although only in men; the authors estimated the population attributable risk of dying because of LLD—that is, the percentage of deaths that could be avoided if no one developed LLD—to be 8.5% (Diniz et al. 2014). Depression also increases the risk of death in patients with coronary heart disease and stroke. Possible explanations for the link between LLD and death include vascular disease; unhealthy behaviors such as tobacco use, binge drinking, or physical inactivity; poor adherence to medical treatment recommendations; or an inflammatory process (Wei et al. 2019).

Elders with depression are also at higher risk of developing coronary heart disease (or having another myocardial infarction), of having a stroke (or another stroke), of falling, of developing diabetes mellitus (or having worse diabetic course), of having more somatic symptoms (stomach problems, shortness of breath, dizziness, pain, and difficulties with eyesight) and of experiencing generally worse physical health (Fiske et al. 2009; Niles and O'Donovan 2019; Stubbs et al. 2016; Wu et al. 2019). Whether treating LLD has an impact on medical morbidity is unclear.

DISABILITY

LLD is a predictor of the onset of disability—that is, problems with carrying out personal or instrumental ADLs—with a roughly 40% increase in risk of developing disability among depressed elders compared with elders without depression (Mendes de Leon and Rajan 2014). The impact of depression on progression of disability is less clear, with conflicting evidence from various studies. The disability associated with LLD also leaves older adults less able to work and more likely to engage in unpaid family roles (e.g., babysitting grandchildren), with adverse financial implications (Snow and Abrams 2016; Zivin et al. 2013). Depression also contributes to physical frailty, which is discussed in greater detail in the subsection "Frailty and Failure to Thrive."

IMPACT ON FAMILY AND OTHER CAREGIVERS

Because of decreased energy, motivation, and ability to carry out ADLs, older adults with depression may need to rely on family members and others for support. Compared with elders without depression, those with LLD receive up to 3 extra hours per week of informal caregiving (Zivin et al. 2013). This in turn takes an emotional and financial toll on caregivers. For example, family caregivers of elders suffering from depression are at higher risk of depression themselves, as well other negative health outcomes (Zivin et al. 2013). In 2016, the cost of unpaid caregiving of elders with either minor depression or MDD in the United States was estimated to be almost $13 billion (Snow and Abrams 2016). Strikingly, LLD can impact family members beyond direct caregivers: for example, young children living in the same household as a depressed elder have more problems with behavior, sleep, attention, and school (Zivin et al. 2013).

Comorbidities

LLD rarely manifests in isolation. About half of older adults with depression also have clinically significant anxiety; cognitive impairment is exceedingly common; excessive alcohol use and substance use disorders may complicate matters; and other medical conditions such as sleep disorders may be present. We provide an overview of these comorbidities next.

ANXIETY

Late-life anxiety is the other major topic of this book and thus will be covered extensively in Chapters 2, 3, 5, and 6. Here we briefly focus on the extensive comorbidity of depression and anxiety, both cross-sectionally and longitudinally. Up to half of elders with depression also have an anxiety disorder, and about one-quarter of those with anxiety also have depression (Beekman et al. 2000). Although much of the literature on this comorbidity specifically refers to generalized anxiety disorder (GAD), older adults with depression are more likely to have comorbid social phobia, panic disorder, and/or agoraphobia than GAD (van der Veen et al. 2015).

GAD tends to be chronic, with onset in early life for about half of older adults; in elders with both GAD and MDD, the onset of GAD usually precedes the onset of MDD (Lenze et al. 2005). Older adults with both depression and anxiety have worse outcomes than those with either one alone, including persistence of depressive symptoms, high rates of depression relapse, more cognitive decline, and higher risk of suicidal ideation or suicide (Lenze and Wetherell 2011). We go into greater detail about the comorbidity between depression and anxiety, including theories about why the two are so highly comorbid, in Chapter 2, "Introduction to Late-Life Anxiety and Related Disorders," subsection "Depression."

COGNITIVE IMPAIRMENT AND DEMENTIA

Cognitive impairment and neuropsychological deficits are common in depression and can be so severe as to mimic dementia—a construct sometimes referred to as *pseudodementia* (Brodaty and Connors 2020).

Cognitive impairment may persist even after successful treatment of LLD, and depression roughly doubles the risk of dementia (Cherbuin et al. 2015).

Both early-onset and late-onset depression are associated with later cognitive impairment or development of dementia. In one large longitudinal study, compared with subjects with no depression, elders who had midlife depressive symptoms were 20% more likely to develop dementia, those with late-onset depression were 70% more likely, and those with depressive symptoms in both midlife and late life were 80% more likely (Barnes et al. 2012). In general, late-onset depression appears to be associated with a higher risk of cognitive decline than early-onset depression. For example, the Whitehall II study, which followed British civil servants over 28 years, found that people who went on to develop dementia were more likely to be depressed 11 years prior to the diagnosis of dementia but not earlier; at the time of diagnosis, people with dementia were 9 times more like to be depressed than were those without dementia (Singh-Manoux et al. 2017). However, it should be noted that at least one study found the opposite, namely, a higher risk of dementia with early-onset depression (Riddle et al. 2017).

The trajectory of symptoms may make a difference, too: for example, older adults with a pattern of "high and increasing" depression symptoms (greater depression severity at baseline, followed by increasing severity over the course of 5 years) have twice the risk of developing dementia than do those with minimal or moderate symptoms (Kaup et al. 2016). The risk that depression confers may be higher for vascular dementia than for dementia due to Alzheimer's disease (Diniz et al. 2013). Depression results in increased risk of progression from mild cognitive impairment (mild neurocognitive disorder) to dementia (major neurocognitive disorder) (Dafsari and Jessen 2020). It is possible that LLD represents a modifiable risk factor for dementia, accounting for 4% of the population-attributable fraction of dementia risk (Livingston et al. 2020).

The exact nature of the relationship between depression and dementia remains unclear, with evidence supporting each of the following possibilities:

- The pathophysiology of recurrent MDD (e.g., HPA axis dysfunction or dysfunctional neural networks) leads to or exacerbates the pathologies that lead to dementia.
- Behaviors associated with recurrent MDD (e.g., substance use, physical inactivity, poor health habits) lead to or exacerbate the pathologies that lead to dementia (e.g., cerebrovascular disease).

- MDD, in particular late-onset depression, that arises prior to dementia reflects an early clinical manifestation of underlying pathology (i.e., cerebrovascular disease or neurodegenerative disease) that will eventually lead to dementia.
- Depression that arises after the onset of dementia is due to the pathological changes associated with dementia and/or represents a psychological reaction (grief) to memory loss, as discussed earlier in the subsections "Neurobiology" and "Vascular Depression."
- MDD and dementia are not causally related but instead have shared risk factors (e.g., genetic liability, social determinants of health, chronic medical problems).
- Depression causes cognitive impairment during a depressive episode but otherwise is not associated with dementia.

These hypotheses are not mutually exclusive, and in a large heterogeneous population of people with depression and dementia, all could be true. Clinicians should take away the following from this discussion: 1) older adults with depression may have significant cognitive impairment, such that they appear to have dementia; 2) when assessing and caring for patients with dementia, it is important to keep in mind the possibility of depression, a potentially reversible cause of impairment; 3) elders experiencing their first episode of depression are at markedly higher risk for developing dementia. The following case illustrates these points further.

CASE EXAMPLE 2: "IT'S JUST NOT LIKE HIM TO FORGET TO PAY HIS BILLS"

Mr. Rodríguez is a 68-year-old retired accountant whose family has become increasingly concerned about his memory and behavior. His two adult daughters first noticed a change 8 months ago, soon after his wife died from ovarian cancer. He stopped showing interest in his usual activities, went to church on Sundays only after his children insisted, and no longer wanted to babysit his grandchildren. He stopped exercising, citing fatigue. He started sleeping excessively and had a hard time getting out of bed in the morning. His diet shifted to mostly junk food, and he gained 10 pounds. He seemed forgetful, was repetitive in his speech, and on a couple of occasions forgot to pay his bills (a new and surprising occurrence, given his background as an accountant). Mr. Rodríguez's daughters thought that he might still be grieving, but his symptoms seemed excessive.

Mr. Rodríguez has no psychiatric history; his medical problems include hypertension (for which he takes a diuretic), hyperglycemia (which does not meet criteria for diabetes), and dyslipidemia (for which he takes a statin). There is no known family history of neuropsychiatric disease. His primary care provider ordered laboratory work (electrolytes, renal function, liver function, thyroid-stimulating hormone, complete blood count) and an electrocardiogram, all of which was normal except for elevated blood sugar. Mr. Rodríguez was referred to a psychiatrist for further evaluation.

On examination, Mr. Rodríguez is mildly disheveled, makes poor eye contact, and appears sullen, crying at times. He denies active suicidal ideation but states, "I wish God would take me away." He denies psychotic and manic symptoms. He worries about his finances and whether he can continue to live alone. He reports rare use of alcohol and no use of illicit substances. He scores 10 out of 15 on the short version of the Geriatric Depression Scale (Yesavage et al. 1982), consistent with moderate to severe depression. Bedside cognitive testing is abnormal, with deficits in memory and executive function. However, Mr. Rodríguez may not have given his full effort during the testing.

You diagnose Mr. Rodríguez as having major depressive disorder, single episode, moderate. To complete the evaluation of other medical etiologies of depression, you order polysomnography to rule out sleep apnea and a test to measure his serum vitamin B_{12} level. You explain to Mr. Rodríguez and his daughters that his cognitive impairment is likely due to depression and should improve with successful treatment of depression. You recommend a trial of sertraline and refer him for cognitive-behavioral therapy. He is then lost to follow-up.

Four years later, Mr. Rodríguez and his daughters return. They report that initially his mood, memory, and functioning improved markedly with the combination of an antidepressant and psychotherapy. He discontinued both after 6 months, and the depression did not recur, at least initially. About 1 year ago, however, his daughters noticed that he was becoming repetitive in his speech again; he got lost driving on two occasions and also got into a minor motor vehicle accident (without injury). He did not seem particularly depressed, just disinterested. His daughters insisted he resume sertraline, but this did not seem to help—in fact, his memory seemed even worse after restarting the medication. He was not interested in psychotherapy and declined all other offers of help. His responses to a recent Patient Health Questionnaire–9 (PHQ-9; Kroenke et al. 2001) were essentially normal, but bedside cognitive testing was worse than 4 years earlier.

You suspect that Mr. Rodríguez has now developed major neurocognitive disorder, and you refer him for neuropsychological assessment and neuroimaging to confirm the diagnosis and help establish the etiology.

SUBSTANCE USE DISORDERS

Problems with alcohol and substance use are common in older adults. The prevalence of at-risk alcohol use (two or more drinks on a usual drinking day in the past 30 days) or binge-drinking (five or more drinks on at least 1 day in the past 30 days) is 28% in older men and 11% in older women (Wu and Blazer 2014). Among older adults, at-risk alcohol use decreases with age and with prescription drug use, a proxy for diminished health (Foster and Patel 2019). In the 2005–2007 National Surveys on Drug Use and Health conducted among community-dwelling individuals in the United States, the prevalence of DSM-IV alcohol abuse and dependence among older adults was 0.9% and 0.6%, respectively (Wu and Blazer 2014); note that in DSM-5 the term *alcohol use disorder* replaces both alcohol abuse and alcohol dependence.

Older adults with greater alcohol use are more likely to have comorbid MDD and more likely to develop new-onset MDD: in a review of studies published between 2005 and 2013, Wu and Blazer (2014) found that about 4% of adults ≥60 years with alcohol use disorder developed MDD over the course of 3 years. Alcohol use disorders were the most common *substance use disorders* among older adults admitted to an inpatient psychiatric unit, constituting 73% of use disorders and 9% of all admissions; MDD was comorbid in 26% of patients with substance use disorders (Dombrowski et al. 2016). In another study, 26% of psychiatric inpatients had substance use disorders (most commonly, cocaine use disorder), and substance use disorders were associated with greater length of stay (Lane et al. 2018). Alcohol use can both contribute to depression and complicate its treatment, including interacting with antidepressants. Clinicians should screen all depressed elders for alcohol use, recognizing that use that does not meet criteria for alcohol use disorder can still be a problem in older adults.

A recent survey of older adults in a geriatrics clinic found that 15% had used cannabis within the past 3 years, and half of them reported daily or weekly use (Yang et al. 2021). Interestingly, 61% reported their first use of cannabis after age 60; 78% reported using cannabis for medical purposes only, including depression, anxiety, and insomnia; less than half had told their health care providers about their use of cannabis (Yang et al. 2021). Older adults who use cannabis and have MDD are more likely to misuse prescription pain relievers than are older adults who use cannabis and do not have MDD (Choi et al. 2021a). Reports to U.S. poison control centers of cannabis toxicity among older adults increased eighteenfold from 2009 to 2019, sometimes with serious consequences such as suicide attempts (Choi et al. 2021b). Older adults who used cannabis in the past year had high rates of depression: 17% in the past year and 32% lifetime (Vacaflor et al. 2020). Suicidal ideation in the past year was found in 14% of older adults who used cannabis combined with other drugs and in 5% of older adults who used only cannabis (compared with 2% of older adults who had never used cannabis) (Vacaflor et al. 2020). With the increasing use of cannabis among older adults, clinicians need to screen their patients for cannabis use and address comorbid depression and cannabis use.

Other substance use disorders in older adults, and their comorbidity with depression, have been less well studied. About 9% of older Americans smoke, and 4% meet criteria for nicotine dependence (Cawkwell et al. 2015; Wu and Blazer 2014). Older adults may be less likely than younger adults to report being interested in quitting smoking, and their primary care providers may be less likely to offer smoking cessation treatment, even though older adults have more success with smoking cessation (Cawkwell et al. 2015; Jordan et al. 2017). The comorbidity of smoking and depression has not been well studied. Older adults who continue to smoke have higher rates of psychological distress than do older adults who quit smoking (Cawkwell et al. 2015). In addition, they increase their cardiovascular risk factors, potentially contributing to vascular depression and potentially dementia in the long term. Given the tremendous benefits of smoking cessation at any age, all older adults presenting with depression should be screened for tobacco use and offered evidence-based smoking cessation techniques.

Illicit substance use is relatively uncommon among older adults, although comorbidity with depression is high. In the review by Wu and Blazer (2014), 7% of older adults with a substance use disorder (other than alcohol use disorder) developed MDD within 3 years. Twenty-seven percent of older adults accessing emergency care for psychiatric conditions had positive urine toxicology for illicit drug use (Wu and Blazer 2014). The opioid epidemic has not spared older adults, with 2.5% of older adults reporting misuse of prescription opioids in the past year; those misusing opioids were more likely to have depression; more likely to have alcohol use disorder; more likely to misuse sedatives or stimulants; and more likely to use tobacco, cocaine, or cannabis (Han et al. 2019).

PERSONALITY DISORDERS

As noted in the section "Clinical Course," certain personality traits (e.g., avoidance coping, psychological inflexibility, neuroticism, harm avoidance) are associated with the development and persistence of LLD. *Personality disorders* are also common, found in about 24%–31% of older adults with depression (Devanand 2002). The most common personality disorders among this group are from cluster C ("anxious") of the DSM-5 classification of personality disorders, specifically, obsessive-compulsive personality disorder and avoidant personality disorder (Devanand 2002). Personality pathology has been associated with worse treatment outcomes in LLD, including longer time to response and lower likelihood of remission (Kiosses et al. 2011). Personality disorders are more associated with early-onset depression than late-onset depression (Devanand 2002).

Interestingly, cluster B ("dramatic") personality disorders such as borderline personality disorder are much less common in older adults with depression than in younger adults with depression. Why? Perhaps withdrawal and estrangement from family and friends replace self-harm behavior and volatile interpersonal relationships, or perhaps patients with these personality disorders are less likely to survive into old age because of suicide or other consequences of high-risk behavior (Devanand 2002). Nevertheless, given their likely history of one or more suicide attempts, their chronic depression and low self-esteem, and their lack of interpersonal supports, elders with comorbid LLD and borderline personality disorder require attentive clinical care.

SLEEP DISORDERS

About 30% of community-dwelling elders report sleep disturbance, which is a risk factor for the onset, exacerbation, and recurrence of depression (Bao et al. 2017). Short sleep duration (6 or fewer hours) is predictive of onset of depression, whereas long sleep duration (more than 9 hours) is not (Sun et al. 2018). Insomnia is also a risk factor for suicide attempts in older adults (Kay et al. 2016). Conversely, depressed elders are 70% more likely to develop problems with sleep than are nondepressed elders (Bao et al. 2017).

Of course, insomnia and hypersomnia are criteria for MDD, so some comorbidity would be expected. Beyond diagnostic overlap, possible mechanisms for this high level of comorbidity include changes in rapid eye movement (REM) sleep associated with aging (e.g., REM dysregulation is a predictor of recurrence of depression), changes in circadian rhythm (phase advance, i.e., going to sleep and waking up earlier), hyperarousal mediated by disturbances in the HPA axis, and structural and functional changes in the brain stem and hypothalamus (Bao et al. 2017). Some antidepressants can have negative effects on sleep, including changes in slow-wave ("deep") sleep and REM sleep (Wichniak et al. 2017), whereas others are used to treat both depression and insomnia (Schroeck et al. 2016). Medications used in the treatment of insomnia, including benzodiazepines, "z-drugs" (zolpidem, zaleplon, and eszopiclone), and suvorexant, may exacerbate depression or suicidal ideation (McCall et al. 2017; Schroeck et al. 2016) and are not indicated for long-term use.

As noted earlier in the subsection "Neurobiology," the possibility of obstructive sleep apnea (OSA) should be considered in the evaluation of older adults with depression. OSA at least doubles the risk of developing depression, perhaps via cerebral hypoperfusion associated with apneic episodes leading to or exacerbating cerebrovascular disease (Kerner and Roose 2016). Treatment of OSA has been found to reduce depressive symptoms in older adults, including in those who do not respond to antidepressants (Kerner and Roose 2016).

FRAILTY AND FAILURE TO THRIVE

Finally, we explore the relationship between frailty, failure to thrive, and depression. The *frailty phenotype* includes having three or more of the following five criteria: 1) weight loss (≥5% of body weight in the past year), 2) exhaustion (positive response to questions regarding effort required for activity), 3) weakness (decreased grip strength), 4) slow gait (>6 seconds to walk 15 feet), and 5) decreased physical activity (measured in calories expended per week) (Fried et al. 2001). Frailty is associated with falls, hospitalizations, disability, and depression—which itself is a risk factor for frailty; in particular, slow gait predicts depression and vice versa (Brown et al. 2016). Frail elders are about four times more likely than nonfrail elders to have depression, with a prevalence of about 40% (Soysal et al. 2017).

There is significant diagnostic overlap between frailty and depression: weight loss, fatigue, and psychomotor slowing represent three of the nine DSM-5 criteria for MDD. In a reanalysis of the Epidemiologic Catchment Area study, 100% of severely depressed elders were considered frail (Brown et al. 2016). LLD and frailty are not synonymous, but they are highly comorbid; for example, a more recent study found that a quarter of depressed adults ≥60 years met the aforementioned Fried criteria for frailty and that roughly half had decreased grip strength, slow gait, or both (Brown et al. 2020). A meta-analysis of studies of elders diagnosed with MDD found that 18% were also frail (Soysal et al. 2017).

Mitochondrial dysfunction (resulting in fatigue and decreased mobility), dopaminergic dysfunction (resulting in cognitive and motor slowing), and chronic inflammation (discussed in the subsection "Neurobiology") have been proposed as mechanisms for the relationship between frailty and depression (Brown et al. 2016). Cerebrovascular disease does not appear to be involved (Brown et al. 2020).

I should note that there is some controversy about the term *failure to thrive* (FTT). Physical frailty is a symptom—perhaps the core symptom—of FTT. FTT is included in the ICD and has been described as "a syndrome of weight loss, decreased appetite and poor nutrition, and inactivity, often accompanied by dehydration, depressive symptoms, impaired immune function, and low cholesterol" (Sarkisian and Lachs 1996, p. 1074). However, there is concern that the imprecision of the term and the implication that FTT is a psychosocial problem (as reflected in the pejorative concept of a "social admission") may lead to delays in care and may perhaps reflect or contribute to ageism (Sarkisian and Lachs 1996; Tsui et al. 2020). In one study of older adults admitted for FTT, 88% were in fact found to have an acute medical condition (Tsui et al. 2020). Sarkisian and Lachs argue that a presumptive diagnosis of FTT should lead to a search for causes of impaired physical functioning, malnutrition, and cognitive decline—as well as identifying and addressing depression.

Summary: Understanding How Depression Arises and Progresses in Older Adults

Depression is a common, disabling, and potentially lethal syndrome in older adults. Neurobiological, psychosocial, cultural, and spiritual factors, as well as social determinants of health, contribute to depression, which can manifest somewhat differently in older adults than in younger adults. Late-onset depression may be a distinct disorder that represents a prodrome of dementia. Late-life depression is comorbid with (and exacerbates) a wide variety of other medical conditions, including anxiety disorders, substance use disorders, sleep disorders, personality disorders, cardiovascular disease, cerebrovascular disease, and neurodegenerative disorders. Suicide is of particular concern among depressed elders, who are also at risk of death from cardiovascular and other medical conditions. Unrecognized or undertreated depression can lead to many other negative outcomes, including worsening medical conditions, physical frailty, disability, and caregiver burden.

KEY POINTS

- Late-life depression (LLD) is common, affecting at least 5%–10% of older adults and up to 48% in some subsets of older adults.

- Depression can manifest differently in older adults than in younger adults, including more somatic symptoms, greater cognitive impairment, and subtle psychotic symptoms (e.g., delusional guilt).

- Older adults with depression follow one of these clinical courses:

  - Earlier onset of major depressive disorder (MDD) or bipolar disorder, with recurrence or chronicity into older adulthood

  - Subclinical depression or anxiety through early adulthood or midlife, worsening into clinical depression in late life

  - Late-life onset of depression that is either a risk factor for or harbinger of dementia. This is related to the construct of vascular depression, that is, depression that arises in the context of cerebrovascular disease and manifests with more executive dysfunction.

  - Depression that arises after the onset of and is presumably due to a neurodegenerative disorder or cerebrovascular disease. This is to be distinguished from apathy (the most common behavioral and psychological symptom of dementia), which does not include the psychological distress associated with depression.

  - Minor depression (not meeting full criteria for MDD) that nevertheless can result in disability and other negative outcomes

- Depression arises in older adults from some combination of the following: genetic and developmental factors (e.g., childhood abuse); personality characteristics; social determinants of health; social and cultural factors, including race, ethnicity, and LGBTQ+ status; stressful life events, including the death of loved ones; dysfunction of the hypothalamic-pituitary-adrenal axis and/or reproductive hormone systems; cerebrovascular disease; neurodegenerative disease; inflammatory processes; use of alcohol and other substances; and dysfunction of neural networks involved in emotion regulation.

- Cognitive impairment and depression are closely linked in older adults. LLD often includes cognitive symptoms, which may be so severe that the elder appears to have dementia. Conversely, Alzheimer's disease and other causes of dementia can cause or contribute to depression. Clinicians evaluating older adults with depression should also assess their cognition; clinicians evaluating people suspected of having dementia should screen for depression.

- Because LLD is comorbid with many other medical conditions, clinicians should also assess for anxiety, use of alcohol and other substances, sleep disorders (especially sleep apnea), and personality disorders.

- In the United States, older men have the highest risk of suicide of any demographic. LLD is also associated with increased cardiovascular mortality and all-cause mortality.

Resources for Patients, Families, and Caregivers

National Suicide Prevention Lifeline

https://suicidepreventionlifeline.org

1-800-273-8255

1-800-799-4889 (TTY)

• Older adults with depression are at especially high risk of suicide.

• The National Suicide Prevention Lifeline provides free, confidential 24/7 support for people in distress and prevention and crisis resources for people in distress and their loved ones.

National Institute of Mental Health (NIMH)

www.nimh.nih.gov/health/publications/older-adults-and-depression/index.shtml

• NIMH is the lead federal agency for research on mental disorders.

• In addition to funding research, NIMH has developed educational materials on a number of topics, including "Older Adults and Depression," available in English and Spanish.

National Institute on Aging (NIA)

www.nia.nih.gov/health/depression-and-older-adults

www.nia.nih.gov/health/mourning-death-spouse

• NIA is a federal agency that studies the nature of aging and conducts research into Alzheimer's disease and related dementias.

• NIA has developed educational materials on a number of topics, including "Depression and Older Adults" and "Mourning the Death of a Spouse."

Depression and Bipolar Support Alliance (DBSA)

www.dbsalliance.org

• DBSA offers educational and support services for people suffering from depression or bipolar disorder and their family members.

• Services are available online 24/7, in local support groups, in audiocasts and videocasts, or via printed materials.

References

Aggarwal NK: Reassessing cultural evaluations in geriatrics: insights from cultural psychiatry. J Am Geriatr Soc 58(11):2191–2196, 2010 20977437

Ahearn EP, Szymanski BR, Chen P, et al: Increased risk of dementia among veterans with bipolar disorder or schizophrenia receiving care in the VA Health System. Psychiatr Serv 71(10):998–1004, 2020 32517643

Alexopoulos GS: Mechanisms and treatment of late-life depression. Transl Psychiatry 9(1):188, 2019 31383842

American Psychiatric Association: Diagnostic and Statistical Manual of Mental Disorders, 4th Edition. Washington, DC, American Psychiatric Association, 1994

American Psychiatric Association: Diagnostic and Statistical Manual of Mental Disorders, 5th Edition. Arlington, VA, American Psychiatric Association, 2013

American Psychiatric Association: Diagnostic and Statistical Manual of Mental Disorders, 5th Edition, Text Revision. Washington, DC, American Psychiatric Association, 2022

Angst J, Gamma A, Sellaro R, et al: Recurrence of bipolar disorders and major depression: a life-long perspective. Eur Arch Psychiatry Clin Neurosci 253(5):236–240, 2003 14504992

Areán PA, Reynolds CF 3rd: The impact of psychosocial factors on late-life depression. Biol Psychiatry 58(4):277–282, 2005 16102545

Aziz R, Steffens DC: What are the causes of late-life depression? Psychiatr Clin North Am 36(4):497–516, 2013 24229653

Balsis S, Cully JA: Comparing depression diagnostic symptoms across younger and older adults. Aging Ment Health 12(6):800–806, 2008 19023732

Bao YP, Han Y, Ma J, et al: Cooccurrence and bidirectional prediction of sleep disturbances and depression in older adults: meta-analysis and systematic review. Neurosci Biobehav Rev 75:257–273, 2017 28179129

Barnes DE, Yaffe K, Byers AL, et al: Midlife vs late-life depressive symptoms and risk of dementia: differential effects for Alzheimer disease and vascular dementia. Arch Gen Psychiatry 69(5):493–498, 2012 22566581

Barry LC, Wakefield DB, Trestman RL, et al: Disability in prison activities of daily living and likelihood of depression and suicidal ideation in older prisoners. Int J Geriatr Psychiatry 32(10):1141–1149, 2017 27650475

Beekman ATF, de Beurs E, van Balkom AJLM, et al: Anxiety and depression in later life: co-occurrence and communality of risk factors. Am J Psychiatry 157(1):89–95, 2000 10618018

Bremmer MA, Deeg DJ, Beekman AT, et al: Major depression in late life is associated with both hypo- and hypercortisolemia. Biol Psychiatry 62(5):479–486, 2007 17481591

Brodaty H, Connors MH: Pseudodementia, pseudo-pseudodementia, and pseudodepression. Alzheimers Dement (Amst) 12(1):e12027, 2020 32318620

Brown PJ, Rutherford BR, Yaffe K, et al: The depressed frail phenotype: the clinical manifestation of increased biological aging. Am J Geriatr Psychiatry 24(11):1084–1094, 2016 27618646

Brown PJ, Roose SP, O'Boyle KR, et al: Frailty and its correlates in adults with late life depression. Am J Geriatr Psychiatry 28(2):145–154, 2020 31734083

Burton R: The Anatomy of Melancholy. New York, New York Review Books Classics, 2001

Byers AL, Yaffe K, Covinsky KE, et al: High occurrence of mood and anxiety disorders among older adults: the National Comorbidity Survey Replication. Arch Gen Psychiatry 67(5):489–496, 2010 20439830

Cai W, Mueller C, Shetty H, et al: Predictors of mortality in people with late-life depression: a retrospective cohort study. J Affect Disord 266:695–701, 2020 32056946

Carrière I, Farré A, Proust-Lima C, et al: Chronic and remitting trajectories of depressive symptoms in the elderly: characterisation and risk factors. Epidemiol Psychiatr Sci 26(2):146–156, 2017 26768574

Cawkwell PB, Blaum C, Sherman SE: Pharmacological smoking cessation therapies in older adults: a review of the evidence. Drugs Aging 32(6):443–451, 2015 26025119

Centers for Disease Control and Prevention: WISQARS—Web-Based Injury Statistics Query and Reporting System. Atlanta, GA, Centers for Disease Control and Prevention, July 1, 2020. Available at: www.cdc.gov/injury/wisqars/index.html. Accessed April 11, 2021.

Chen P, Dols A, Rej S, Sajatovic M: Update on the epidemiology, diagnosis, and treatment of mania in older-age bipolar disorder. Curr Psychiatry Rep 19(8):46, 2017 28647815

Cheong EV, Sinnott C, Dahly D, et al: Adverse childhood experiences (ACEs) and later-life depression: perceived social support as a potential protective factor. BMJ Open 7(9):e013228, 2017 28864684

Cherbuin N, Kim S, Anstey KJ: Dementia risk estimates associated with measures of depression: a systematic review and meta-analysis. BMJ Open 5(12):e008853, 2015 26692556

Chihuri S, Mielenz TJ, DiMaggio CJ, et al: Driving cessation and health outcomes in older adults. J Am Geriatr Soc 64(2):332–341, 2016 26780879

Choi NG, DiNitto DM, Choi BY: Prescription pain reliever use and misuse among cannabis users aged 50+ years. Clin Gerontol 44(1):53–65, 2021a 32374215

Choi NG, Marti CN, DiNitto DM, et al: Cannabis and synthetic cannabinoid poison control center cases among adults aged 50+, 2009–2019. Clin Toxicol (Phila) 59(4):334–342, 2021b 32840426

Conner KO, Copeland VC, Grote NK, et al: Barriers to treatment and culturally endorsed coping strategies among depressed African-American older adults. Aging Ment Health 14(8):971–983, 2010 21069603

Cuevas-Esteban J, Iglesias-González M, Rubio-Valera M, et al: Prevalence and characteristics of catatonia on admission to an acute geriatric psychiatry ward. Prog Neuropsychopharmacol Biol Psychiatry 78:27–33, 2017 28533149

Dafsari FS, Jessen F: Depression-an underrecognized target for prevention of dementia in Alzheimer's disease. Transl Psychiatry 10(1):160, 2020 32433512

Devanand DP: Comorbid psychiatric disorders in late life depression. Biol Psychiatry 52(3):236–242, 2002 12182929

Devanand DP: Dysthymic disorder in the elderly population. Int Psychogeriatr 26(1):39–48, 2014 24152873

Dilworth-Anderson P, Gibson BE: The cultural influence of values, norms, meanings, and perceptions in understanding dementia in ethnic minorities. Alzheimer Dis Assoc Disord 16(suppl 2):S56–S63, 2002 12351916

Diniz BS, Butters MA, Albert SM, et al: Late-life depression and risk of vascular dementia and Alzheimer's disease: systematic review and meta-analysis of community-based cohort studies. Br J Psychiatry 202(5):329–335, 2013 23637108

Diniz BS, Reynolds CF 3rd, Butters MA, et al: The effect of gender, age, and symptom severity in late-life depression on the risk of all-cause mortality: the Bambuí Cohort Study of Aging. Depress Anxiety 31(9):787–795, 2014 24353128

Dombrowski D, Norrell N, Holroyd S: Substance use disorders in elderly admissions to an academic psychiatric inpatient service over a 10-year period. J Addict 2016:4973018, 2016 27840765

Fiske A, Wetherell JL, Gatz M: Depression in older adults. Annu Rev Clin Psychol 5:363–389, 2009 19327033

Flores-Flores O, Zevallos-Morales A, Carrión I, et al: "We can't carry the weight of the whole world": illness experiences among Peruvian older adults with symptoms of depression and anxiety. Int J Ment Health Syst 14:49, 2020 32670400

Fornaro M, Solmi M, Stubbs B, et al: Prevalence and correlates of major depressive disorder, bipolar disorder and schizophrenia among nursing home residents without dementia: systematic review and meta-analysis. Br J Psychiatry 216(1):6–15, 2020 30864533

Foster J, Patel S: Prevalence of simultaneous use of alcohol and prescription medication in older adults: findings from a cross-sectional survey (Health Survey for England 2013). BMJ Open 9(6):e023730, 2019 31256017

Fried LP, Tangen CM, Walston J, et al: Frailty in older adults: evidence for a phenotype. J Gerontol A Biol Sci Med Sci 56(3):M146–M156, 2001 11253156

Gallagher D, Mhaolain AN, Greene E, et al: Late life depression: a comparison of risk factors and symptoms according to age of onset in community dwelling older adults. Int J Geriatr Psychiatry 25(10):981–987, 2010 19998316

Georgakis MK, Thomopoulos TP, Diamantaras AA, et al: Association of age at menopause and duration of reproductive period with depression after menopause: a systematic review and meta-analysis. JAMA Psychiatry 73(2):139–149, 2016 26747373

Geerlings MI, Gerritsen L: Late-life depression, hippocampal volumes, and hypothalamic-pituitary-adrenal axis regulation: a systematic review and meta-analysis. Biol Psychiatry 82(5):339–350, 2017 28318491

Gournellis R, Oulis P, Howard R: Psychotic major depression in older people: a systematic review. Int J Geriatr Psychiatry 29(8):789–796, 2014 25191689

Han BH, Sherman SE, Palamar JJ: Prescription opioid misuse among middle-aged and older adults in the United States, 2015–2016. Prev Med 121:94–98, 2019 30763631

Hirshbein LD: Gender, age, and diagnosis: the rise and fall of involutional melancholia in American psychiatry, 1900–1980. Bull Hist Med 83(4):710–745, 2009 20061671

Jordan H, Hidajat M, Payne N, et al: What are older smokers' attitudes to quitting and how are they managed in primary care? An analysis of the cross-sectional English Smoking Toolkit Study. BMJ Open 7(11):e18150, 2017 29146649

Kaplan LM, Vella L, Cabral E, et al: Unmet mental health and substance use treatment needs among older homeless adults: results from the HOPE HOME Study. J Community Psychol 47(8):1893–1908, 2019 31424102

Katon WJ, Fan MY, Lin EH, et al: Depressive symptom deterioration in a large primary care-based elderly cohort. Am J Geriatr Psychiatry 14(3):246–254, 2006 16505129

Katz S: Assessing self-maintenance: activities of daily living, mobility, and instrumental activities of daily living. J Am Geriatr Soc 31(12):721–727, 1983 6418786

Kaup AR, Byers AL, Falvey C, et al: Trajectories of depressive symptoms in older adults and risk of dementia. JAMA Psychiatry 73(5):525–531, 2016 26982217

Kay DB, Dombrovski AY, Buysse DJ, et al: Insomnia is associated with suicide attempt in middle-aged and older adults with depression. Int Psychogeriatr 28(4):613–619, 2016 26552935

Kerner NA, Roose SP: Obstructive sleep apnea is linked to depression and cognitive impairment: evidence and potential mechanisms. Am J Geriatr Psychiatry 24(6):496–508, 2016 27139243

Kessler RC, Berglund P, Demler O, et al: Lifetime prevalence and age-of-onset distributions of DSM-IV disorders in the National Comorbidity Survey Replication. Arch Gen Psychiatry 62(6):593–602, 2005 15939837

Kiosses DN, Leon AC, Areán PA: Psychosocial interventions for late-life major depression: evidence-based treatments, predictors of treatment outcomes, and moderators of treatment effects. Psychiatr Clin North Am 34(2):377–401, viii, 2011 21536164

König H, König HH, Konnopka A: The excess costs of depression: a systematic review and meta-analysis. Epidemiol Psychiatr Sci 29:e30, 2019 30947759

Kroenke K, Spitzer RL, Williams JB: The PHQ-9: validity of a brief depression severity measure. J Gen Intern Med 16(9):606–613, 2001 11556941

Kupfer DJ, Frank E, Phillips ML: Major depressive disorder: new clinical, neurobiological, and treatment perspectives. Lancet 379(9820):1045–1055, 2012 22189047

Laird KT, Krause B, Funes C, et al: Psychobiological factors of resilience and depression in late life. Transl Psychiatry 9(1):88, 2019 30765686

Lane SD, da Costa SC, Teixeira AL, et al: The impact of substance use disorders on clinical outcomes in older-adult psychiatric inpatients. Int J Geriatr Psychiatry 33(2):e323–e329, 2018 29044798

Lee YY, Stockings EA, Harris MG, et al: The risk of developing major depression among individuals with subthreshold depression: a systematic review and meta-analysis of longitudinal cohort studies. Psychol Med 49(1):92–102, 2019 29530112

Lenze EJ, Wetherell JL: A lifespan view of anxiety disorders. Dialogues Clin Neurosci 13(4):381–399, 2011 22275845

Lenze EJ, Mulsant BH, Mohlman J, et al: Generalized anxiety disorder in late life: lifetime course and comorbidity with major depressive disorder. Am J Geriatr Psychiatry 13(1):77–80, 2005 15653943

Livingston G, Huntley J, Sommerlad A, et al: Dementia prevention, intervention, and care: 2020 report of the Lancet Commission. Lancet 396(10248):413–446, 2020 32738937

Luppa M, Sikorski C, Luck T, et al: Age- and gender-specific prevalence of depression in latest-life—systematic review and meta-analysis. J Affect Disord 136(3):212–221, 2012a 21194754

Luppa M, Sikorski C, Motzek T, et al: Health service utilization and costs of depressive symptoms in late life—a systematic review. Curr Pharm Des 18(36):5936–5957, 2012b 22681171

Lyness JM, Heo M, Datto CJ, et al: Outcomes of minor and subsyndromal depression among elderly patients in primary care settings. Ann Intern Med 144(7):496–504, 2006 16585663

Mansour R, Tsamakis K, Rizos E, et al: Late-life depression in people from ethnic minority backgrounds: Differences in presentation and management. J Affect Disord 264:340–347, 2020 32056770

Martínez-Cengotitabengoa M, Carrascón L, O'Brien JT, et al: Peripheral inflammatory parameters in late-life depression: a systematic review. Int J Mol Sci 17(12):2022, 2016 27918465

McCall WV, Benca RM, Rosenquist PB, et al: Hypnotic medications and suicide: risk, mechanisms, mitigation, and the FDA. Am J Psychiatry 174(1):18–25, 2017 27609243

Meeks TW, Vahia IV, Lavretsky H, et al: A tune in "A minor" can "B major": a review of epidemiology, illness course, and public health implications of subthreshold depression in older adults. J Affect Disord 129(1–3):126–142, 2011 20926139

Mendes de Leon CF, Rajan KB: Psychosocial influences in onset and progression of late life disability. J Gerontol B Psychol Sci Soc Sci 69(2):287–302, 2014 24389123

Miao X, Fan B, Li R, et al: Network analysis of depression-related transcriptomic profiles. Neuromolecular Med 21(2):143–149, 2019 30825116

Miller AH, Haroon E, Raison CL, et al: Cytokine targets in the brain: impact on neurotransmitters and neurocircuits. Depress Anxiety 30(4):297–306, 2013 23468190

Morin RT, Insel P, Nelson C, et al: Latent classes of cognitive functioning among depressed older adults without dementia. J Int Neuropsychol Soc 25(8):811–820, 2019 31232250

Munro CA, Longmire CF, Drye LT, et al: Cognitive outcomes after sertaline treatment in patients with depression of Alzheimer disease. Am J Geriatr Psychiatry 20(12):1036–1044, 2012 23032478

Musliner KL, Munk-Olsen T, Eaton WW, et al: Heterogeneity in long-term trajectories of depressive symptoms: patterns, predictors and outcomes. J Affect Disord 192:199–211, 2016 26745437

Niles AN, O'Donovan A: Comparing anxiety and depression to obesity and smoking as predictors of major medical illnesses and somatic symptoms. Health Psychol 38(2):172–181, 2019 30556708

Okura T, Plassman BL, Steffens DC, et al: Prevalence of neuropsychiatric symptoms and their association with functional limitations in older adults in the United States: the aging, demographics, and memory study. J Am Geriatr Soc 58(2):330–337, 2010 20374406

Olin JT, Schneider LS, Katz IR, et al: Provisional diagnostic criteria for depression of Alzheimer disease. Am J Geriatr Psychiatry 10(2):125–128, 2002 11925273

Pickett YR, Bazelais KN, Bruce ML: Late-life depression in older African Americans: a comprehensive review of epidemiological and clinical data. Int J Geriatr Psychiatry 28(9):903–913, 2013 23225736

Rashidi-Ranjbar N, Miranda D, Butters MA, et al: Evidence for structural and functional alterations of frontal-executive and corticolimbic circuits in late-life depression and relationship to mild cognitive impairment and dementia: a systematic review. Front Neurosci 14:253, 2020 32362808

Rhee TG, Capistrant BD, Schommer JC, et al: Effects of the 2009 USPSTF depression screening recommendation on diagnosing and treating mental health conditions in older adults: a difference-in-differences analysis. J Manag Care Spec Pharm 24(8):769–776, 2018 30058984

Riddle M, Potter GG, McQuoid DR, et al: Longitudinal cognitive outcomes of clinical phenotypes of late-life depression. Am J Geriatr Psychiatry 25(10):1123–1134, 2017 28479153

Ridout KK, Ridout SJ, Price LH, et al: Depression and telomere length: a meta-analysis. J Affect Disord 191:237–247, 2016 26688493

Sadavoy J, Meier R, Ong AY: Barriers to access to mental health services for ethnic seniors: the Toronto study. Can J Psychiatry 49(3):192–199, 2004 15101502

Sajatovic M, Strejilevich SA, Gildengers AG, et al: A report on older-age bipolar disorder from the International Society for Bipolar Disorders Task Force. Bipolar Disord 17(7):689–704, 2015 26384588

Sarkisian CA, Lachs MS: "Failure to thrive" in older adults. Ann Intern Med 124(12):1072–1078, 1996 8633822

Schaakxs R, Comijs HC, Lamers F, et al: Associations between age and the course of major depressive disorder: a 2-year longitudinal cohort study. Lancet Psychiatry 5(7):581–590, 2018 29887519

Scholtz M: Hippocrates' aphorisms. Cal West Med 55(3):140, 1941

Schroeck JL, Ford J, Conway EL, et al: Review of safety and efficacy of sleep medicines in older adults. Clin Ther 38(11):2340–2372, 2016 27751669

Seitz D, Purandare N, Conn D: Prevalence of psychiatric disorders among older adults in long-term care homes: a systematic review. Int Psychogeriatr 22(7):1025–1039, 2010 20522279

Seyfried LS, Kales HC, Ignacio RV, et al: Predictors of suicide in patients with dementia. Alzheimers Dement 7(6):567–573, 2011 22055973

Shear MK: Clinical practice. Complicated grief. N Engl J Med 372(2):153–160, 2015 25564898

Simon NM, Shear MK, Reynolds CF, et al: Commentary on evidence in support of a grief-related condition as a DSM diagnosis. Depress Anxiety 37(1):9–16, 2020 31916663

Singh-Manoux A, Dugravot A, Fournier A, et al: Trajectories of depressive symptoms before diagnosis of dementia: a 28-year follow-up study. JAMA Psychiatry 74(7):712–718, 2017 28514478

Snow CE, Abrams RC: The indirect costs of late-life depression in the united states: a literature review and perspective. Geriatrics (Basel) 1(4):30, 2016 31022823

Sonsin-Diaz N, Gottesman RF, Fracica E, et al: Chronic systemic inflammation is associated with symptoms of late-life depression: the ARIC Study. Am J Geriatr Psychiatry 28(1):87–98, 2020 31182350

Soysal P, Veronese N, Thompson T, et al: Relationship between depression and frailty in older adults: a systematic review and meta-analysis. Ageing Res Rev 36:78–87, 2017 28366616

Stubbs B, Stubbs J, Gnanaraj SD, et al: Falls in older adults with major depressive disorder (MDD): a systematic review and exploratory meta-analysis of prospective studies. Int Psychogeriatr 28(1):23–29, 2016 26234532

Sun Y, Shi L, Bao Y, et al: The bidirectional relationship between sleep duration and depression in community-dwelling middle-aged and elderly individuals: evidence from a longitudinal study. Sleep Med 52:221–229, 2018 29861378

Swartz C, Galang RL: Adverse outcome with delay in identification of catatonia in elderly patients. Am J Geriatr Psychiatry 9(1):78–80, 2001 11156756

Tai-Seale M, McGuire T, Colenda C, et al: Two-minute mental health care for elderly patients: inside primary care visits. J Am Geriatr Soc 55(12):1903–1911, 2007 18081668

Taylor MA, Fink M: Catatonia in psychiatric classification: a home of its own. Am J Psychiatry 160(7):1233–1241, 2003 12832234

Tsang RS, Mather KA, Sachdev PS, et al: Systematic review and meta-analysis of genetic studies of late-life depression. Neurosci Biobehav Rev 75:129–139, 2017 28137459

Tsui C, Kim K, Spencer M: The diagnosis "failure to thrive" and its impact on the care of hospitalized older adults: a matched case-control study. BMC Geriatr 20(1):62, 2020 32059639

United Nations, Department of Economic and Social Affairs, Population Division: World Population Ageing 2017—highlights (ST/ESA/SER.A/397). New York, United Nations, 2017. Available at: www.un.org/en/development/desa/population/publications/pdf/ageing/WPA2017_Highlights.pdf. Accessed May 13, 2021.

University of Ottawa: Activities of Daily Living (ADL). Ottawa, Canada, University of Ottawa, 2011. Available at: http://archive.is/20130628054204/http://www.medicine.uottawa.ca/sim/data/Disability_ADL_e.htm. Accessed August 23, 2020.

Vacaflor BE, Beauchet O, Jarvis GE, et al: Mental health and cognition in older cannabis users: a review. Can Geriatr J 23(3):242–249, 2020 32904776

van der Veen DC, van Zelst WH, Schoevers RA, et al: Comorbid anxiety disorders in late-life depression: results of a cohort study. Int Psychogeriatr 27(7):1157–1165, 2015 25370017

Verkaik R, Francke AL, van Meijel B, et al: Comorbid depression in dementia on psychogeriatric nursing home wards: which symptoms are prominent? Am J Geriatr Psychiatry 17(7):565–573, 2009 19554671

Vyas CM, Donneyong M, Mischoulon D, et al: Association of race and ethnicity with late-life depression severity, symptom burden, and care. JAMA Netw Open 3(3):e201606, 2020 32215634

Walaszek A: Behavioral and Psychological Symptoms of Dementia. Washington, DC, American Psychiatric Association Publishing, 2019

Walther A, Breidenstein J, Miller R: Association of testosterone treatment with alleviation of depressive symptoms in men: a systematic review and meta-analysis. JAMA Psychiatry 76(1):31–40, 2019 30427999

Ward EC, Mengesha MM, Issa F: Older African American women's lived experiences with depression and coping behaviours. J Psychiatr Ment Health Nurs 21(1):46–59, 2014 23742034

Wei J, Hou R, Zhang X, et al: The association of late-life depression with all-cause and cardiovascular mortality among community-dwelling older adults: systematic review and meta-analysis. Br J Psychiatry 215(2):449–455, 2019 30968781

Wichniak A, Wierzbicka A, Walecka M, et al: Effects of antidepressants on sleep. Curr Psychiatry Rep 19(9):63, 2017 28791566

Wu LT, Blazer DG: Substance use disorders and psychiatric comorbidity in mid and later life: a review. Int J Epidemiol 43(2):304–317, 2014 24163278

Wu MH, Chang SM, Chou FH: Systematic literature review and meta-analysis of filial piety and depression in older people. J Transcult Nurs 29(4):369–378, 2018 29308707

Wu QE, Zhou AM, Han YP, et al: Poststroke depression and risk of recurrent stroke: a meta-analysis of prospective studies. Medicine (Baltimore) 98(42):e17235, 2019 31626084

Yang KH, Kaufmann CN, Nafsu R, et al: Cannabis: an emerging treatment for common symptoms in older adults. J Am Geriatr Soc 69(1):91–97, 2021 33026117

Yarns BC, Abrams JM, Meeks TW, et al: The mental health of older LGBT adults. Curr Psychiatry Rep 18(6):60, 2016 27142205

Yesavage JA, Brink TL, Rose TL, et al: Development and validation of a geriatric depression screening scale: a preliminary report. J Psychiatr Res 17(1):37–49, 1982 7183759

Zhao Q-F, Tan L, Wang H-F, et al: The prevalence of neuropsychiatric symptoms in Alzheimer's disease: systematic review and meta-analysis. J Affect Disord 190:264–271, 2016 26540080

Zivin K, Wharton T, Rostant O: The economic, public health, and caregiver burden of late-life depression. Psychiatr Clin North Am 36(4):631–649, 2013 24229661

CHAPTER 2

Introduction to Late-Life Anxiety and Related Disorders

Lisa L. Boyle, M.D., M.P.H.

PRÉCIS

Although anxiety disorders are the most common mental health disorders, including in later life, they are less studied than mood disorders. Anxiety is ubiquitous and serves an evolutionary function to mobilize responses and defend against threats in the environment; however, when it is severe or maladaptive for the situational context, it is associated with high levels of disability and suffering. Older adults with anxiety disorders experience fear, worry, somatic symptoms, avoidance, and other maladaptive behaviors. Because anxiety tends to be chronic, most older adults first experience symptoms starting in adolescence and young adulthood. Biological, psychological, and social factors contribute to anxiety disorders in late life. Several medical conditions have been associated with anxiety. Conversely, anxiety disorders have been associated with medical problems, other psychiatric disorders, and overall worse outcomes; a particularly complex relationship exists among depression, anxiety, cognitive impairment, and dementia. Late-life anxiety is underrecognized and undertreated. Earlier and more accurate identification and diagnosis can help patients receive appropriate management and access to resources to alleviate unnecessary suffering, promote improved functioning and health, and reduce health care costs.

Public Health Impact of Late-Life Anxiety and Related Disorders

Anxiety is the most common mental health disorder, including among older adults. Given the complexity and heterogeneity of the older adult population, it takes more effort and time to assess anxiety in older adults compared with younger patients. Older adults generally have more extensive histories, have more comorbid health conditions, and are prescribed more medications—making assessment and management more challenging. Stigma associated with mental illness may prevent older adults from seeking mental health care. Ageism—for example, when patients, families, or providers attribute pathological anxiety symptoms to manifestations of normal aging—can also be a barrier.

Anxiety in late life is often underrecognized and undertreated (Calleo et al. 2009; Mohlman et al. 2012). Older adults may report anxiety symptoms less accurately than do younger adults (Wetherell et al. 2009). For example, cognitive impairment may impair some older adults' ability to report anxiety symptoms. Older adults may report somatic concerns without recognizing that they are also experiencing the psychological symptoms of anxiety, attributing the symptoms to other somatic concerns or comorbid health conditions. Because anxiety symptoms can overlap with symptoms of other medical conditions, older adults may attribute anxiety to or have trouble distinguishing it from their medical conditions.

The public health consequences of anxiety include increased distress and suffering, increased disability, and increased health care costs. For example, panic symptoms among primary care patients are associated with increased risk of disability and use of mental health services compared with those without panic. Even subthreshold panic and anxiety symptoms increase risk for marital distress, loss of work, and utilization of mental health services (Olfson et al. 1996).

These consequences will be covered in more detail later in this chapter as we discuss each specific anxiety disorder.

Etiology of Anxiety

Anxiety is a universal response to stress. It is characterized by the subjective experiences of worry and fear, and it encompasses cognitive, emotional, and physical symptoms. Bateson et al. (2011) proposed that anxiety is an evolutionary function that allows humans to survive threats in the environment (see Table 2–1).

Table 2–1. Adaptive functions of anxiety

Anxiety symptoms	Function
Hypervigilance (easy startle, increased sensitivity to noise)	Can mobilize threat response easily and quickly
Insomnia	Persistent alertness
Restlessness, increased heart rate	Body is prepared to mobilize for action
Preferential attention to threatening cues	Aware of threats sooner
Interpreting ambiguous signals as threatening	Lower likelihood of missing possible threats
Aversion to ambiguity	Avoidance of situations when level of threat is not certain

Source. Adapted from Bateson et al. 2011.

Whether anxiety is adaptive or maladaptive depends on context, including the threat level and one's vulnerability. Higher levels of anxiety are protective if one is in a situation with a high level of threat (e.g., walking through a field of land mines) or if one is more vulnerable (e.g., injured and unable to run from threats). In these scenarios, absence of or low levels of anxiety could place an individual at higher risk of not being able to monitor and respond to threats in the environment. For example, an older adult who is relatively vulnerable because of physical frailty, disability limiting her ability to care for herself, and limited resources (living alone on a fixed income) may understandably worry about how to continue to live independently in her home.

Engaging the fight-or-flight response to respond to an attack can increase one's chance of surviving threatening situations. If one's threshold for mobilizing a response is set too low, then there will be more false alarms; however, if the threshold is set too high, there will be more misses. Ideally, the threshold for mobilizing a threat would match the likelihood of threat and individual vulnerability (Bateson et al. 2011).

Considering the developmental challenges that older adults face in the later years of life, experiencing some anxiety could be considered a normal response to certain situations (Hellwig and Domschke 2019). For example, anxiety may be a reaction to threats to one's health or facing one's mortality or to being isolated or lonely because of grief and loss of social supports as one ages.

Diagnosing an anxiety disorder necessitates understanding the context of the symptoms and determining whether the symptoms are excessive and cause significant distress or functional impairment. Anxiety has a broad differential diagnosis because it can be a symptom of various disorders, including depression, bipolar disorder, psychotic disorders, neurocognitive disorders, somatic symptom disorders, substance use disorders, and trauma disorders. Psychiatric comorbidity is common: individuals diagnosed with a specific anxiety disorder are often diagnosed with other psychiatric disorders as well.

The development of an anxiety disorder in later life is complex and multifactorial, including influences from biological, environmental, and psychological factors. Hellwig and Domschke (2019) proposed a model of late-life anxiety arising from these interconnected factors (Figure 2–1). The next subsection, which covers neurobiological etiologies of late-life anxiety disorders, borrows heavily from their review.

NEUROBIOLOGY

Family history of anxiety or mood disorder is a risk factor for all anxiety disorders in older adults (Beekman et al. 1998). In younger adults, the heritability of anxiety disorders ranges from 32% for generalized anxiety disorder (GAD) to 67% for agoraphobia; genetic contributions may become even more significant after age 60 (Hellwig and Domschke 2019).

Late-life anxiety disorders and neurocognitive disorders may have shared genetic influences. For example, older adults with elevated levels of amyloid-β who were also carriers of the *APOE* ε4 allele (a risk factor for Alzheimer's disease) were more anxious than those without the ε4 allele. In another study, being an ε4 allele carrier was associated with anxiety only in those subjects who had amyloid deposition in subcortical regions of the brain (Hellwig and Domschke 2019). There has been conflicting evidence about the association of polymorphisms of the *SLCA64* gene (which encodes for serotonin transporter): no association was found in one study, whereas a pharmacogenetic study found that polymorphisms moderated the response to escitalopram of older adults with GAD (Hellwig and Domschke 2019). Using functional neuroimaging, Hesse et al. (2011) demonstrated reduced availability of central serotonin transporter in limbic regions of the brain in treatment-naïve individuals with late-onset obsessive-compulsive disorder (OCD) but not early-onset OCD, with possible links to *SLCA64* polymorphisms.

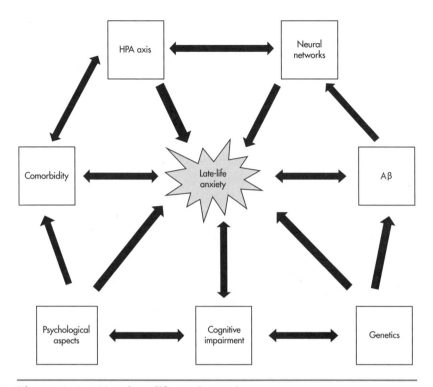

Figure 2–1. How late-life anxiety arises.

See text for details. HPA=hypothalamic-pituitary-adrenal; Aβ=amyloid-β.
Source. Adapted from Hellwig and Domschke 2019.

Studies have demonstrated structural and functional changes in the brain associated with late-life anxiety. Some of the key areas involve the prefrontal system (e.g., orbitofrontal cortex, inferior frontal gyrus, and anterior cingulate cortex) and limbic system. In a study of late-life GAD, changes involving reduced thickness of the cortex were demonstrated in the orbitofrontal cortex, the inferior frontal gyrus, and the anterior cingulate cortex; higher severity of worry symptoms were seen with changes in the orbitofrontal cortex, anterior cingulate cortex, and putamen gray matter (Hellwig and Domschke 2019). Functional neuro-imaging studies have demonstrated abnormal interactions between limbic areas (which activate fear responses) and prefrontal areas (which help regulate emotional responses) (Hellwig and Domschke 2019). Abnormal cortical-subcortical circuits may be particularly important in the development of OCD. The orbitofrontal cortex, which helps regulate motivation and emotional responses, is abnormal on neuroimaging and autopsy examination of neuron densities in patients with OCD compared with control subjects (de Oliveira et al. 2019).

Older adults with anxiety disorders can have abnormal stress hormone regulation; unfortunately, few studies examine the relationship between age-related hypothalamic-pituitary-adrenal (HPA) axis changes and late-life anxiety (Hellwig and Domschke 2019). Following stress, elevated cortisol can persist for longer periods of time in older adults with anxiety compared with those without anxiety (Chaudieu et al. 2008). Elevated cortisol is associated with the diagnosis of late-life GAD and with GAD symptom severity (Mantella et al. 2008). Salivary cortisol levels are reduced in older adults with GAD treated with escitalopram; in one study, a combination of cognitive-behavioral therapy and escitalopram resulted in lower peak cortisol levels in older adults with GAD (Hellwig and Domschke 2019).

Menopause can be associated with anxiety and panic attacks, and estradiol has been implicated in fear learning and fear extinction. However, studies of the effects of hormone replacement therapy on anxiety in postmenopausal women have been mixed (Hellwig and Domschke 2019).

PSYCHOSOCIAL, PSYCHOLOGICAL, AND PERSONALITY FACTORS

Several psychosocial stressors have been investigated as risk factors for anxiety disorders in older adults, focusing on developmental challenges that are more commonly encountered with aging. Specifically, social isolation and loneliness have been shown to be associated with more severe anxiety in late life, including increased risk for hospitalizations due to anxiety (Hellwig and Domschke 2019).

Psychological and personality risk factors for depression and anxiety in older adults frequently overlap. Higher levels of neurotic personality traits have been associated with higher risk for both anxiety and depression in older adults (Gale et al. 2011). Individuals with neurotic personality traits are more prone to experiencing negative emotions and feelings such as anxiety and depression and respond more negatively to routine stressors. Moreover, a large community sample of older adults revealed that panic disorder, social anxiety disorder, and GAD were more likely in individuals with certain types of personality disorders, including schizotypal, borderline, and narcissistic personality disorders (Hellwig and Domschke 2019).

One cognitive theory of anxiety disorders involves *selective attention.* People prone to anxiety disorders tend to focus more of their attention on negative stimuli. Interestingly, studies have shown that healthy older adults are more likely than younger cohorts to focus their attention on positive stimuli. A study examining older adults with GAD found that older patients with GAD focused attention preferentially directed toward negative stimuli and less preferentially toward positive stimuli, whereas older adults without GAD had the opposite pattern of selective attention (Cabrera et al. 2020). Having an external locus of control is a risk factor for any anxiety disorder, including GAD, phobic disorder, and panic disorder, in late life (Beekman et al. 1998).

CULTURAL AND SPIRITUAL FACTORS

Cultural and spiritual factors impact individual and societal beliefs and behaviors; thus, they can have a profound influence on how individuals or groups perceive, express, or cope with illness. Cultural and spiritual factors can also influence how individuals or a group access, engage with, or utilize health care services. Further review of cultural and spiritual influences on anxiety and depression in older adults is presented in Chapter 6, "Comprehensive Cultural Assessment of the Older Adult With Depression and Anxiety." Overall, the literature focusing on cultural influences on the manifestations of anxiety in late life is limited.

Individuals are born into a specific culture; however, these influences may change over a lifetime, especially if a person is exposed to other cultures. For example, relocating to live in another country through immigration is associated with a myriad of exposures to life changes and stressors and adjustment to new culture or acculturation. Zisberg (2017) conducted a prospective study of older adults without cognitive disorders who were hospitalized on medical units in Israel to better understand the role of culture and acculturation on anxiety. Differences in anxiety, but not depression, were found across groups, with Russian-born immigrants (both recently and remotely immigrated) experiencing higher anxiety compared with native Israelis and veteran immigrants from other countries. Women immigrants were more likely to express higher anxiety compared with men, whereas gender differences were not found in the nonimmigrant group (Zisberg 2017).

Religion and spiritual beliefs can also impact health through such factors as social supports and perceived connectedness and existential beliefs about life, death, suffering, and values. Religious beliefs have been shown to mediate the relationship between death anxiety (fear of dying or worries about what happens after death) and depression in older adults, with higher levels of death anxiety and religious doubt increasing risk for depression (Willis et al. 2019). Additionally, race moderated these relationships: Black older adults with religious doubt were at higher risk for more severe depressive symptoms when compared with white older adults. These findings are consistent with other studies that demonstrate that religiosity is associated with well-being in Black older adults (Krause 2003). Huang et al. (2012) also demonstrated that religious involvement had a moderating effect on the impacts of both anxiety and depression on quality of life in older adults; in those seeking psychiatric care, older patients who engaged more in religious activities reported less anxiety and better quality of life compared with those who had less religious engagement.

The relationship between these risk factors and anxiety disorders in general and specific anxiety disorders is illustrated in Table 2–2. We cover social determinants of health in Chapter 6.

MEDICAL FACTORS

Several physical health conditions have been associated with increased risk for anxiety. Because people generally develop chronic health conditions as they age, the differential diagnosis of anxiety in an older adult must include physical health conditions that can cause anxiety (Table 2–3). Anxiety and physical health conditions can have a bidirectional relationship in older adults, with some medical conditions increasing risk of anxiety and anxiety itself increasing risk of medical conditions (Mohlman et al. 2012). In a sample of community-dwelling older adults, several physical health conditions (arthritis; back pain; migraine; allergies; cataracts; and gastrointestinal, lung, and heart disease) were associated with higher risk for developing any anxiety disorder (the odds ratio ranged from 1.66 to 2.82) (El-Gabalawy et al. 2011). In a survey of 4,219 older adults from the Health and Retirement Study, the number of medical comorbidities increased risk for anxiety, with a 2.3 times elevated risk if an older adult had three or more medical conditions (Gould et al. 2016). In a study examining adjustment disorder with anxiety in later life, the most common life stressors reported (29% of participants) were personal illness or health problems (Arbus et al. 2014).

Epidemiology

Anxiety is the most common mental health disorder in both mixed-age populations (Kessler et al. 2005) and older adult populations (Gum et al. 2009; Reynolds et al. 2015). In general, the prevalence of anxiety disorders in older adults is less than the prevalence in younger adults, and

Table 2–2.   Risk factors for late-life anxiety

Factor	Any anxiety disorder	GAD	Phobia	Panic disorder	OCD
Stress related					
Recent life events	√	√	√	√	√
Partner loss	√	√	√	√	
Chronic physical illness	√	√	√	√	√
Functional limitations	√	√	√	√	√
Subjective health fair or poor	√	√	√	√	√
Vulnerability					
Female sex	√	√	√	√	
Low education	√	√	√	√	√
Unmarried	√	√	√	√	√
External locus of control	√	√	√	√	
Family history	√	√	√	√	√
Early life stressors	√	√	√	√	√
Social networks					
Smaller contact network	√		√		
Less emotional support received			√		
Less emotional support provided			√		
Loneliness	√	√	√	√	√

Note.   GAD=generalized anxiety disorder; OCD=obsessive-compulsive disorder.
Source.   Adapted from Beekman et al. 1998.

rates decrease with age (Byers et al. 2010; Canuto et al. 2018; Flint 1994; Gum et al. 2009; Reynolds et al. 2015). However, with an aging population around the world, we should expect that the absolute number of older adults with anxiety disorders will increase over time.

The prevalence of anxiety disorders and anxiety symptoms in late life varies depending on the population surveyed, with higher prevalence in clinical settings (1%–28% for anxiety disorders, 15%–56% for

Table 2–3. Medical conditions associated with anxiety

Medical condition	Anxiety disorder	Clinical pearls
Cardiovascular disease		
Congestive heart failure (CHF)	• Anxiety symptoms are present in up to 60% of CHF patients.	• Depression is more frequently and better studied than anxiety in CHF.
Coronary artery disease (CAD)	• Patients with CAD have approximately 5% and 15% 12-month prevalence for anxiety disorders and subthreshold anxiety, respectively • Approximately 10% of patients with CAD meet criteria for GAD. • 10%–50% of patients with CAD have panic disorder.	• Depression is more frequently and better studied than anxiety in CAD. • CAD patients with subthreshold and threshold anxiety are more likely to have hypertension and depression. • GAD is associated with poorer prognosis, independent of depression, in patients with CAD. • Anxiety is high in patients with noncardiac chest pain (21%–53%).
Neoplastic disease		
Cancer	• 15%–23% of cancer patients have anxiety • 69%–79% experience anxiety during later stages of disease.	• Approximately 25%–50% of patients treated for breast cancer experience anxiety (less for radiation therapy than for chemotherapy). • Anxiety can persist in cancer survivors and spouses of survivors (almost 50% of spouses).

Table 2–3. Medical conditions associated with anxiety *(continued)*

Medical condition	Anxiety disorder	Clinical pearls
Endocrine disease		
Diabetes mellitus	• Unspecified anxiety, specific phobia, GAD, and social phobia are most reported among diabetic patients. • 15%–73% have subthreshold anxiety. • 1.4%–15.6% have anxiety disorder.	
Thyroid disorders	• Both hypothyroidism and hyperthyroidism increase severity of anxiety.	• Treatment for both clinical hypothyroidism and hyperthyroidism to achieve euthyroid states improved anxiety symptoms and quality of life; there was less improvement in subclinical conditions (Gulseren et al. 2006).
Neurological disease		
Stroke	• 18%–25% of patients have anxiety disorders following a stroke. • GAD and phobic disorders are most common.	• Age and gender were not risk factors for anxiety after stroke in most studies.
Traumatic brain injury (TBI)	• 10% of patients experienced comorbid anxiety and depression following TBI, and half of those with anxiety also had depression.	
Mild cognitive impairment (MCI)	• 11%–75% of patients with MCI have symptoms of anxiety.	

Table 2–3. Medical conditions associated with anxiety (*continued*)

Medical condition	Anxiety disorder	Clinical pearls
Neurological disease (*continued*)		
Multiple sclerosis (MS)	• 32% of patients with MS have anxiety disorders, and >50% have symptoms of anxiety. • 26% have health anxiety.	
Respiratory disease		
Chronic obstructive pulmonary disease (COPD)	• GAD or PD is present in 34% of patients with COPD. • Prevalence of GAD is 3× higher and prevalence of panic disorder is 5× higher in patients with COPD than in the general population. • Anxiety disorder is present in up to 51%, and anxiety symptoms are present in up to 74% of patients with COPD.	• Comorbid anxiety leads to more disability, lower quality of life, lower functional status, and more hospitalizations for COPD exacerbation. • <30% of COPD patients with anxiety disorder were diagnosed.
Acute respiratory distress syndrome (ARDS)	• 23%–48% of ARDS survivors have anxiety following discharge from the intensive care unit.	
Other		
End-stage renal disease	• Up to 38% of patients with renal disease have anxiety symptoms.	
AIDS	• 8%–34% of AIDS patients have anxiety symptoms.	

Table 2–3. Medical conditions associated with anxiety *(continued)*

Medical condition	Anxiety disorder	Clinical pearls
Limb amputation(s)	• Approximately 25%–50% of limb amputees have anxiety.	

Note. GAD=generalized anxiety disorder; PD=panic disorder.
Source. Adapted from Brenes 2003; Grenier et al. 2012; Gulseren et al. 2006; Kunik et al. 2005; Osborn et al. 2017; Remes et al. 2016; Tully et al. 2013; Yohannes et al. 2010.

symptoms) compared with community settings (1.2%–15% for anxiety disorders, 15%–52.3% for symptoms). In addition, rates vary depending on the diagnostic criteria and methods used to measure anxiety (Bryant et al. 2008).

Estimates of 12-month prevalence of anxiety disorders in community-dwelling older adults range from 7% to 17%, higher than that of mood disorders (2.6%–5%). Similar to findings in younger populations, female elders have higher rates of anxiety disorders than do male elders (Beekman et al. 1998; Byers et al. 2010; Canuto et al. 2018; Flint 1994; Gum et al. 2009; Reynolds et al. 2015). The most common anxiety disorders (lifetime prevalence) are specific phobia (15.6%), social phobia (10.7%), separation anxiety disorder (6.7%), PTSD (5.7%), GAD (4.3%), panic disorder with or without agoraphobia (3.8%), agoraphobia with or without panic disorder (2.5%), and OCD (2.3%) (Kessler et al. 2012).

Subsyndromal or subthreshold anxiety (anxiety that does not meet full diagnostic criteria) is common. For example, in a community sample of older adults ($N=2,784$), the 12-month prevalence of clinically significant anxiety that did not meet diagnostic criteria for a disorder in older adults was estimated to be 26%, compared with 5.6% meeting diagnostic criteria for any anxiety disorder (Grenier et al. 2011a).

ETHNIC AND SEXUAL MINORITY ELDERS

In a systematic review of mixed-age epidemiological studies, anxiety disorders were less fequent in East Asia and highest in North America and North Africa/Middle East. Across the globe, specific phobia and GAD have the highest lifetime prevalence and panic disorder has the lowest (Remes et al. 2016). Studies of the prevalence of anxiety among older adults from diverse ethnic/racial groups in the United States have had mixed results. For example, the National Comorbidity Study Replication (NCS-R) did not find differences in prevalence of anxiety disorders across racial/ethnic groups in adults 55 years old and older (Byers et al. 2010). On the other hand, the National Institute of Mental Health Collaborative Psychiatric Epidemiology Surveys of adults 50 years old and older reported lower 12-month and lifetime prevalence of anxiety in Asian and Afro-Caribbean populations than in Latino and non-Latino whites, with some nuances depending on the specific anxiety disorder and when comparing U.S.-born with immigrant populations (Jimenez et al. 2010). The lifetime prevalence of anxiety disorders in LGBTQ+ older adults is 24%–33%, with a past-year prevalence of 4% (Yarns et al. 2016). We cover cultural factors in late-life psychiatric disorders in greater detail in Chapter 6.

PRIMARY CARE PATIENTS

The prevalence of anxiety disorders in primary care is high, with at least 20% of patients meeting criteria for at least one anxiety disorder. In a study of 965 patients in primary care, the most common disorders were PTSD (8.6%), GAD (7.6%), panic disorder (6.8%), and social anxiety disorder (6.2%); remarkably, 41% of patients with an anxiety disorder were not receiving treatment (Kroenke et al. 2007). Subthreshold anxiety is also common in primary care, with approximately 6.6% of a mixed-age primary care population in one study reporting anxiety symptoms and 10% reporting panic symptoms (Olfson et al. 1996).

RESIDENTS OF SKILLED NURSING FACILITIES

In a systematic review of prevalence studies conducted in nursing home populations, GAD (0.9%–11.2%) and specific phobias (1%–14%) were the most common anxiety disorders, followed by panic disorder (0.9%–5%), OCD (5%), agoraphobia (2.1%–4%), and social phobia (0.6%); overall, anxiety disorders were found in 3.2%–20% of residents (Creighton et al. 2016). Clinically significant anxiety symptoms (prevalence of 6.5%–58.4%) were more common than anxiety disorders (3.2%–20%) (Creighton et al. 2016). Although both anxiety disorders and subthreshold anxiety disorders are common, they are underreported by nursing staff (Creighton et al. 2018).

HOME HEALTH CARE RECIPIENTS

A study of older adults receiving home health care services found that anxiety was less common than one might anticipate given the study population's high level of disability, with only 3.6% having mild or moderate anxiety symptoms and 64% reporting no anxiety symptoms at all. Having major depression or a recent fall increased the risk of experiencing anxiety symptoms. It is unclear whether the relatively low rates reported were reflective of unique protective factors associated with the home health setting or limitations of the assessment methods (Jayasinghe et al. 2013).

Clinical Presentation

Anxiety is a core feature of many psychiatric disorders. In this section, we focus on GAD, panic disorder and agoraphobia (now distinct disorders in DSM-5; American Psychiatric Association 2013), specific phobia (including fear of falling), social anxiety disorder (social phobia), posttraumatic stress disorder (now categorized as a trauma- and stressor-related disorder in DSM-5), and OCD (now categorized as an obsessive-compulsive and related disorder). See Table 2–4 for an overview. Substance/medication-induced anxiety disorder and anxiety disorder due to another medical condition are covered in the discussion of the assessment of late-life anxiety disorders in Chapter 3, "Assessment of Late-Life Depression and Anxiety." We do not cover separation anxiety disorder and selective mutism (both DSM-5 anxiety disorders) in this book, given the dearth of information in older adults.

Table 2–4. Clinical features of anxiety disorders

Disorder	Clinical features
Specific phobia	Fear or anxiety about a specific object or situation that leads to active avoidance; intense fear or anxiety when exposed to the object or situation
Social anxiety disorder (social phobia)	Fear or anxiety about social situations exposing one to potential scrutiny by others and fear that one will act in a way that will be negatively perceived by others, leading to avoidance of social situations; intense fear or anxiety when exposed to social situations
Panic disorder	Recurrent unexpected panic attacks with persistent worry about additional panic attacks and/or maladaptive behavior change related to the attack
Agoraphobia	Marked fear or anxiety related to using public transportation, being in open and/or enclosed spaces, standing in line or being in a crowd, and/or being outside of one's home, leading to avoidant behaviors or requiring the presence of a companion; intense fear or anxiety when exposed
Generalized anxiety disorder	Persistent and excessive anxiety and worry that is difficult to control and is associated with physical symptoms
Substance/medication-induced anxiety disorder	Panic attacks or anxiety that develop during or soon after substance intoxication or withdrawal or after exposure to medication that can cause anxiety (not exclusively during a delirium)
Anxiety disorder due to another medical condition	Panic attacks or anxiety that are the direct pathophysiological sequelae of another medical condition (not exclusively during a delirium)

Source. Adapted from American Psychiatric Association 2013; Canuto et al. 2018; Kessler et al. 2012.

To meet criteria for a DSM-5 anxiety disorder, a patient's fear, anxiety, or avoidance symptoms must lead to "clinically significant distress or impairment in social, occupational, or other important areas of functioning" (American Psychiatric Association 2013). Compared with younger adults, determining impact on social or occupational functioning can be more challenging because older adults may not have as many opportunities to socialize or work.

Subsyndromal or subthreshold anxiety is common in late life, but older adults may not endorse the severity or the number of symptoms required by DSM-5 to make a diagnosis. DSM-5 criteria were not developed specifically for older adults, leading to potential challenges in applying these criteria in this population. Mohlman et al. (2012) summarized the challenges of applying DSM criteria for late-life anxiety disorders:

- Age-related differences exist in manifestation of anxiety.
- Recognizing and reporting symptoms can be more challenging in older adults because of the complexity associated with comorbid depression, cognitive disorders, and other medical illnesses.
- Recognizing excessive symptoms of fear or worry or assessing significant impairment from these symptoms can be difficult with elders compared with younger cohorts.
- Older adults may also experience avoidant behaviors that are maladaptive in the context of facing challenges associated with aging itself (Table 2–5).

GENERALIZED ANXIETY DISORDER

GAD is the most common anxiety disorder in older adults (Bryant et al. 2008). GAD is characterized by excessive worry that is difficult to control. In addition, patients experience some combination of feeling restless or being "keyed up," fatigue, problems with concentration, irritability, muscle tension, and sleep disturbance. As with all DSM-5 diagnoses, these symptoms should cause significant distress or impaired functioning to meet the diagnostic threshold (American Psychiatric Association 2013). Box 2–1 lists the full DSM-5 criteria for GAD.

Most older adults with GAD have lived with this chronic, remitting condition for much of their lives, although a fair number have late-life onset. GAD in late life tends to be highly comorbid with other psychiatric disorders: more than 50% of older adults with GAD also have mood or other anxiety disorders, and 25% have a personality disorder (Mackenzie et al. 2011). A common temporal pattern of comorbidity is

Table 2–5.   Examples of maladaptive behaviors associated with age-specific challenges

Behavior	Fear
Avoidance behaviors	
Leaving home when dark or going out alone	Being a victim of a crime
Avoiding physical activity or exercise	Falling or vertigo
Avoiding public transportation	Falling
Not driving	Having a car accident or getting lost due to slowed reactions or not being able to see
Avoidance of socializing	Not being able to hear or being embarrassed
Not walking or using hearing aids	Being perceived as old or frail
Not speaking with adult children	Arguments or conflicts over differing political or other belief systems
Not seeking or accepting help	Being a burden or becoming dependent
Not buying essential supplies	Becoming destitute
Not discarding old or unnecessary items	Not having the items if needed in the future
Not taking classes or joining book clubs	Being perceived as stupid
Excessive behaviors	
Monitoring health (e.g., blood pressure, blood sugar, heart rate, bowel movements)	Illness
Checking finances	Not having enough money to live
Checking on family members' health and wellness	Something bad happening to loved ones
Becoming too involved with activities; staying too busy	Being idle leading to not being able to control worry

Source.   Adapted from Mohlman et al. 2012.

for major depressive episodes to complicate long-standing GAD, with GAD symptoms persisting even after remission of depression (Lenze et al. 2005).

Box 2–1.   DSM-5 Diagnostic Criteria for Generalized Anxiety
Disorder

A. Excessive anxiety and worry (apprehensive expectation), occurring more days than not for at least 6 months, about a number of events or activities (such as work or school performance).

B. The individual finds it difficult to control the worry.

C. The anxiety and worry are associated with three (or more) of the following six symptoms (with at least some symptoms having been present for more days than not for the past 6 months):

Note: Only one item is required in children.

1. Restlessness or feeling keyed up or on edge.
2. Being easily fatigued.
3. Difficulty concentrating or mind going blank.
4. Irritability.
5. Muscle tension.
6. Sleep disturbance (difficulty falling or staying asleep, or restless, unsatisfying sleep).

D. The anxiety, worry, or physical symptoms cause clinically significant distress or impairment in social, occupational, or other important areas of functioning.

E. The disturbance is not attributable to the physiological effects of a substance (e.g., a drug of abuse, a medication) or another medical condition (e.g., hyperthyroidism).

F. The disturbance is not better explained by another mental disorder (e.g., anxiety or worry about having panic attacks in panic disorder, negative evaluation in social anxiety disorder [social phobia], contamination or other obsessions in obsessive-compulsive disorder, separation from attachment figures in separation anxiety disorder, reminders of traumatic events in posttraumatic stress disorder, gaining weight in anorexia nervosa, physical complaints in somatic symptom disorder, perceived appearance flaws in body dysmorphic disorder, having a serious illness in illness anxiety disorder, or the content of delusional beliefs in schizophrenia or delusional disorder).

Source.   Reprinted from American Psychiatric Association: *Diagnostic and Statistical Manual of Mental Disorders,* 5th Edition, Arlington, VA, American Psychiatric Association, 2013. Copyright © 2013 American Psychiatric Association. Used with permission.

Compared with younger adults with GAD, older patients generally report more sleep disturbance, pursue less reassurance seeking, and experience more severe depression. Moreover, older adults with GAD, when compared with younger adults, struggle with more worry-related disability despite relatively less severe GAD symptoms. Worry tends to be focused on concerns about personal health and family well-being in older adults, whereas younger adults tend to think more about their future and worry about other people's health (Altunoz et al. 2018). Older adults with GAD generally report more alcohol use than do those without GAD, although frequency of use is relatively low. Older adults with GAD who drink a moderate amount of alcohol tend to report less severe worry, anxiety, and insomnia (Ivan et al. 2014).

Anxiety symptoms can overlap with somatic symptoms, leading older adults to seek medical care. Unfortunately, only 34% of older patients with GAD have their anxiety symptoms recognized in primary care (Calleo et al. 2009). Because GAD symptoms can overlap with other conditions, such as depression and other chronic health conditions, identifying GAD when working in settings with older adults who may have some of these other conditions can be challenging. Older adults in primary care with GAD are more likely to have diabetes and gastrointestinal problems, which suggests that older adults presenting with these conditions could benefit from being screened for anxiety (Wetherell et al. 2010). There is conflicting evidence about whether anxiety symptoms or physical symptoms are more sensitive for detecting GAD in older adults (Miloyan and Pachana 2015; Wetherell et al. 2010). Moreover, physical symptoms are associated with additional adverse outcomes such as distress and occupational and functional disability, whereas worry symptoms are associated only with distress (Miloyan and Pachana 2015).

GAD in late life can have a significant impact on quality of life and functioning. When compared with older adults without anxiety, older adults with GAD have higher levels of disability, have worse health-related quality of life, and use more health care services, even without other psychiatric comorbidities. When controlling for medical comorbidity and depressive symptoms, higher levels of anxiety are associated with more disability and lower health-related quality of life; lower self-efficacy and fewer social supports are also associated with worse quality of life (Mackenzie et al. 2011; Porensky et al. 2009; Shrestha et al. 2015). Older adults with GAD have low rates of seeking treatment for their GAD (Mackenzie et al. 2011).

PANIC DISORDER AND AGORAPHOBIA

Panic disorder is characterized by recurrent unexpected *panic attacks* accompanied by one or both of the following: anticipatory anxiety about experiencing future panic attacks or the consequences of the attacks and/or maladaptive behavior in response to the panic attacks (e.g., avoiding new situations over concern of having more panic attacks) (American Psychiatric Association 2013). A panic attack is defined as the sudden onset of symptoms of severe fear or discomfort that peak within minutes and encompass some combination of symptoms listed in Box 2–2. Panic attacks can be associated with any other mental disorder (e.g., GAD with panic attacks, major depressive disorder with panic attacks) and other medical conditions (e.g., coronary artery disease, chronic obstructive pulmonary disease). In a primary care sample, approximately 42% of patients who reported panic symptoms met criteria for another psychiatric disorder (most commonly major depressive disorder and alcohol use disorder) (Olfson et al. 1996).

Box 2–2.   DSM-5 Diagnostic Criteria for Panic Disorder

A. Recurrent unexpected panic attacks. A panic attack is an abrupt surge of intense fear or intense discomfort that reaches a peak within minutes, and during which time four (or more) of the following symptoms occur:

Note: The abrupt surge can occur from a calm state or an anxious state.

1. Palpitations, pounding heart, or accelerated heart rate.
2. Sweating.
3. Trembling or shaking.
4. Sensations of shortness of breath or smothering.
5. Feelings of choking.
6. Chest pain or discomfort.
7. Nausea or abdominal distress.
8. Feeling dizzy, unsteady, light-headed, or faint.
9. Chills or heat sensations.
10. Paresthesias (numbness or tingling sensations).
11. Derealization (feelings of unreality) or depersonalization (being detached from oneself).
12. Fear of losing control or "going crazy."
13. Fear of dying.

Note: Culture-specific symptoms (e.g., tinnitus, neck soreness, headache, uncontrollable screaming or crying) may be seen. Such symptoms should not count as one of the four required symptoms.

B. At least one of the attacks has been followed by 1 month (or more) of one or both of the following:

1. Persistent concern or worry about additional panic attacks or their consequences (e.g., losing control, having a heart attack, "going crazy").
2. A significant maladaptive change in behavior related to the attacks (e.g., behaviors designed to avoid having panic attacks, such as avoidance of exercise or unfamiliar situations).

C. The disturbance is not attributable to the physiological effects of a substance (e.g., a drug of abuse, a medication) or another medical condition (e.g., hyperthyroidism, cardiopulmonary disorders).

D. The disturbance is not better explained by another mental disorder (e.g., the panic attacks do not occur only in response to feared social situations, as in social anxiety disorder; in response to circumscribed phobic objects or situations, as in specific phobia; in response to obsessions, as in obsessive-compulsive disorder; in response to reminders of traumatic events, as in posttraumatic stress disorder; or in response to separation from attachment figures, as in separation anxiety disorder).

Source.   Reprinted from American Psychiatric Association: *Diagnostic and Statistical Manual of Mental Disorders,* 5th Edition, Arlington, VA, American Psychiatric Association, 2013. Copyright © 2013 American Psychiatric Association. Used with permission.

Panic disorder tends to develop early in life. The frequency of panic disorder decreases with age, and panic disorder is less common in older adults (1%) compared with other anxiety disorders (Beekman et al. 1998). Moreover, panic disorder tends to be less severe in older adults compared with those who are younger. Compared with younger adults, older adults tend to have fewer panic symptoms, lower anxiety and arousal symptoms, milder severity of comorbid depressive symptoms, and higher functioning (Sheikh et al. 2004). With an age cutoff of 27 years differentiating early- and late-onset panic disorder, individuals with early-onset panic disorder tend to be younger and female and to have comorbid agoraphobia, history of childhood trauma and traumatic life events, and higher suicide attempt rates compared with individuals who have late-onset panic disorder (Tibi et al. 2013). Differences in younger versus older populations with panic disorder may be due to biological changes of aging in the brain that alter fear and stress responses and psychosocial differences involving degree of supports and coping strategies (Sheikh et al. 2004).

DSM-5 uncoupled panic disorder and *agoraphobia*, recognizing that they are two distinct disorders. Agoraphobia is defined by persistent, severe, and culturally excessive fear or anxiety of two or more of the five scenarios listed in Box 2–3. Individuals with agoraphobia can experience a high level of disability due to severe avoidance of these situations or due to extreme fear when facing the situations. Agoraphobia in older adults has not been well studied.

Box 2–3.   DSM-5 Diagnostic Criteria for Agoraphobia

A. Marked fear or anxiety about two (or more) of the following five situations:

1. Using public transportation (e.g., automobiles, buses, trains, ships, planes).
2. Being in open spaces (e.g., parking lots, marketplaces, bridges).

3. Being in enclosed places (e.g., shops, theaters, cinemas).
4. Standing in line or being in a crowd.
5. Being outside of the home alone.

B. The individual fears or avoids these situations because of thoughts that escape might be difficult or help might not be available in the event of developing panic-like symptoms or other incapacitating or embarrassing symptoms (e.g., fear of falling in the elderly; fear of incontinence).

C. The agoraphobic situations almost always provoke fear or anxiety.

D. The agoraphobic situations are actively avoided, require the presence of a companion, or are endured with intense fear or anxiety.

E. The fear or anxiety is out of proportion to the actual danger posed by the agoraphobic situations and to the sociocultural context.

F. The fear, anxiety, or avoidance is persistent, typically lasting for 6 months or more.

G. The fear, anxiety, or avoidance causes clinically significant distress or impairment in social, occupational, or other important areas of functioning.

H. If another medical condition (e.g., inflammatory bowel disease, Parkinson's disease) is present, the fear, anxiety, or avoidance is clearly excessive.

I. The fear, anxiety, or avoidance is not better explained by the symptoms of another mental disorder—for example, the symptoms are not confined to specific phobia, situational type; do not involve only social situations (as in social anxiety disorder); and are not related exclusively to obsessions (as in obsessive-compulsive disorder), perceived defects or flaws in physical appearance (as in body dysmorphic disorder), reminders of traumatic events (as in posttraumatic stress disorder), or fear of separation (as in separation anxiety disorder).

Note: Agoraphobia is diagnosed irrespective of the presence of panic disorder. If an individual's presentation meets criteria for panic disorder and agoraphobia, both diagnoses should be assigned.

Panic disorder can occur with or without agoraphobia, and agoraphobia can occur without panic disorder (Wittchen et al. 2010). In fact, 46%–85% of people in the community with agoraphobia do not have panic disorder, although this number is likely lower in clinical samples (Wittchen et al. 2010). When the two disorders are comorbid, panic attacks develop before agoraphobia in approximately 50% of people. Individuals with panic disorder and agoraphobia have the most severe disability, whereas having panic attacks (without meeting criteria for panic disorder) is associated with less disability; agoraphobia without panic and panic disorder without agoraphobia results in disability severity somewhere in between

(Wittchen et al. 2010). Individuals who have agoraphobia without panic disorder are less likely to receive specialty mental health services compared with individuals with panic disorder (Wittchen et al. 2010).

SPECIFIC PHOBIA, INCLUDING FEAR OF FALLING

Specific phobia is characterized by marked fear or anxiety about a specific object or situation, which is actively avoided or endured with intense fear or anxiety (American Psychiatric Association 2013). Specific phobia is the second most common anxiety disorder in older adults (Beekman et al. 1998). The most frequent fears among older adults with specific phobia are situational and are related to the natural environment. Most older adults with specific phobia fail to recognize the excessiveness of their fears (Grenier et al. 2011b).

Older adults are more likely than younger adults to experience fear of falling (FOF), which may or may not meet criteria for specific phobia or agoraphobia. In a large study of community-dwelling elders, 54% reported FOF and 38% reported avoidance of activities; note that subjects were not assessed for the diagnosis of specific phobia or agoraphobia (Zijlstra et al. 2007). Although FOF can develop in the absence of a history of falls (Denkinger et al. 2015), a history of falls increases sixfold the risk for developing FOF (Kim and So 2013). Several risk factors for FOF have been recognized (Table 2–6), with a higher number of risk factors increasing risk for FOF (Oh-Park et al. 2011). In more severe cases, older adults with FOF avoid leaving their homes altogether (Arfken et al. 1994). The following case illustrates FOF superimposed on preexisting GAD.

CASE EXAMPLE 1: "MY WIFE WANTS ME TO GET OUT MORE—BUT WHAT IF I FALL DOWN?"

Mr. Young is a 74-year-old remarried veteran who presents to a geriatric psychiatry clinic on referral from his neurologist for management of anxiety. He is accompanied by his wife, and they both report that he has had long-standing anxiety and was diagnosed with GAD as a young adult. He characterizes his symptoms as challenges with controlling worries. For example, when his children were in high school and were late getting home from after-school activities, his mind would automatically jump to catastrophic worries that there had been an accident or some other tragedy. He would then not be able to stop worrying about this possibility and would have to repeatedly call his children to check

Table 2–6. Risk factors for fear of falling

Sociodemographic factors	Health factors	Functional factors
Older age	History of falls and higher frequency of falls	Increased dependence on activities of daily living/ increased disability
Female sex		
Lower household income	Multimorbid health conditions	
Black/minority ethnic group	Frailty (difficulty rising from a chair)	Use of a walking aid
Lower education	Being less mobile and less physically active	Difficulty using public transportation
	Poor balance/gait	
	Higher body mass index	
	Depression	
	Pain	
	Lower perceived health	
	Polypharmacy	

Source. Adapted from Hoang et al. 2017; Kim and So 2013; Kocic et al. 2017; Kumar et al. 2014; Lee et al. 2017; Patel et al. 2014; Rivasi et al. 2020.

in for reassurance that they were OK. These symptoms often took a lot of his energy such that he often experienced fatigue, difficulties concentrating, severe muscle pain, and headaches, and his first wife complained that he was persistently irritable and difficult to live with. They divorced, and he lived alone for several years. During that time, he continued to cope with his worries by frequently checking in for reassurance; however, he never brought up these concerns with his primary care physician and never sought formal mental health services.

About 5 years ago, Mr. Young's primary care physician noted an asymmetrical resting tremor and bradykinesia and referred Mr. Young to see a neurologist, who diagnosed him with Parkinson's disease. Since diagnosis, he has had progressive challenges with his balance and has considerably restricted his activities. When asked why, he endorses that he does not feel steady on his feet and that he has had several falls. He anticipates that he will fall again, which frightens him, so he prefers to remain at home and to avoid activities that could cause him to fall. This has caused considerable strain on Mr. Young's wife and other family members because he no longer participates in any family activities outside the home and has not been to church, an activity he used to enjoy immensely, for the past 2 years. He recognizes that these fears are limiting him but does not perceive that he can change. His neurologist recognizes that he had preexisting GAD and initiates a trial of a selective serotonin reuptake inhibitor, which results in some improvement in his symptoms. However, his fear of falling does not respond to the antidepressant, and his neurologist refers him to both physical therapy and geriatric psychiatry for additional assessment and recommendations for management of his fear of falling.

SOCIAL ANXIETY DISORDER (SOCIAL PHOBIA)

Social anxiety disorder, also known as *social phobia,* is characterized by fear or worry that arises in social situations associated with potentially being judged by others, such as social interactions, being observed by others, or performing for an audience. The central fear is of behaving in a way or exhibiting anxiety symptoms that others will perceive negatively, leading to avoidance of social interactions or enduring them with marked anxiety (American Psychiatric Association 2013). Applying the DSM-5 social phobia criteria (which removed the DSM-IV requirement that individuals perceive their fear as unreasonable) resulted in a doubling of 1-month prevalence rates, from 2.5% to 5.1%, in a geriatric population (Karlsson et al. 2016). Late-life social phobia is often comorbid with other psychiatric conditions. Interestingly, however, it does not appear to negatively affect quality of life or health services utilization to the same extent as other anxiety disorders (Cairney et al. 2007; Chou 2009).

POSTTRAUMATIC STRESS DISORDER

Although PTSD has been reconceptualized as a trauma- and stressor-related disorder, its emotional core remains excessive anxiety, so we cover it here. The DSM-5 criteria (Box 2–4) are descriptive and comprehensive. Approximately 90% of older adults have had exposure to at least one traumatic experience over their lifetime, including military combat, unexpected death, or serious injury or illness of someone close or oneself (Kuwert et al. 2013). PTSD prevalence decreases with age, and older adults report fewer traumatic experiences, less severe illness, and fewer psychiatric comorbidities compared with younger cohorts, although mental health-related quality of life is similar (Reynolds et al. 2016).

Box 2–4.   DSM-5 Diagnostic Criteria for Posttraumatic Stress Disorder

---

Note: The following criteria apply to adults, adolescents, and children older than 6 years. For children 6 years and younger, see corresponding criteria below.

A. Exposure to actual or threatened death, serious injury, or sexual violence in one (or more) of the following ways:

1. Directly experiencing the traumatic event(s).
2. Witnessing, in person, the event(s) as it occurred to others.
3. Learning that the traumatic event(s) occurred to a close family member or close friend. In cases of actual or threatened death of a family member or friend, the event(s) must have been violent or accidental.

4. Experiencing repeated or extreme exposure to aversive details of the traumatic event(s) (e.g., first responders collecting human remains; police officers repeatedly exposed to details of child abuse).

Note: Criterion A4 does not apply to exposure through electronic media, television, movies, or pictures, unless this exposure is work related.

B. Presence of one (or more) of the following intrusion symptoms associated with the traumatic event(s), beginning after the traumatic event(s) occurred:

1. Recurrent, involuntary, and intrusive distressing memories of the traumatic event(s).

   Note: In children older than 6 years, repetitive play may occur in which themes or aspects of the traumatic event(s) are expressed.

2. Recurrent distressing dreams in which the content and/or affect of the dream are related to the traumatic event(s).

   Note: In children, there may be frightening dreams without recognizable content.

3. Dissociative reactions (e.g., flashbacks) in which the individual feels or acts as if the traumatic event(s) were recurring. (Such reactions may occur on a continuum, with the most extreme expression being a complete loss of awareness of present surroundings.)

   Note: In children, trauma-specific reenactment may occur in play.

4. Intense or prolonged psychological distress at exposure to internal or external cues that symbolize or resemble an aspect of the traumatic event(s).

5. Marked physiological reactions to internal or external cues that symbolize or resemble an aspect of the traumatic event(s).

C. Persistent avoidance of stimuli associated with the traumatic event(s), beginning after the traumatic event(s) occurred, as evidenced by one or both of the following:

1. Avoidance of or efforts to avoid distressing memories, thoughts, or feelings about or closely associated with the traumatic event(s).

2. Avoidance of or efforts to avoid external reminders (people, places, conversations, activities, objects, situations) that arouse distressing memories, thoughts, or feelings about or closely associated with the traumatic event(s).

D. Negative alterations in cognitions and mood associated with the traumatic event(s), beginning or worsening after the traumatic event(s) occurred, as evidenced by two (or more) of the following:

1. Inability to remember an important aspect of the traumatic event(s) (typically due to dissociative amnesia and not to other factors such as head injury, alcohol, or drugs).

2. Persistent and exaggerated negative beliefs or expectations about oneself, others, or the world (e.g., "I am bad," "No one can be trusted," "The world is completely dangerous," "My whole nervous system is permanently ruined").
3. Persistent, distorted cognitions about the cause or consequences of the traumatic event(s) that lead the individual to blame himself/herself or others.
4. Persistent negative emotional state (e.g., fear, horror, anger, guilt, or shame).
5. Markedly diminished interest or participation in significant activities.
6. Feelings of detachment or estrangement from others.
7. Persistent inability to experience positive emotions (e.g., inability to experience happiness, satisfaction, or loving feelings).

E. Marked alterations in arousal and reactivity associated with the traumatic event(s), beginning or worsening after the traumatic event(s) occurred, as evidenced by two (or more) of the following:

1. Irritable behavior and angry outbursts (with little or no provocation) typically expressed as verbal or physical aggression toward people or objects.
2. Reckless or self-destructive behavior.
3. Hypervigilance.
4. Exaggerated startle response.
5. Problems with concentration.
6. Sleep disturbance (e.g., difficulty falling or staying asleep or restless sleep).

F. Duration of the disturbance (Criteria B, C, D, and E) is more than 1 month.

G. The disturbance causes clinically significant distress or impairment in social, occupational, or other important areas of functioning.

H. The disturbance is not attributable to the physiological effects of a substance (e.g., medication, alcohol) or another medical condition.

Specify whether:

With dissociative symptoms: The individual's symptoms meet the criteria for posttraumatic stress disorder, and in addition, in response to the stressor, the individual experiences persistent or recurrent symptoms of either of the following:

1. **Depersonalization:** Persistent or recurrent experiences of feeling detached from, and as if one were an outside observer of, one's mental processes or body (e.g., feeling as though one were in a dream; feeling a sense of unreality of self or body or of time moving slowly).

2. **Derealization:** Persistent or recurrent experiences of unreality of surroundings (e.g., the world around the individual is experienced as unreal, dreamlike, distant, or distorted).

Note: To use this subtype, the dissociative symptoms must not be attributable to the physiological effects of a substance (e.g., blackouts, behavior during alcohol intoxication) or another medical condition (e.g., complex partial seizures).

Specify if:

With delayed expression: If the full diagnostic criteria are not met until at least 6 months after the event (although the onset and expression of some symptoms may be immediate).

Posttraumatic Stress Disorder for Children 6 Years and Younger

A. In children 6 years and younger, exposure to actual or threatened death, serious injury, or sexual violence in one (or more) of the following ways:

 1. Directly experiencing the traumatic event(s).
 2. Witnessing, in person, the event(s) as it occurred to others, especially primary caregivers.

    Note: Witnessing does not include events that are witnessed only in electronic media, television, movies, or pictures.

 3. Learning that the traumatic event(s) occurred to a parent or caregiving figure.

B. Presence of one (or more) of the following intrusion symptoms associated with the traumatic event(s), beginning after the traumatic event(s) occurred:

 1. Recurrent, involuntary, and intrusive distressing memories of the traumatic event(s).

    Note: Spontaneous and intrusive memories may not necessarily appear distressing and may be expressed as play reenactment.

 2. Recurrent distressing dreams in which the content and/or affect of the dream are related to the traumatic event(s).

    Note: It may not be possible to ascertain that the frightening content is related to the traumatic event.

 3. Dissociative reactions (e.g., flashbacks) in which the child feels or acts as if the traumatic event(s) were recurring. (Such reactions may occur on a continuum, with the most extreme expression being a complete loss of awareness of present surroundings.) Such trauma-specific reenactment may occur in play.

 4. Intense or prolonged psychological distress at exposure to internal or external cues that symbolize or resemble an aspect of the traumatic event(s).

 5. Marked physiological reactions to reminders of the traumatic event(s).

C. One (or more) of the following symptoms, representing either persistent avoidance of stimuli associated with the traumatic event(s) or negative alterations in cognitions and mood associated with the traumatic event(s), must be present, beginning after the event(s) or worsening after the event(s):

Persistent Avoidance of Stimuli

1. Avoidance of or efforts to avoid activities, places, or physical reminders that arouse recollections of the traumatic event(s).
2. Avoidance of or efforts to avoid people, conversations, or interpersonal situations that arouse recollections of the traumatic event(s).

Negative Alterations in Cognitions

3. Substantially increased frequency of negative emotional states (e.g., fear, guilt, sadness, shame, confusion).
4. Markedly diminished interest or participation in significant activities, including constriction of play.
5. Socially withdrawn behavior.
6. Persistent reduction in expression of positive emotions.

D. Alterations in arousal and reactivity associated with the traumatic event(s), beginning or worsening after the traumatic event(s) occurred, as evidenced by two (or more) of the following:

1. Irritable behavior and angry outbursts (with little or no provocation) typically expressed as verbal or physical aggression toward people or objects (including extreme temper tantrums).
2. Hypervigilance.
3. Exaggerated startle response.
4. Problems with concentration.
5. Sleep disturbance (e.g., difficulty falling or staying asleep or restless sleep).

E. The duration of the disturbance is more than 1 month.

F. The disturbance causes clinically significant distress or impairment in relationships with parents, siblings, peers, or other caregivers or with school behavior.

G. The disturbance is not attributable to the physiological effects of a substance (e.g., medication or alcohol) or another medical condition.

Specify whether:

With dissociative symptoms: The individual's symptoms meet the criteria for posttraumatic stress disorder, and the individual experiences persistent or recurrent symptoms of either of the following:

1. **Depersonalization:** Persistent or recurrent experiences of feeling detached from, and as if one were an outside observer of, one's mental processes or body (e.g., feeling as though one were in a dream; feeling a sense of unreality of self or body or of time moving slowly).
2. **Derealization:** Persistent or recurrent experiences of unreality of surroundings (e.g., the world around the individual is experienced as unreal, dreamlike, distant, or distorted).

Note: To use this subtype, the dissociative symptoms must not be attributable to the physiological effects of a substance (e.g., blackouts) or another medical condition (e.g., complex partial seizures).

Specify if:

With delayed expression: If the full diagnostic criteria are not met until at least 6 months after the event (although the onset and expression of some symptoms may be immediate).

Source. Reprinted from American Psychiatric Association: *Diagnostic and Statistical Manual of Mental Disorders,* 5th Edition, Arlington, VA, American Psychiatric Association, 2013. Copyright © 2013 American Psychiatric Association. Used with permission.

The most common trauma reported by older women with PTSD in a nationally representative survey was physical and/or sexual assault, often occurring decades earlier in life (Cook and Simiola 2017). Veterans, the most studied population of older adults with PTSD, are more likely than nonveterans to have PTSD, and female Vietnam War veterans have higher rates (13.5% current prevalence and 16.9% lifetime prevalence) than were reported previously (Cook and Simiola 2017). PTSD often is comorbid with depression and other anxiety disorders (Kuwert et al. 2013). Older adults with prolonged trauma exposure have more severe PTSD symptoms compared with those exposed to brief trauma (Shrira et al. 2017). In a study of older adults exposed to the natural disaster of Hurricane Ike, the risk of PTSD was associated with increased exposure to the hurricane and experiencing dissociative symptoms (e.g., feeling disconnected from one's body, blanking out) and/or autonomic activation symptoms (e.g., trembling, shaking, heart palpitations, sweaty palms) during the exposure (Pietrzak et al. 2012c).

OBSESSIVE-COMPULSIVE DISORDER

OCD is diagnosed when an individual has obsessions, compulsions, or both. *Obsessions* are recurrent thoughts, urges, or images that are intrusive, unwanted, and anxiety-provoking or distressing. *Compulsions* are repetitive behaviors or mental acts that someone is compelled to do in response to the obsession. The level of insight about the truth of OCD beliefs varies from good to poor to delusional. The full criteria are listed in Box 2–5.

Box 2–5.   DSM-5 Diagnostic Criteria for Obsessive-Compulsive Disorder

---

A. Presence of obsessions, compulsions, or both:

Obsessions are defined by (1) and (2):

1. Recurrent and persistent thoughts, urges, or images that are experienced, at some time during the disturbance, as intrusive and unwanted, and that in most individuals cause marked anxiety or distress.

2. The individual attempts to ignore or suppress such thoughts, urges, or images, or to neutralize them with some other thought or action (i.e., by performing a compulsion).

Compulsions are defined by (1) and (2):

1. Repetitive behaviors (e.g., hand washing, ordering, checking) or mental acts (e.g., praying, counting, repeating words silently) that the individual feels driven to perform in response to an obsession or according to rules that must be applied rigidly.
2. The behaviors or mental acts are aimed at preventing or reducing anxiety or distress, or preventing some dreaded event or situation; however, these behaviors or mental acts are not connected in a realistic way with what they are designed to neutralize or prevent, or are clearly excessive.
   Note: Young children may not be able to articulate the aims of these behaviors or mental acts.

B. The obsessions or compulsions are time-consuming (e.g., take more than 1 hour per day) or cause clinically significant distress or impairment in social, occupational, or other important areas of functioning.
C. The obsessive-compulsive symptoms are not attributable to the physiological effects of a substance (e.g., a drug of abuse, a medication) or another medical condition.
D. The disturbance is not better explained by the symptoms of another mental disorder (e.g., excessive worries, as in generalized anxiety disorder; preoccupation with appearance, as in body dysmorphic disorder; difficulty discarding or parting with possessions, as in hoarding disorder; hair pulling, as in trichotillomania [hair-pulling disorder]; skin picking, as in excoriation [skin-picking] disorder; stereotypies, as in stereotypic movement disorder; ritualized eating behavior, as in eating disorders; preoccupation with substances or gambling, as in substance-related and addictive disorders; preoccupation with having an illness, as in illness anxiety disorder; sexual urges or fantasies, as in paraphilic disorders; impulses, as in disruptive, impulse-control, and conduct disorders; guilty ruminations, as in major depressive disorder; thought insertion or delusional preoccupations, as in schizophrenia spectrum and other psychotic disorders; or repetitive patterns of behavior, as in autism spectrum disorder).

Specify if:

With good or fair insight: The individual recognizes that obsessive-compulsive disorder beliefs are definitely or probably not true or that they may or may not be true.
With poor insight: The individual thinks obsessive-compulsive disorder beliefs are probably true.
With absent insight/delusional beliefs: The individual is completely convinced that obsessive-compulsive disorder beliefs are true.

Source.   Reprinted from American Psychiatric Association: *Diagnostic and Statistical Manual of Mental Disorders,* 5th Edition, Arlington, VA, American Psychiatric Association, 2013. Copyright © 2013 American Psychiatric Association. Used with permission.

Although the prevalence of OCD in community-dwelling elders is relatively low, it may be higher in those residing in nursing homes (Calamari et al. 2012). OCD may follow one of several trajectories: chronic persistent illness that starts early in life; subclinical OCD early in life that becomes threshold OCD following stressors of late life such as loss of a significant other or serious health problems; or onset of OCD late in life, usually associated with neurological disorders (Calamari et al. 2012).

Unfortunately, OCD may not be recognized until several years after onset, perhaps because of high levels of comorbidity. In the NCS-R, 90% of people with lifetime OCD met criteria for another psychiatric disorder, including other anxiety disorders (76%), mood disorders (63%), and substance use disorders (39%) (Ruscio et al. 2010). In late life, hypochondriasis is a common comorbidity (Calamari et al. 2012). In clinical practice, health-related obsessions are commonly encountered in geriatric patients.

HOARDING DISORDER

Hoarding disorder is defined by difficulties discarding or parting with possessions, regardless of value, due to a need to save the items and distress caused by discarding them. These symptoms culminate in excessive clutter of active living areas that limits their actual use. If there is not significant clutter, it is because of interventions of others. Hoarding leads to clinically significant distress or functional impairment (American Psychiatric Association 2013). Community prevalence studies are limited, but in available studies, hoarding is more common in later life, and symptoms tend to be more severe in older compared with younger populations (Calamari et al. 2012; Mohlman et al. 2012). Hoarding disorder is also associated with comorbid dementia and other serious mental disorders.

Clinical Course

AGE AT ONSET

The onset of most anxiety disorders is usually in adolescence or early adulthood, although many older adults with GAD have late-life onset. The median age at onset is 15–17 years for phobias, 23 years for panic disorder, and 30 years for GAD (Kessler et al. 2012). GAD may have a bimodal onset, with roughly 25%–50% of older adults with GAD developing the condition later in life (Chou 2009; Lenze et al. 2005; Zhang et al. 2015a). Risk factors for late-onset GAD include female sex, recent adverse life events, and chronic physical (e.g., respiratory, cardiac, dyslipidemia, cognitive impairment) and mental (e.g., depression, phobia) disorders (Zhang et al. 2015b). Older adults with early-onset GAD are more likely to have other comorbid anxiety disorders, are less likely to have other comorbid medical conditions, and have better health-related quality of life compared with adults with late-onset GAD (Chou 2009).

In a 20-year study following Israeli war veterans, approximately 16.5% of veterans had delayed-onset PTSD, with the majority experiencing some PTSD symptoms prior to the delayed PTSD onset. Longer lag times to the onset of PTSD were associated with milder PTSD severity (Horesh et al. 2013).

The mean age at onset of OCD is 20 years (Kessler et al. 2005). Fewer than 9% of people develop OCD after age 40 years, although older women appear to have a second peak onset of OCD after age 64 (Calamari et al. 2012; Frydman et al. 2014). Risk factors for developing OCD after age 40 include being female, having a history of subclinical OCD symptoms for at least a decade, having PTSD after age 40, and pregnancy (Frydman et al. 2014).

PROGNOSIS

Anxiety disorders tend to be persistent and chronic; 39%–52% of older adults with anxiety disorders experience persistent or remitting symptoms over the course of 3–6 years (Sami and Nilforooshan 2015). Predictors of persistence of anxiety disorders in general include poorer mental health–related quality of life; more comorbid medical conditions; neurotic personality traits; and more comorbid mental disorders, including personality disorders and mood disorders (Mackenzie et al. 2014; Sami and Nilforooshan 2015). In a study of 1,994 older adults, poor physical health–related quality of life and history of lifetime suicide attempts predicted persistence of panic disorder, and treatment-seeking for social phobia predicted persistence of social phobia (Mackenzie et al. 2014). Poorer reported mental health–related quality of life and comorbid mental health disorders, Axis II personality disorder, and mood disorders predicted persistence of any anxiety disorder in older adults (Mackenzie et al. 2014).

Older adults with anxiety disorders may transition to depression or mixed anxiety and depression over time. Relapse rates are high in older adults with mixed anxiety and depression—up to 74% after 3 years. Predictors of persistent anxiety in older adults with comorbid depressive disorder include higher degree of worry symptoms and less cognitive inhibitory control (Spinhoven et al. 2017).

Over time, the severity and frequency of panic symptoms and functional impairment of panic disorder decrease with age (Sheikh et al. 2004). Agoraphobia is a risk marker for poorer prognosis and lower chance of remission in panic disorder (Wittchen et al. 2010). FOF has a persistent clinical course in approximately 60% of cases (Oh-Park et al. 2011). Social phobia in older adults may not be as persistent as seen in other anxiety disorders: in one study of 612 older adults, only 11% still met criteria after 5 years of follow-up (Karlsson et al. 2010). PTSD can have a variable clinical course over time, with some patients having persistent and chronic symptoms and others experiencing remission and recurrence later in life (Chopra et al. 2014; Cook and Simiola 2017). In one study, approximately 50% of older adults with PTSD experienced a persistent course of illness (Byers et al. 2014).

Consequences and Complications

SUICIDE ATTEMPTS

The evaluation and management of suicidal ideation is covered in greater detail in Chapter 4, "Suicide Risk Reduction in Older Adults." In studies of mixed-age populations, more than 70% of individuals with a lifetime history of suicide attempt had an anxiety disorder (Nepon et al. 2010). Panic disorder and PTSD have the strongest associations with suicide attempts, especially when comorbid with personality disorders (Nepon et al. 2010). In a retrospective study of individuals admitted for depression or anxiety disorders, there was an almost eightfold increase in suicides in those with anxious depression over the course of more than 20 years (Sami and Nilforooshan 2015).

Individuals with early-onset panic disorder (age 27 years or younger) attempt suicide more frequently when compared with those with late-onset panic disorder (Tibi et al. 2013). Veterans with trauma history and PTSD report more mental distress and suicidal ideation and are more likely to die than patients without trauma or those who are exposed to trauma but do not have PTSD symptoms (Durai et al. 2011). Older men with PTSD have a threefold increased likelihood of a lifetime history of suicide attempt compared with those without PTSD (Pietrzak et al. 2012b). In general, older adults with an anxiety disorder are less likely to experience suicidal ideation than are younger adults with an anxiety disorder—nevertheless, screening for suicidal ideation, as discussed in Chapter 4, is critical (Raposo et al. 2014).

MORBIDITY AND OTHER CAUSES OF DEATH

Anxiety disorders in later life can have a profound impact on an individual's quality of life. For example, GAD is associated with lower health-related quality of life (Porensky et al. 2009). Older adults with panic disorder have lower reported health-related quality of life (Chou 2010). PTSD increases risk for poorer health and disability (Cook and Simiola 2017) and poorer mental health–related quality of life (Chopra et al. 2014). Having a higher number of anxiety symptoms has been associated with lower health-related quality of life in individuals with comorbid neurological disorders, including lower physical health–related quality of life in patients with migraines and lower mental health–related quality of life in patients with epilepsy, migraine, multiple sclerosis, stroke, or Parkinson's disease (Prisnie et al. 2018).

Moreover, anxiety disorders are a risk factor for comorbid medical problems and multimorbidity, perhaps even more so than depressive disorders (Gould et al. 2016). In a longitudinal study of more than 10,000 older adults, any lifetime history of anxiety disorder or PTSD was associated with increased risk of developing a gastrointestinal disorder (El-Gabalawy et al. 2014). In another longitudinal study of more than 32,000 subjects with coronary artery disease (CAD), the presence of GAD was associated with higher risk for developing CAD, and improvement in GAD symptoms lowered the risk of developing CAD (Liu et al. 2019). Older adults with an anxiety disorder or subthreshold anxiety generally have more chronic medical conditions and are more likely to be taking a benzodiazepine compared with older adults without anxiety symptoms (Grenier et al. 2011a). Older adults with either subthreshold or specific phobia have more chronic physical health problems and are more likely to use benzodiazepines compared with those without anxiety (Grenier et al. 2011b). PTSD is associated with increased risk for cardiovascular disease and other related cardiovascular risk factors (Kuwert et al. 2013). Older adults with PTSD have higher rates of hypertension, angina and other heart disease, stomach ulcers, and arthritis (Pietrzak et al. 2012a).

Anxiety disorders are associated with increased risk for falls. This relationship is especially found in men, with anxiety disorders associated with a threefold increased risk of falls in men but not women (Holloway et al. 2016). FOF is a risk factor for falls, disability, and mortality (Chang et al. 2017; Gazibara et al. 2017; Makino et al. 2018). Anxiety in the context of comorbid medical illness leads to worse rehabilitation outcomes in older adults (Yohannes et al. 2000).

In a mixed-ethnic population of community-dwelling older adults, high levels of anxiety were associated with increased mortality from all causes, including cardiovascular causes and cancer (Ostir and Goodwin 2006). A few studies have demonstrated a lack of association between anxiety and increased mortality; in one study, older anxious men had increased mortality when compared with older anxious women, but the men also had more physical conditions and ischemic heart disease (Sami and Nilforooshan 2015).

DISABILITY

Anxiety symptoms and anxiety disorders are associated with increased disability and impairment of activities of daily living (Brenes et al. 2005; Dong et al. 2020). In a primary care mixed-age population, having an anxiety disorder was associated with increased functional impairment in areas related to mental health, social and role functioning, physical functioning, and pain compared with those without anxiety disorders (Kroenke et al. 2007). GAD in later life is associated with higher levels of disability (Porensky et al. 2009). FOF has been associated with increased risk for disability (Makino et al. 2018). Chronic PTSD in older adults increases risk for disability threefold compared with older adults without PTSD (Byers et al. 2014). Specifically, in older veterans with PTSD, actual and self-reported physical functioning, daily activity functioning, and general health are poorer (Hall et al. 2014). OCD is a debilitating and pervasive disorder, with two-thirds of individuals reporting severe disability in several aspects of functioning (Ruscio et al. 2010).

HEALTH CARE UTILIZATION

Caring for older adults with anxiety can be challenging because without additional assessment and tests it may not be readily apparent that somatic concerns are caused by anxiety. Therefore, anxiety in older adults can lead to increased use of medical services to work up somatic symptoms associated with anxiety.

Some studies have found that anxiety disorders and symptoms are associated with increased use of non–mental health care and decreased use of mental health care, and assessment of health care costs for anxiety disorders go mostly toward costs related to somatic concerns. However, a systematic review of the relationship of anxiety and health care utilization and costs specifically in older adults revealed a paucity of studies, with mixed quality and conflicting findings: some studies reported that anxiety was associated with higher utilization and costs, and others did not establish an association (Hohls et al. 2018). In a study of primary care patients ages 85 and older, those with anxiety had 31% more health care costs than did those without anxiety over a period of 6 months (Hohls et al. 2019c). However, when controlling for predisposing, enabling, and need characteristics, anxiety symptoms were not a risk factor for health care utilization or costs, whereas multimorbidity, cognitive impairment, and functional impairment were risk factors.

In one study, GAD in older adults was shown to increase health care utilization (Porensky et al. 2009) and use of radiology services, independent of medical comorbidity, when compared with those with and without other psychiatric disorders (Calleo et al. 2009). Older adults with panic disorder or panic attacks use more emergency services and have higher outpatient, inpatient, and overall health care costs than do those without panic disorder (Chou 2010; Hohls et al. 2019a, 2019b).

In a population of community-dwelling older adults in a government-run health care system, older adults with anxiety had higher total health care (outpatient and inpatient) costs. Approximately $80 million per 1,000,000 older adult population could be attributable to excess annual adjusted health care costs due to anxiety and $119.8 million for comorbid anxiety and depression (Vasiliadis et al. 2013).

Among older adults with mood and anxiety disorders in the NCS-R study, mental health services were underutilized, with estimates that 70% who met criteria were not using services (Byers et al. 2012). Several risk factors for not using mental health services were identified: minority race/ethnic group status, discomfort with discussing personal issues, marital status of married or cohabitating, middle rather than high income, mild disorders, having no chronic pain concerns, and low perceived cognitive impairment. OCD seems to be an exception: individuals with the most severe OCD are the most likely to receive mental health treatment for an anxiety disorder (Ruscio et al. 2010).

FAMILY AND OTHER CAREGIVERS

Caring for an older adult with mental illness can be fulfilling and rewarding, but it also can be challenging, stressful, and time-consuming. Anxiety disorders lead to maladaptive behaviors such as frequent checking behaviors or reassurance seeking and avoidance that can cause increased dependence on other family and care partners. These maladaptive behaviors and avoidance are experienced across a variety of anxiety disorders.

Caregiving for a dependent older adult can increase risk for caregiver stress, anxiety, and depression. Studies suggest that caregiver anxiety varies depending on type of care, duration of care, and other characteristics of the care recipient; additionally, the caregiver's characteristics can affect risk for developing anxiety. Risk factors for developing anxiety while providing care for dependent older adults include denial and self-blame; protective factors include planning, acceptance, humor coping strategies (Pérez-Cruz et al. 2019), and mastery (i.e., sense of being in control) and caregiving competence (Chan et al. 2018).

Comorbidities

DEPRESSION

Anxiety and depression are often comorbid. Twenty-six percent of older adults with anxiety disorders have comorbid depression, and almost 48% of older adults with depression have a comorbid anxiety disorder (Beekman et al. 2000). van der Veen and colleagues (2015) examined factors associated with comorbid anxiety disorder in older adults with major depression; they identified approximately 39% of older adults with major depressive disorder as having comorbid anxiety disorders (in descending order of prevalence: social phobia, panic disorder with and without agoraphobia, agoraphobia, and GAD). In this study, risk factors for comorbid anxiety disorders in older adults with major depression included younger age, female sex, and having more severe depressive symptoms; moreover, different risk factor profiles were associated with different anxiety disorders comorbid with major depressive disorder (e.g., higher depressive symptoms and early trauma were associated with panic disorder; personality traits of neuroticism, extroversion, and conscientiousness were associated with social phobia) (van der Veen et al. 2015). Anxiety is a risk factor for developing depressive symptoms and for recurrence of depressive symptoms in older adults (Potvin et al. 2013).

Various theories to explain the relationship between anxiety and depression have been hypothesized, including anxiety as a prodrome of depression; anxiety as a vulnerability factor for depression; and anxiety and depression possibly existing on a continuum, with anxiety at one point of the spectrum and depression at another. Certain personality traits such as neuroticism have been tied to both anxiety and depression, and models for persistent anxiety leading to abnormal hypothalamic-pituitary-adrenal axis stress hormones leading to depression have also been postulated (Potvin et al. 2013).

In older adults, lifetime history of panic disorder is associated with major depressive disorder (Chou 2010). Older adults with specific phobia or subthreshold symptoms also have more comorbid depression (Grenier et al. 2011b). PTSD in older adults, when compared with older adults with trauma but without PTSD symptoms, increases risk for several psychiatric comorbid disorders, including depression, other anxiety disorders, drug use, and some personality disorders (Pietrzak et al. 2012b). Approximately 63% of patients with OCD also have a mood disorder (Ruscio et al. 2010).

COGNITIVE IMPAIRMENT AND DEMENTIA

The relationship between anxiety and cognitive impairment is complex. In Chapter 1, "Introduction to Late-Life Depression," we discussed the relationship between depression and cognitive impairment (see Figure 1–2). As with depression, high levels of anxiety can interfere with one's ability to concentrate or focus. This can lead to challenges with registering information from one's environment to be accessed later. People who worry excessively can ruminate and thus appear distractible. Studies have demonstrated that anxiety disorders increase risk for cognitive disorders, and cognitive disorders can manifest with and/or lead to anxiety, representing a bidirectional relationship (Mohlman et al. 2012). Studies employing functional neuroimaging looking at amyloid-β suggest that there may be a shared biological mechanism between the development of anxiety and cognitive impairment. Moreover, both anxiety and cognitive impairment are considered prognostic factors that worsen outcomes in individuals who have cognitive and anxiety disorders, respectively (Hellwig and Domschke 2019).

Older adults with PTSD have been found to have more memory impairment and impaired learning compared with control subjects (Scott Mackin et al. 2012). Incidence and prevalence of dementia is higher in veterans with PTSD compared with those without PTSD, an effect amplified in former prisoners of war (Meziab et al. 2014; Qureshi et al. 2010). Combat veterans with PTSD have more cognitive impairment than Holocaust survivors with PTSD (Schuitevoerder et al. 2013). Although the literature is somewhat contradictory, it does appear that PTSD is a risk factor for developing dementia (Kang et al. 2019; Kuring et al. 2020; Yaffe et al. 2010).

In older adults, severe FOF has been associated with higher risk of developing cognitive decline (Noh et al. 2019). Patients with OCD exhibit impairments in cognitive functioning, with patients with early-onset OCD having more problems with visuospatial construction and memory and patients with late-onset OCD demonstrating more executive dysfunction (i.e., problems with cognitive flexibility, organization, and verbal fluency) (Kim et al. 2020).

Anxiety behaviors related to dementia can be explained by the progressively lowered stress threshold model. This model proposes that there is a mismatch between environmental stressors and the ability of the person with dementia to adapt to those stressors; anxious behaviors develop as the individual with progressive cognitive impairment approaches her or his stress threshold (Walaszek 2019). In patients who have preserved insight, anxiety can be a response to experiences of cognitive impairment and functional challenges (e.g., feeling confused or forgetting can lead to fear or worry) and is a common behavioral or psychological symptom of dementia, with estimated prevalence of 39% in patients with Alzheimer's disease (Walaszek 2019). When an older adult experiences cognitive challenges, he or she may also struggle to access usual cognitive coping strategies for managing stressors or anxiety symptoms. Therefore, it can become much more difficult for the person to cope with or self-manage fear or worry symptoms in the setting of comorbid cognitive impairment, leading to either new onset or exacerbation of clinically significant anxiety symptoms.

Clinical presentations of anxiety as part of behavioral and psychological symptoms of dementia can include the following: uncontrollable worry, repetitive speech, anxiety at being separated from one's caregiver(s), becoming agitated when the caregiver is not in sight, and avoidant behaviors (e.g., being too afraid to leave one's home, go to new places, try new activities, or talk to new people). Individuals with dementia can experience catastrophic reactions, which manifest as a sudden display of emotions such as tearfulness, anger, or fearfulness that is disproportionate to the context of the situation. It often is more challenging for caregivers to provide reassurance to someone with dementia; forgetfulness can make it difficult to sustain reassurance (Walaszek 2019). Anxiety may be a part of a dementia prodrome, with the cognitive impairment coming later—therefore, if an older adult presents with new-onset anxiety, the clinician should consider the possibility of neurocognitive disorder in the differential diagnosis.

We illustrate the interaction between anxiety and cognitive impairment in the following case example.

CASE EXAMPLE 2: "I DON'T KNOW WHY I WORRY SO MUCH—I JUST DO"

Mr. Zapata is a 79-year-old widowed father of two adult sons who has a history of major depressive disorder. He presents to the geriatric psychiatry clinic on referral by his primary care physician for concerns about depression. He reports that he has not been able to do his usual activities for the past 2 months, so he has been neglecting grooming and other household tasks. Every morning, he wakes up with dread. He finds it challenging to get out of bed to start the day and therefore spends hours in bed, although he reports he cannot sleep. He has lost 15 pounds because of a combination of poor appetite and insufficient energy to prepare meals. He has lost interest and pleasure in his usual routines and has been isolating at home. His sons have expressed concerns about his depression and contacted his primary care physician. Mr. Zapata acknowledges that he has had similar episodes in the past, but this time has been the worst he has experienced. He also endorses persistent worries that he will not be able to shake this depression and that something bad is going to happen. He reports he cannot stop thinking that something is terribly wrong with him and he will not be able to continue to take care of himself in his home. He has been more irritable, tense, and fatigued and complains that his memory is "shot." He reports that he has periods when his anxiety and fear are so intense that his heart races and his entire body starts shaking, and he feels as if he cannot catch his breath. During these periods, he fears that he is about to die. He denies suicidal ideation or history of past attempts. He has presented to the emergency department for these symptoms three times in the past 3 months, and workup has been unremarkable. He has been to his primary care physician for various physical complaints almost weekly for the past month, and he responds to reassurance in the moment but then repeatedly calls the clinic with concerns that something is wrong.

Mr. Zapata is diagnosed with recurrent major depressive disorder with anxious distress, and various antidepressants are tried. However, his depression does not respond to a selective serotonin reuptake inhibitor, and he is unable to tolerate a serotonin-norepinephrine reuptake inhibitor. He experiences partial response to a tricyclic antidepressant, but symptoms and functional impairment persist, and he agrees to pursue electroconvulsive therapy. His depressive symptoms improve significantly, and he achieves remission following a course of electroconvulsive therapy. However, he continues to experience severe symptoms of excessive worry and recurrent panic attacks.

Mr. Zapata finds it challenging to work with a therapist to identify triggers or approaches other than behavioral activation that he might try to help him cope with his anxiety. In the moment, he struggles with initiating cognitive or behavioral strategies that he developed with the therapist in sessions. He continues to experience significant cognitive impairment and reports a high degree of anxiety about his ability to continue to care for himself independently.

Formal neuropsychometric testing confirms amnestic memory impairment and executive dysfunction. The treatment team formulates that Mr. Zapata's persistent anxiety is not responsive to usual cognitive behavioral and antidepressant interventions, likely because of an underlying neurocognitive disorder that challenges his ability to engage in usual coping strategies. They recommend bringing in additional in-home resources or transitioning to a higher level of care to better meet Mr. Zapata's need for increased structure and support.

SUBSTANCE USE DISORDERS

Individuals with anxiety disorders may turn to alcohol, illicit substances such as cannabis or heroin, or prescribed opioids or sedative-hypnotics to try to reduce anxiety. In clinical practice, excessive use of alcohol or other substances may be a manifestation of avoidant behaviors in PTSD and other anxiety disorders. PTSD in older adults may not be recognized until after the older adult stops drinking or on retirement, when the individual no longer uses coping strategies to distract or avoid and instead begins to pursue alternative ways of managing PTSD symptoms.

In general, there is a paucity of literature that examines alcohol and substance use disorders in older adults and their relationship to psychiatric comorbidities. Wu and Blazer (2014) presented one of the most comprehensive reviews of psychiatric comorbidity studies in alcohol and substance use disorders in older adults. They reported results of cross-sectional studies, including the following:

- Approximately 31% of past-year benzodiazepine-dependent older adults had mood or anxiety disorders.
- Among opioid-dependent older adults, 30% had comorbid GAD, 28% had PTSD, and 47% had a mood disorder or an anxiety disorder.
- Among older alcohol users, prevalence of anxiety disorder stratified by alcohol use risk was 1.4% for elders at low risk of alcohol use, 2.3% for those at moderate risk, and 8.8% for those at high risk.
- Anxiety disorders increased risk for benzodiazepine dependence in older adults.

In a study by Pietrzak et al. (2012b), PTSD in older adults was associated with higher risk of comorbid drug use disorders but not alcohol use disorders; Another smaller study found that PTSD increases risk of alcohol use disorders later in life (Davidson et al. 1990). Thirty-nine percent of patients with OCD have comorbid substance use disorders (Ruscio et al. 2010).

SOMATIZATION

Somatoform disorders were reorganized into *somatic symptom and related disorders* in DSM-5 (American Psychiatric Association 2013). Individuals who had previously met criteria for hypochondriasis—a preoccupation with or excessive fear of having a serious illness—now generally meet criteria for *somatic symptom disorder* (approximately 75%) or *illness anxiety disorder* (approximately 25%) (Aan de Stegge et al. 2018). Because this reclassification took place fairly recently, most literature about older adults focuses on hypochondriasis and health anxiety.

Somatic symptom disorder occurs when an individual experiences, for at least 6 months, one or more somatic symptoms causing distress or disruption in daily life and has excessive thoughts, feelings, or behaviors associated with these symptoms or worries about health with at least one of the following problems: excessive thoughts about the seriousness of the symptoms, high levels of anxiety about health or symptoms, and/or excessive effort devoted to these symptoms or concerns. Somatic symptom disorder with predominant pain replaces the condition formerly referred to as pain disorder (American Psychiatric Association 2013).

Illness anxiety disorder is defined by worry about having or acquiring a serious illness in the absence of somatic symptoms, or, if present, the somatic symptoms experienced are mild. To meet the criteria, if the patient has medical comorbidities or has risk for such, the worry should be excessive. The individual experiences a high degree of health anxiety and has a low threshold for feeling alarmed about his or her own health. Excessive health-related behaviors include excessive surveillance, reassurance seeking, or checking for illness or maladaptive avoidance of health-related appointments. These distorted beliefs and maladaptive behaviors have been present for at least 6 months, and patients with illness anxiety disorder can be specified by either care-seeking or care-avoidant types (American Psychiatric Association 2013).

Worry about health is more frequent in older adults because of a higher risk of having comorbid health conditions and vulnerabilities associated with aging. In addition, multimorbidity is a risk factor for anxiety. Generally, health anxiety is conceptualized along a spectrum, with milder forms being adaptive because they prompt individuals toward self-care, whereas at its most extreme (e.g., hypochondriasis), it is maladaptive, with high levels of disability and poor quality of life (El-Gabalawy et al. 2013). It is estimated that up to 20% of medically ill populations have significant health anxiety. Age is a risk factor, with an average age at onset of hypochondriasis of 57 years; being female is another risk factor (El-Gabalawy et al. 2013). Hypochondriasis shares similar features with panic disorder and OCD, but comorbidity with GAD has not been established. It is frequently associated with depression as well (El-Gabalawy et al. 2013).

Summary: Understanding How Anxiety Arises and Progresses in Older Adults

As people age, the manifestations of anxiety can be quite varied. Although the prevalence of anxiety disorders is lower in geriatric populations when compared with younger populations, anxiety and related disorders remain the most common mental disorders in late life. For most older adults, anxiety disorders start early in life and are chronic, either persistent or remitting and recurring; in a minority of patients, onset of anxiety disorders is later in life. Differences can arise in presentations of anxiety and related disorders depending on whether onset was early or later in life. The most common anxiety disorders that manifest later in life are GAD and fear of falling. Usually, the severity of anxiety disorders is milder as one ages; however, subsyndromal and syndromal anxiety and related disorders often cause disability and other complications, including multimorbidity with other health conditions and other psychiatric comorbidities such as depression, neurocognitive disorders, and substance use disorders. Anxiety carries profound costs for the individual, the family and care partners, health care systems, and society.

KEY POINTS

- Anxiety and related disorders and symptoms are the most common mental health problems experienced by older adults and are associated with poorer cognitive, mental, and physical health and functional outcomes.

- Except for fear of falling, anxiety and related disorders are more prevalent and severe in younger adults than in older adults.

- In most cases, anxiety and related disorders start early in life. Generalized anxiety disorder (GAD) is an exception, with a bimodal pattern of onset. Approximately 25%–50% of GAD cases develop later in life.

- The relationship between anxiety and comorbid medical conditions is bidirectional, so potential medical etiologies for new-onset anxiety in an older adult should be considered.

Resources for Patients, Families, and Caregivers

Anxiety and Depression Association of America

https://adaa.org

- The Anxiety and Depression Association of America is a non-profit organization that works to improve the quality of lives of people living with anxiety and depressive disorders and their families by providing free education and additional resources.
- The website includes information on anxiety in older adults.

Health in Aging

www.healthinaging.org

- The Health in Aging website is provided through the American Geriatrics Society's Health in Aging Foundation.
- This website provides updated educational and other supportive resources for older adults and their caregivers. It covers a range of health issues, including late-life anxiety.

Mental Health America website

www.mhanational.org

- Mental Health America is a community-based nonprofit organization that supports individuals living with mental illness through advocacy, education, and other resources.
- The website includes a section on anxiety in older adults.

References

Aan de Stegge BM, Tak LM, Rosmalen JGM, et al: Death anxiety and its association with hypochondriasis and medically unexplained symptoms: a systematic review. J Psychosom Res 115:58–65, 2018 30470318

Altunoz U, Kokurcan A, Kirici S, et al: Clinical characteristics of generalized anxiety disorder: older vs. young adults. Nord J Psychiatry 72(2):97–102, 2018 29065768

American Psychiatric Association: Diagnostic and Statistical Manual of Mental Disorders, 5th Edition. Arlington, VA, American Psychiatric Association, 2013

Arbus C, Hergueta T, Duburcq A, et al: Adjustment disorder with anxiety in old age: comparing prevalence and clinical management in primary care and mental health care. Eur Psychiatry 29(4):233–238, 2014 23769681

Arfken CL, Lach HW, Birge SJ, et al: The prevalence and correlates of fear of falling in elderly persons living in the community. Am J Public Health 84(4):565–570, 1994 8154557

Bateson M, Brilot B, Nettle D: Anxiety: an evolutionary approach. Can J Psychiatry 56(12):707–715, 2011 22152639

Beekman ATF, Bremmer MA, Deeg DJH, et al: Anxiety disorders in later life: a report from the Longitudinal Aging Study Amsterdam. Int J Geriatr Psychiatry 13(10):717–726, 1998 9818308

Beekman ATF, de Beurs E, van Balkom AJLM, et al: Anxiety and depression in later life: co-occurrence and communality of risk factors. Am J Psychiatry 157(1):89–95, 2000 10618018

Brenes GA: Anxiety and chronic obstructive pulmonary disease: prevalence, impact, and treatment. Psychosom Med 65(6):963–970, 2003 14645773

Brenes GA, Guralnik JM, Williamson JD, et al: The influence of anxiety on the progression of disability. J Am Geriatr Soc 53(1):34–39, 2005 15667373

Bryant C, Jackson H, Ames D: The prevalence of anxiety in older adults: methodological issues and a review of the literature. J Affect Disord 109(3):233–250, 2008 18155775

Byers AL, Yaffe K, Covinsky KE, et al: High occurrence of mood and anxiety disorders among older adults: the National Comorbidity Survey Replication. Arch Gen Psychiatry 67(5):489–496, 2010 20439830

Byers AL, Arean PA, Yaffe K: Low use of mental health services among older Americans with mood and anxiety disorders. Psychiatr Serv 63(1):66–72, 2012 22227762

Byers AL, Covinsky KE, Neylan TC, et al: Chronicity of posttraumatic stress disorder and risk of disability in older persons. JAMA Psychiatry 71(5):540–546, 2014 24647756

Cabrera I, Brugos D, Montorio I: Attentional biases in older adults with generalized anxiety disorder. J Anxiety Disord 71:102207, 2020 32145484

Cairney J, McCabe L, Veldhuizen S, et al: Epidemiology of social phobia in later life. Am J Geriatr Psychiatry 15(3):224–233, 2007 17213375

Calamari JE, Pontarelli NK, Armstrong KM, et al: Obsessive-compulsive disorder in late life. Cogn Behav Pract 19(1):136–150, 2012

Calleo J, Stanley MA, Greisinger A, et al: Generalized anxiety disorder in older medical patients: diagnostic recognition, mental health management and service utilization. J Clin Psychol Med Settings 16(2):178–185, 2009 19152056

Canuto A, Weber K, Baertschi M, et al: Anxiety disorders in old age: psychiatric comorbidities, quality of life, and prevalence according to age, gender, and country. Am J Geriatr Psychiatry 26(2):174–185, 2018 29031568

Chan EY, Glass G, Chua KC, et al: Relationship between mastery and caregiving competence in protecting against burden, anxiety and depression among caregivers of frail older adults. J Nutr Health Aging 22(10):1238–1245, 2018 30498832

Chang HT, Chen HC, Chou P: Fear of falling and mortality among community-dwelling older adults in the Shih-Pai study in Taiwan: a longitudinal follow-up study. Geriatr Gerontol Int 17(11):2216–2223, 2017 28060445

Chaudieu I, Beluche I, Norton J, et al: Abnormal reactions to environmental stress in elderly persons with anxiety disorders: evidence from a population study of diurnal cortisol changes. J Affect Disord 106(3):307–313, 2008 17727959

Chopra MP, Zhang H, Pless Kaiser A, et al: PTSD is a chronic, fluctuating disorder affecting the mental quality of life in older adults. Am J Geriatr Psychiatry 22(1):86–97, 2014 24314889

Chou KL: Age at onset of generalized anxiety disorder in older adults. Am J Geriatr Psychiatry 17(6):455–464, 2009 19472431

Chou KL: Panic disorder in older adults: evidence from the national epidemiologic survey on alcohol and related conditions. Int J Geriatr Psychiatry 25(8):822–832, 2010 19946867

Cook JM, Simiola V: Trauma and PTSD in older adults: prevalence, course, concomitants and clinical considerations. Curr Opin Psychol 14:1–4, 2017 28813305

Creighton AS, Davison TE, Kissane DW: The prevalence of anxiety among older adults in nursing homes and other residential aged care facilities: a systematic review. Int J Geriatr Psychiatry 31(6):555–566, 2016 26552603

Creighton AS, Davison TE, Kissane DW: The prevalence, reporting, and treatment of anxiety among older adults in nursing homes and other residential aged care facilities. J Affect Disord 227:416–423, 2018 29154158

Davidson JR, Kudler HS, Saunders WB, Smith RD: Symptom and comorbidity patterns in World War II and Vietnam veterans with posttraumatic stress disorder. Compr Psychiatry 31(2):162–170, 1990 2311383

de Oliveira KC, Grinberg LT, Hoexter MQ, et al: Layer-specific reduced neuronal density in the orbitofrontal cortex of older adults with obsessive-compulsive disorder. Brain Struct Funct 224(1):191–203, 2019 30298291

Denkinger MD, Lukas A, Nikolaus T, et al: Factors associated with fear of falling and associated activity restriction in community-dwelling older adults: a systematic review. Am J Geriatr Psychiatry 23(1):72–86, 2015 24745560

Dong L, Freedman VA, Mendes de Leon CF: The association of comorbid depression and anxiety symptoms with disability onset in older adults. Psychosom Med 82(2):158–164, 2020 31688675

Durai UN, Chopra MP, Coakley E, et al: Exposure to trauma and posttraumatic stress disorder symptoms in older veterans attending primary care: comorbid conditions and self-rated health status. J Am Geriatr Soc 59(6):1087–1092, 2011 21649614

El-Gabalawy R, Mackenzie CS, Shooshtari S, Sareen J: Comorbid physical health conditions and anxiety disorders: a population-based exploration of prevalence and health outcomes among older adults. Gen Hosp Psychiatry 33(6):556–564, 2011 21908055

El-Gabalawy R, Mackenzie CS, Thibodeau MA, et al: Health anxiety disorders in older adults: conceptualizing complex conditions in late life. Clin Psychol Rev 33(8):1096–1105, 2013 24091001

El-Gabalawy R, Mackenzie CS, Pietrzak RH, et al: A longitudinal examination of anxiety disorders and physical health conditions in a nationally representative sample of U.S. older adults. Exp Gerontol 60:46–56, 2014 25245888

Flint AJ: Epidemiology and comorbidity of anxiety disorders in the elderly. Am J Psychiatry 151(5):640–649, 1994 8166303

Frydman I, do Brasil PE, Torres AR, et al: Late-onset obsessive-compulsive disorder: risk factors and correlates. J Psychiatr Res 49:68–74, 2014 24267559

Gale CR, Sayer AA, Cooper C, et al: Factors associated with symptoms of anxiety and depression in five cohorts of community-based older people: the HALCyon (Healthy Ageing across the Life Course) Programme. Psychol Med 41(10):2057–2073, 2011 21349224

Gazibara T, Kurtagic I, Kisic-Tepavcevic D, et al: Falls, risk factors and fear of falling among persons older than 65 years of age. Psychogeriatrics 17(4):215–223, 2017 28130862

Gould CE, O'Hara R, Goldstein MK, et al: Multimorbidity is associated with anxiety in older adults in the Health and Retirement Study. Int J Geriatr Psychiatry 31(10):1105–1115, 2016 27441851

Grenier S, Préville M, Boyer R, et al: The impact of DSM-IV symptom and clinical significance criteria on the prevalence estimates of subthreshold and threshold anxiety in the older adult population. Am J Geriatr Psychiatry 19(4):316–326, 2011a 21427640

Grenier S, Schuurmans J, Goldfarb M, et al: The epidemiology of specific phobia and subthreshold fear subtypes in a community-based sample of older adults. Depress Anxiety 28(6):456–463, 2011b 21400642

Grenier S, Potvin O, Hudon C, et al: Twelve-month prevalence and correlates of subthreshold and threshold anxiety in community-dwelling older adults with cardiovascular diseases. J Affect Disord 136(3):724–732, 2012 22055425

Gum AM, King-Kallimanis B, Kohn R: Prevalence of mood, anxiety, and substance-abuse disorders for older Americans in the national comorbidity survey-replication. Am J Geriatr Psychiatry 17(9):769–781, 2009 19700949

Gulseren S, Gulseren L, Hekimsoy Z, et al: Depression, anxiety, health-related quality of life, and disability in patients with overt and subclinical thyroid dysfunction. Arch Med Res 37(1):133–139, 2006 16314199

Hall KS, Beckham JC, Bosworth HB, et al: PTSD is negatively associated with physical performance and physical function in older overweight military Veterans. J Rehabil Res Dev 51(2):285–295, 2014 24933726

Hellwig S, Domschke K: Anxiety in late life: an update on pathomechanisms. Gerontology 65(5):465–473, 2019 31212285

Hesse S, Stengler K, Regenthal R, et al: The serotonin transporter availability in untreated early onset and late-onset patients with obsessive-compulsive disorder. Int J Neuropsychopharmacol 14(5):606–617, 2011 21232166

Hoang OTT, Jullamate P, Piphatvanitcha N, et al: Factors related to fear of falling among community-dwelling older adults. J Clin Nurs 26(1–2):68–76, 2017 27723217

Hohls JK, König HH, Raynik YI, et al: A systematic review of the association of anxiety with health care utilization and costs in people aged 65 years and older. J Affect Disord 232:163–176, 2018 29494900

Hohls JK, König HH, Heider D, et al: Longitudinal association between panic disorder and health care costs in older adults. Depress Anxiety 36(12):1135–1142, 2019a 31609044

Hohls JK, Wild B, Heider D, et al: Association of generalized anxiety symptoms and panic with health care costs in older age—results from the ESTHER cohort study. J Affect Disord 245:978–986, 2019b 30562680

Hohls JK, König HH, van den Bussche H, et al: Association of anxiety symptoms with health care use and costs in people aged 85 and over. Int J Geriatr Psychiatry 34(5):765–776, 2019c 30821399

Holloway KL, Williams LJ, Brennan-Olsen SL, et al: Anxiety disorders and falls among older adults. J Affect Disord 205:20–27, 2016 27391268

Horesh D, Solomon Z, Keinan G, et al: The clinical picture of late-onset PTSD: a 20-year longitudinal study of Israeli war veterans. Psychiatry Res 208(3):265–273, 2013 23294854

Huang CY, Hsu MC, Chen TJ: An exploratory study of religious involvement as a moderator between anxiety, depressive symptoms and quality of life outcomes of older adults. J Clin Nurs 21(5–6):609–619, 2012 21470323

Ivan MC, Amspoker AB, Nadorff MR, et al: Alcohol use, anxiety, and insomnia in older adults with generalized anxiety disorder. Am J Geriatr Psychiatry 22(9):875–883, 2014 23973253

Jayasinghe N, Rocha LP, Sheeran T, et al: Anxiety symptoms in older home health care recipients: prevalence and associates. Home Health Care Serv Q 32(3):163–177, 2013 23937710

Jimenez DE, Alegría M, Chen CN, et al: Prevalence of psychiatric illnesses in older ethnic minority adults. J Am Geriatr Soc 58(2):256–264, 2010 20374401

Kang B, Xu H, McConnell ES: Neurocognitive and psychiatric comorbidities of posttraumatic stress disorder among older veterans: a systematic review. Int J Geriatr Psychiatry 34(4):522–538, 2019 30588665

Karlsson B, Sigström R, Waern M, et al: The prognosis and incidence of social phobia in an elderly population: a 5-year follow-up. Acta Psychiatr Scand 122(1):4–10, 2010 20384601

Karlsson B, Sigström R, Östling S, et al: DSM-IV and DSM-5 prevalence of social anxiety disorder in a population sample of older people. Am J Geriatr Psychiatry 24(12):1237–1245, 2016 27720603

Kessler RC, Chiu WT, Demler O, et al: Prevalence, severity, and comorbidity of 12-month DSM-IV disorders in the National Comorbidity Survey Replication. Arch Gen Psychiatry 62(6):617–627, 2005 15939839

Kessler RC, Petukhova M, Sampson NA, et al: Twelve-month and lifetime prevalence and lifetime morbid risk of anxiety and mood disorders in the United States. Int J Methods Psychiatr Res 21(3):169–184, 2012 22865617

Kim S, So WY: Prevalence and correlates of fear of falling in Korean community-dwelling elderly subjects. Exp Gerontol 48(11):1323–1328, 2013 24001938

Kim T, Kwak S, Hur JW, et al: Neural bases of the clinical and neurocognitive differences between early and late-onset obsessive–compulsive disorder. J Psychiatry Neurosci 45(4):234–242, 2020 31765115

Kocic M, Stojanovic Z, Lazovic M, et al: Relationship between fear of falling and functional status in nursing home residents aged older than 65 years. Geriatr Gerontol Int 17(10):1470–1476, 2017 27576941

Krause N: A preliminary assessment of race differences in the relationship between religious doubt and depressive symptoms. Rev Relig Res 45(2):93–115, 2003

Kroenke K, Spitzer RL, Williams JBW, et al: Anxiety disorders in primary care: prevalence, impairment, comorbidity, and detection. Ann Intern Med 146(5):317–325, 2007 17339617

Kumar A, Carpenter H, Morris R, et al: Which factors are associated with fear of falling in community-dwelling older people? Age Ageing 43(1):76–84, 2014 24100619

Kunik ME, Roundy K, Veazey C, et al: Surprisingly high prevalence of anxiety and depression in chronic breathing disorders. Chest 127(4):1205–1211, 2005 15821196

Kuring JK, Mathias JL, Ward L: Risk of dementia in persons who have previously experienced clinically significant depression, anxiety, or PTSD: a systematic review and meta-analysis. J Affect Disord 274:247–261, 2020 32469813

Kuwert P, Pietrzak RH, Glaesmer H: Trauma and posttraumatic stress disorder in older adults. CMAJ 185(8):685, 2013 23339159

Lee J, Choi M, Kim CO: Falls, a fear of falling and related factors in older adults with complex chronic disease. J Clin Nurs 26(23–24):4964–4972, 2017 28793363

Lenze EJ, Mulsant BH, Mohlman J, et al: Generalized anxiety disorder in late life: lifetime course and comorbidity with major depressive disorder. Am J Geriatr Psychiatry 13(1):77–80, 2005 15653943

Liu H, Tian Y, Liu Y, et al: Relationship between major depressive disorder, generalized anxiety disorder and coronary artery disease in the US general population. J Psychosom Res 119:8–13, 2019 30947822

Mackenzie CS, Reynolds K, Chou KL, et al: Prevalence and correlates of generalized anxiety disorder in a national sample of older adults. Am J Geriatr Psychiatry 19(4):305–315, 2011 21427639

Mackenzie CS, El-Gabalawy R, Chou KL, et al: Prevalence and predictors of persistent versus remitting mood, anxiety, and substance disorders in a national sample of older adults. Am J Geriatr Psychiatry 22(9):854–865, 2014 23800537

Makino K, Makizako H, Doi T, et al: Impact of fear of falling and fall history on disability incidence among older adults: prospective cohort study. Int J Geriatr Psychiatry 33(4):658–662, 2018 29231272

Mantella RC, Butters MA, Amico JA, et al: Salivary cortisol is associated with diagnosis and severity of late-life generalized anxiety disorder. Psychoneuroendocrinology 33(6):773–781, 2008 18407426

Meziab O, Kirby KA, Williams B, et al: Prisoner of war status, posttraumatic stress disorder, and dementia in older veterans. Alzheimers Dement 10(3)(suppl):S236–S241, 2014 24924674

Miloyan B, Pachana NA: Clinical significance of worry and physical symptoms in late-life generalized anxiety disorder. Int J Geriatr Psychiatry 30(12):1186–1194, 2015 25703435

Mohlman J, Bryant C, Lenze EJ, et al: Improving recognition of late life anxiety disorders in Diagnostic and Statistical Manual of Mental Disorders, Fifth Edition: observations and recommendations of the Advisory Committee of the Lifespan Disorders Work Group. Int J Geriatr Psychiatry 27(6):549–556, 2012 21773996

Nepon J, Belik SL, Bolton J, et al: The relationship between anxiety disorders and suicide attempts: findings from the National Epidemiologic Survey on Alcohol and Related Conditions. Depress Anxiety 27(9):791–798, 2010 20217852

Noh HM, Roh YK, Song HJ, et al: Severe fear of falling is associated with cognitive decline in older adults: a 3-year prospective study. J Am Med Dir Assoc 20(12):1540–1547, 2019 31351857

Oh-Park M, Xue X, Holtzer R, et al: Transient versus persistent fear of falling in community-dwelling older adults: incidence and risk factors. J Am Geriatr Soc 59(7):1225–1231, 2011 21718266

Olfson M, Broadhead WE, Weissman MM, et al: Subthreshold psychiatric symptoms in a primary care group practice. Arch Gen Psychiatry 53(10):880–886, 1996 8857864

Osborn AJ, Mathias JL, Fairweather-Schmidt AK, et al: Anxiety and comorbid depression following traumatic brain injury in a community-based sample of young, middle-aged and older adults. J Affect Disord 213:214–221, 2017 27919428

Ostir GV, Goodwin JS: High anxiety is associated with an increased risk of death in an older tri-ethnic population. J Clin Epidemiol 59(5):534–540, 2006 16632143

Patel KV, Phelan EA, Leveille SG, et al: High prevalence of falls, fear of falling, and impaired balance in older adults with pain in the United States: findings from the 2011 National Health and Aging Trends Study. J Am Geriatr Soc 62(10):1844–1852, 2014 25283473

Pérez-Cruz M, Parra-Anguita L, López-Martínez C, et al: Coping and anxiety in caregivers of dependent older adult relatives. Int J Environ Res Public Health 16(9):1651, 2019 31083624

Pietrzak RH, Goldstein RB, Southwick SM, et al: Physical health conditions associated with posttraumatic stress disorder in U.S. older adults: results from wave 2 of the National Epidemiologic Survey on Alcohol and Related Conditions. J Am Geriatr Soc 60(2):296–303, 2012a 22283516

Pietrzak RH, Goldstein RB, Southwick SM, et al: Psychiatric comorbidity of full and partial posttraumatic stress disorder among older adults in the United States: results from wave 2 of the National Epidemiologic Survey on Alcohol and Related Conditions. Am J Geriatr Psychiatry 20(5):380–390, 2012b 22522959

Pietrzak RH, Southwick SM, Tracy M, et al: Posttraumatic stress disorder, depression, and perceived needs for psychological care in older persons affected by Hurricane Ike. J Affect Disord 138(1–2):96–103, 2012c 22285792

Porensky EK, Dew MA, Karp JF, et al: The burden of late-life generalized anxiety disorder: effects on disability, health-related quality of life, and health-care utilization. Am J Geriatr Psychiatry 17(6):473–482, 2009 19472438

Potvin O, Bergua V, Swendsen J, et al: Anxiety and 10-year risk of incident and recurrent depressive symptomatology in older adults. Depress Anxiety 30(6):554–563, 2013 23532935

Prisnie JC, Sajobi TT, Wang M, et al: Effects of depression and anxiety on quality of life in five common neurological disorders. Gen Hosp Psychiatry 52:58–63, 2018 29684713

Qureshi SU, Kimbrell T, Pyne JM, et al: Greater prevalence and incidence of dementia in older veterans with posttraumatic stress disorder. J Am Geriatr Soc 58(9):1627–1633, 2010 20863321

Raposo S, El-Gabalawy R, Erickson J, et al: Associations between anxiety disorders, suicide ideation, and age in nationally representative samples of Canadian and American adults. J Anxiety Disord 28(8):823–829, 2014 25306089

Remes O, Brayne C, van der Linde R, et al: A systematic review of reviews on the prevalence of anxiety disorders in adult populations. Brain Behav 6(7):e00497, 2016 27458547

Reynolds K, Pietrzak RH, El-Gabalawy R, et al: Prevalence of psychiatric disorders in U.S. older adults: findings from a nationally representative survey. World Psychiatry 14(1):74–81, 2015 25655161

Reynolds K, Pietrzak RH, Mackenzie CS, et al: Post-traumatic stress disorder across the adult lifespan: findings from a nationally representative survey. Am J Geriatr Psychiatry 24(1):81–93, 2016 26706912

Rivasi G, Kenny RA, Ungar A, et al: Predictors of fear of falling in community-dwelling older adults. J Am Med Dir Assoc 21(5):615–620, 2020 31610994

Ruscio AM, Stein DJ, Chiu WT, et al: The epidemiology of obsessive-compulsive disorder in the National Comorbidity Survey Replication. Mol Psychiatry 15(1):53–63, 2010 18725912

Sami MB, Nilforooshan R: The natural course of anxiety disorders in the elderly: a systematic review of longitudinal trials. Int Psychogeriatr 27(7):1061–1069, 2015 25192470

Schuitevoerder S, Rosen JW, Twamley EW, et al: A meta-analysis of cognitive functioning in older adults with PTSD. J Anxiety Disord 27(6):550–558, 2013 23422492

Scott Mackin R, Lesselyong JA, Yaffe K: Pattern of cognitive impairment in older veterans with posttraumatic stress disorder evaluated at a memory disorders clinic. Int J Geriatr Psychiatry 27(6):637–642, 2012 22213461

Sheikh JI, Swales PJ, Carlson EB, et al: Aging and panic disorder: phenomenology, comorbidity, and risk factors. Am J Geriatr Psychiatry 12(1):102–109, 2004 14729565

Shrira A, Shmotkin D, Palgi Y, et al: Older adults exposed to ongoing versus intense time-limited missile attacks: differences in symptoms of posttraumatic stress disorder. Psychiatry 80(1):64–78, 2017 28409718

Shrestha S, Stanley MA, Wilson NL, et al: Predictors of change in quality of life in older adults with generalized anxiety disorder. Int Psychogeriatr 27(7):1207–1215, 2015 25497362

Spinhoven P, van der Veen DC, Voshaar RCO, et al: Worry and cognitive control predict course trajectories of anxiety in older adults with late-life depression. Eur Psychiatry 44:134–140, 2017 28641215

Tibi L, van Oppen P, Aderka IM, et al: Examining determinants of early and late age at onset in panic disorder: an admixture analysis. J Psychiatr Res 47(12):1870–1875, 2013 24084228

Tully PJ, Cosh SM, Baune BT: A review of the affects of worry and generalized anxiety disorder upon cardiovascular health and coronary heart disease. Psychol Health Med 18(6):627–644, 2013 23324073

van der Veen DC, van Zelst WH, Schoevers RA, et al: Comorbid anxiety disorders in late-life depression: results of a cohort study. Int Psychogeriatr 27(7):1157–1165, 2015 25370017

Vasiliadis HM, Dionne PA, Préville M, et al: The excess healthcare costs associated with depression and anxiety in elderly living in the community. Am J Geriatr Psychiatry 21(6):536–548, 2013 23567409

Walaszek A: Behavioral and Psychological Symptoms of Dementia. Washington, DC, American Psychiatric Association Publishing, 2019

Wang X, Cui D, Wang Z, et al: Cross-sectional comparison of the clinical characteristics of adults with early onset and late-onset obsessive compulsive disorder. J Affect Disord 136(3):498–504, 2012 22119088

Wetherell JL, Petkus AJ, McChesney K, et al: Older adults are less accurate than younger adults at identifying symptoms of anxiety and depression. J Nerv Ment Dis 197(8):623–626, 2009 19684501

Wetherell JL, Ayers CR, Nuevo R, et al: Medical conditions and depressive, anxiety, and somatic symptoms in older adults with and without generalized anxiety disorder. Aging Ment Health 14(6):764–768, 2010 20635235

Willis KD, Nelson T, Moreno O: Death anxiety, religious doubt, and depressive symptoms across race in older adults. Int J Environ Res Public Health 16(19):3645, 2019 31569371

Wittchen HU, Gloster AT, Beesdo-Baum K, et al: Agoraphobia: a review of the diagnostic classificatory position and criteria. Depress Anxiety 27(2):113–133, 2010 20143426

Wu LT, Blazer DG: Substance use disorders and psychiatric comorbidity in mid and later life: a review. Int J Epidemiol 43(2):304–317, 2014 24163278

Yaffe K, Vittinghoff E, Lindquist K, et al: Posttraumatic stress disorder and risk of dementia among US veterans. Arch Gen Psychiatry 67(6):608–613, 2010 20530010

Yarns BC, Abrams JM, Meeks TW, et al: The mental health of older LGBT adults. Curr Psychiatry Rep 18(6):60, 2016 27142205

Yohannes AM, Baldwin RC, Connolly MJ: Depression and anxiety in elderly outpatients with chronic obstructive pulmonary disease: prevalence, and validation of the BASDEC screening questionnaire. Int J Geriatr Psychiatry 15(12):1090–1096, 2000 11180464

Yohannes AM, Willgoss TG, Baldwin RC, et al: Depression and anxiety in chronic heart failure and chronic obstructive pulmonary disease: prevalence, relevance, clinical implications and management principles. Int J Geriatr Psychiatry 25(12):1209–1221, 2010 20033905

Zhang X, Norton J, Carrière I, et al: Generalized anxiety in community-dwelling elderly: prevalence and clinical characteristics. J Affect Disord 172:24–29, 2015a 25451391

Zhang X, Norton J, Carrière I, et al: Risk factors for late-onset generalized anxiety disorder: results from a 12-year prospective cohort (the ESPRIT study). Transl Psychiatry 5:e536, 2015b 25826111

Zijlstra GAR, van Haastregt JCM, van Eijk JTM, et al: Prevalence and correlates of fear of falling, and associated avoidance of activity in the general population of community-living older people. Age Ageing 36(3):304–309, 2007 17379605

Zisberg A: Anxiety and depression in older patients: the role of culture and acculturation. Int J Equity Health 16(1):177, 2017 28978328

CHAPTER 3

Assessment of Late-Life Depression and Anxiety

Rebecca M. Radue, M.D.

PRÉCIS

Effectively addressing depression and anxiety in older adults begins with a comprehensive assessment. In this chapter, we review medical conditions, medications, and substances that can contribute to or cause depression and anxiety, as well as psychological, cultural, and social considerations. We discuss laboratory testing that may be useful in the assessment of late-life depression and anxiety. We review validated tools to help assess substance use, suicide risk, cognition, depressive and anxiety symptoms, and functional status. We present two frameworks—biopsychosocial-spiritual formulation and the Wisconsin Star Method—by which we may organize comprehensive assessment that will inform treatment planning.

Predisposing, Precipitating, and Perpetuating Factors

MEDICAL CONDITIONS

We begin our discussion of assessing older adults with depression and anxiety by first reviewing other medical conditions that can manifest with symptoms of depression or anxiety. Table 3–1 summarizes the discussion in this subsection.

Medical illness in general is associated with greater risk for and higher prevalence of depressive and anxiety disorders in late life, and there are specific considerations depending on individual comorbid diagnoses. It's also important to consider the stigma faced by older adults within the health care system, especially those perceived as having mental health concerns. Often, what may appear to be symptoms of a psychiatric disorder may instead be symptoms of a general medical condition, or the depressive or anxiety disorder may be due to the older adult's general medical condition (Gleason et al. 2013). Older adults being evaluated for depression or anxiety should have a comprehensive assessment that considers all medical possibilities, as we detail in the section "Laboratory, Imaging, and Other Assessments."

Vascular disease is intimately connected to depression and anxiety. In 1997, Alexopoulos and colleagues first described *vascular depression*, using an MRI study showing cerebrovascular disease correlating phenotypically in a subset of depressed elders (Alexopoulos et al. 1997; Krishnan et al. 1997). This relationship between cerebrovascular disease and depression has been studied in detail over the ensuing decades (e.g., Krishnan et al. 1997; Sneed et al. 2008; Taylor et al. 2013). Vascular depression is thought to be characterized by the presence of small vessel ischemic disease observable on MRI, and older adults who suffer a frank stroke also have a very high risk of developing depressive symptoms, with a prevalence rate around 20% for poststroke depression (Robinson 2003). For a detailed discussion of vascular depression, see Chapter 1, "Introduction to Late-Life Depression," in particular the subsection "Vascular Depression."

This connection between vascular disease and depression extends throughout the body. Myocardial infarction and coronary artery disease are strongly associated with the development of major depressive disorder (MDD): 16%–18% of patients hospitalized after a myocardial infarction will develop major depression, with an additional third of patients experiencing clinically significant depressive symptoms within the following year (Gleason et al. 2013). Cardiac procedures such as catheterization and

Table 3–1. Medical conditions to consider when assessing anxiety or depression in older adults

Medical condition	Symptoms overlapping with anxiety or depressive disorder	Diagnostic clues
Cardiovascular disease		
Anemia	Low energy; poor sleep	Recommended standard laboratory workup; presence of dyspnea on exertion may be a clue that this is not simple depression
Pulmonary embolism	Panic, anxiety	Tachycardia, chest pain with respirations, signs of deep venous thrombosis (usually in the legs)
Heart failure	Low energy; may have anxiety symptoms with decreased oxygenation	History of cardiovascular disease history; history of hypertension or dyspnea; depending on type, may have edema, orthopnea, exertional intolerance, persistent productive cough
Arrhythmia	Anxiety, panic	History of hypertension, cardiovascular disease, or valvular heart disease; presence of abnormal vital signs, palpitations, dyspnea, or exertional symptoms
Neurological disease		
Parkinson's disease	Masked facies (facial appearance of being depressed), psychomotor retardation (bradykinesia)	Other parkinsonian signs—resting tremor, shuffling gait
Subdural hematoma	Any alteration in behavior, ability to concentrate, and cognition and potentially mood depending on location	History of falls; taking an anticoagulation medication; note that older adults may not remember hitting their head

Table 3–1. Medical conditions to consider when assessing anxiety or depression in older adults *(continued)*

Medical condition	Symptoms overlapping with anxiety or depressive disorder	Diagnostic clues
Neurological disease *(continued)*		
Seizures (including temporal lobe epilepsy)	Panic, anxiety	Aura preceding symptoms, unresponsive episodes followed by lethargy or confusion, automatisms
Endocrine disease		
Hypothyroidism	Low energy, depressed mood, psychomotor retardation	Dry skin, cold intolerance, constipation, nonpitting edema, weight gain
Hyperthyroidism or Thyrotoxicosis	Episodic or continuous anxiety, panic	Tremor, heat intolerance, weight loss, palpitations, possibly goiter and dysphagia
Diabetes mellitus (particularly hypoglycemia)	Episodic anxiety, panic	Diaphoresis, tremor, hunger with episodes
Pheochromocytoma	Episodic anxiety and panic	Episodic extreme hypertension
Addison's disease	Low mood, low motivation, low appetite and weight loss; essentially any depressive (and more rarely anxiety) symptom	Hyperpigmentation, hypotension, hypoglycemia, digestive issues
Cushing's disease	Depressive and anxiety symptoms broadly, irritability	"Moon face" and "buffalo hump," abdominal striae and thinning of skin, acne

Table 3–1. Medical conditions to consider when assessing anxiety or depression in older adults *(continued)*

Medical condition	Symptoms overlapping with anxiety or depressive disorder	Diagnostic clues
Metabolic disease		
Hypovitaminosis B_{12} and other B vitamins	Low energy, depressive symptoms	Neuropathy, anemias
Hypercalcemia	Sleep disturbance, fatigue, poor concentration, possibly anxiety	Often due to hyperparathyroidism but can have varied other causes; remember "bones, stones, abdominal groans, and psychic moans"; long-term lithium use can precipitate this
Infectious disease		
Neurosyphilis (general paresis)	Mood changes, behavioral changes, psychosis	Other neuropsychiatric sequelae possible
Lyme disease	Various neuropsychiatric symptoms, including depressive and anxiety symptoms	Location where Lyme is prevalent or travel to such an area, evidence of tick bite or subsequent rash, myalgia and migratory joint pain and swelling
HIV	Various neuropsychiatric symptoms, with depressive symptoms being most common	Recurrent infection and signs of immunodeficiency
COVID-19	Delirium; may be complicated by depression, anxiety or PTSD	Sudden onset of mental status changes, especially in an older adult living in a nursing home or assisted living facility

Table 3–1. Medical conditions to consider when assessing anxiety or depression in older adults (continued)

Medical condition	Symptoms overlapping with anxiety or depressive disorder	Diagnostic clues
Genetic disease		
MTHFR deficiency	Depressive symptoms, possibly anxiety symptoms	Elevated serum homocysteine levels
CADASIL	Depressive symptoms, cognitive impairment	Other signs of cerebrovascular disease and stroke, focal neurological signs
Neoplastic disease		
Malignancy	Low appetite and weight loss, low energy; may have depressed mood	Signs more specific to the type of cancer; localizing pain, skin changes, changes in bowel or bladder function, unusual lumps or bumps
Sleep and respiratory disease		
Sleep apnea (obstructive most common, but also central, mixed)	Depressive or anxiety symptoms broadly but especially sleep disturbance and low energy or nighttime panic (associated with apnea/hypopnea and subsequent hyperarousal leading to awakening)	Positive STOP-BANG screen for OSA (Nagappa et al. 2015); see text for discussion
Lung disease (COPD, asthma, others)	Anxiety, panic, or conversely depressive symptoms of low energy especially	History of tobacco use or occupational exposures; dyspnea, wheezing, cough

Note. CADASIL = cerebral autosomal dominant arteriopathy with subcortical infarcts and leukoencephalopathy; COPD = chronic obstructive pulmonary disease; COVID-19 = coronavirus SARS-CoV-2 disease; MTHFR = methyltetrahydrofolate reductase; OSA = obstructive sleep apnea.

cardiac surgery such as coronary artery bypass grafting are in and of themselves associated with an increased risk for subsequent development of depression (Carney and Freedland 2003). Depression and vascular disease can coexist, but it is important to not miss that a cardiovascular condition can mimic symptoms of depression or anxiety. For example, patients with heart failure of all types might present with fatigue, low energy, poor appetite, and other symptoms of depression. A cardiac arrhythmia, valvular heart disease, or pulmonary embolism can mimic anxiety symptoms.

In addition to stroke, other neurological diseases are highly associated with depression and anxiety. For example, in Parkinson's disease, more than 50% of patients will experience clinically significant depression (Reijnders et al. 2008), and more than 30% will experience clinically significant anxiety (Dissanayaka et al. 2014). Up to 50% of patients with multiple sclerosis will experience depression (Patten et al. 2017). Epilepsy is of special concern as well, with a systematic review and meta-analysis reporting a 23.1% prevalence and 2.77 odds ratio of active depression in persons with epilepsy compared with those without epilepsy (Fiest et al. 2013). Other studies suggest that anxiety disorders are highly prevalent as well, present in more than 15% of people with epilepsy, with panic disorder being the most common (Wiglusz et al. 2018). Patients with seizures (e.g., as seen in temporal lobe epilepsy) can also present with psychiatric symptoms (Bessey et al. 2018). Traumatic brain injury is also a risk factor for development of anxiety and depressive disorders (Vaishnavi et al. 2009).

We point out these facts in the assessment chapter because clinicians evaluating an older adult for a depressive disorder should not miss neurological comorbidities, including Parkinson's disease. For example, the book's editor, a geriatric psychiatrist, was able to diagnose Parkinson's disease in an older adult referred for depression who denied depressive symptoms but whose family insisted that the patient looked terribly depressed (because of the masked facies of parkinsonism). As a geriatric and general psychiatrist working with veterans, I also want to point out the importance of screening for lifetime traumatic brain injury. In addition, clinicians should screen for falls when evaluating an older adult. Falls, as we know, are common in older adults (as is fear of falling), and such symptoms as decreased energy, trouble concentrating, and poor sleep could conceivably be due to a subdural hematoma from one or more falls with head injury. Older adults may not present for an emergency department evaluation after such a fall; they may not even recall hitting their head or may think nothing of it.

Endocrine disorders are also associated with depression and anxiety and may mimic depressive or anxiety disorders. Thyroid disease, including both hypothyroidism and hyperthyroidism, has a well-established connection with psychiatric illness (Bunevicius and Prange 2010). Diabetes mellitus and states of hyperglycemia and hypoglycemia have also been associated with an increased risk for depressive and anxiety disorders, and hypoglycemic patients in particular can present with anxiety symptoms (Blazer et al. 2002). Hyperparathyroidism and hypercalcemia are also linked to psychiatric illness; the old adage "bones, stones, abdominal groans, and psychic moans" can help clinicians remember the symptoms of hypercalcemia. Hyperparathyroidism may result from long-term lithium treatment (Parks et al. 2017). Pheochromocytoma is a "zebra" that can certainly manifest along with panic symptoms and is crucial not to miss (Alguire et al. 2018). Addison's disease and Cushing's disease may also go undetected and should remain on the differential diagnosis for depression and anxiety. Fortunately, both of these diseases have fairly clear physical manifestations that should clue in the clinician to their presence (Anglin et al. 2006; Rasmussen et al. 2015).

Although diseases and syndromes due to genetic mutation typically manifest earlier in life, there are two important considerations for the older population. Hyperhomocysteinemia can arise in a variety of ways and has been linked to cognitive impairment and other neuropsychiatric sequelae. In older adults, this usually occurs because of a deficiency of vitamin B_6 (pyridoxine), B_9 (folate), or B_{12} (cyanocobalamin); however, it is conceivable that an older adult has a milder inborn error of metabolism that leads to gradual accumulation of homocysteine such that consequent disease might not manifest or might not be detected until later life (Folstein et al. 2007). One such error that is becoming more a focus of study and treatment is a polymorphism resulting in decreased function of methyltetrahydrofolate reductase (MTHFR). Emerging data indicate that mutations in MTHFR and related genes along this folate metabolism pathway are implicated in depressive and other psychiatric disorders and may be a focus of assessment and treatment, including in older adults (Wan et al. 2018). We discuss the utility of genomic testing in treatment-resistant depression in Chapter 5, "Management of Late-Life Depression and Anxiety," subsection "Efficacy of Antidepressants."

Another genetic disease to consider in late-life depression is cerebral autosomal dominant arteriopathy with subcortical infarcts and leukoencephalopathy (CADASIL). Patients with this condition present with progressive cerebrovascular disease, strokes, and resultant vascular dementia, but they often present with depression along the disease course, or even as a first symptom, with 6% presenting first with depression in one study (Taylor and Doody 2008). Psychiatric symptoms are estimated to be present in up to 30% of these patients. Although the illness typically has onset in midlife, some patients do not have onset until after age 60 (Park et al. 2017; Taylor and Doody 2008).

Depression and anxiety are also strongly connected with cancer, with high rates of depression and anxiety among those living with cancer (Cordella and Poiani 2014). A diagnosis of cancer and the stress of treatment can certainly precipitate depression or anxiety in an older adult. The first symptoms of malignancy might also be psychiatric, or symptoms such as weight loss, poor appetite, and fatigue might be misattributed to psychiatric illness.

Sleep and respiratory disorders are also associated with depressive and anxiety disorders and symptoms. The most pertinent sleep disorder for the older population is sleep apnea, most specifically the obstructive type, although central and mixed apneas should also be considered. Treating sleep apnea can lead to remission of concurrent depressive or anxiety symptoms in many cases. Chronic obstructive pulmonary disease (COPD) and other lung diseases can also lead to and overlap with depressive and anxiety disorders (Economou et al. 2018). It should also be noted that presence of obstructive sleep apnea (OSA), even when treated with continuous positive airway pressure, may predict worse response to antidepressant treatment for late-life depression (Waterman et al. 2016). We recommend using the STOP-BANG questionnaire to screen for OSA: **S**noring (yes/no), **T**iredness (yes/no), **O**bserved apnea (yes/no), high blood **P**ressure (yes/no), **B**MI >35, **A**ge >50, **N**eck circumference >40 cm, and male **G**ender. Presence of three or more positives is 90%–96% sensitive for detecting OSA (Nagappa et al. 2015).

Infectious disease should also be considered when evaluating the depressed or anxious older adult. Although neurosyphilis more commonly manifests in neurocognitive sequelae and psychosis, it is possible for affected patients to present with mood disturbance or anxious distress (Gatchel et al. 2015; Bharwani and Hershey 1998). There is also evidence linking untreated Lyme disease with neuropsychiatric symptoms, including anxiety and depressive symptoms (Gerstenblith and Stern 2014). HIV infection is also associated with high rates of depressive illness across age groups, and HIV-positive patients can present with other neuropsychiatric symptoms (Nanni et al. 2015).

Assessment for these potential conditions is covered in greater detail in the subsection "Laboratory, Imaging, and Other Assessment."

ALCOHOL, OTHER SUBSTANCES, AND MEDICATIONS

The contributions of substances and medications should be considered in the assessment of the anxious or depressed older adult. Substance use disorders are often overlooked in older adults. Alcohol is the most common substance of abuse and the most prevalent substance use disorder in this population, but as their patient's age increases, clinicians become less likely to discuss alcohol use (Duru et al. 2010). Substance use disorders, including alcohol use disorder, in older adults may carry over from younger years, or it may develop later in life. High-risk drinking continues to increase among older adults in the United States, with men at greater risk than women for harmful consumption, but with rates of heavy drinking increasing faster in women than in men (Breslow et al. 2017). Comorbid substance use disorders, especially alcohol use disorder, are risk factors and possible causes of depression or anxiety, and they also point to a poorer prognosis for meaningful remission and recovery from depression or anxiety (Barry and Blow 2016; Le Roux et al. 2016). The good news that makes it all the more important to diagnose substance use disorders in older adults is that older patients are just as likely to benefit from treatment as younger adults, if not even more so (Yarnell et al. 2020). Therefore, these are "do not miss" diagnoses.

Substance use is especially concerning in older adults in part because of physiological differences in metabolism of substances, which leads to increased adverse effects at lower equivalent doses than for younger adults. Even when there is no substantial evidence of frank decreased metabolism (as with alcohol), the consequences of substance use disorders have been demonstrated to be more severe for older adults than for their younger counterparts. Older adults also have greater burden of comorbid health conditions and medications with which substances can interact and interfere (Lehmann and Fingerhood 2018).

Table 3–2 outlines the various validated instruments that can be used to aid in assessment of substance use disorders in older adults, with a focus on alcohol. All of these instruments are in the public domain, and none requires a fee for use. We do not recommend using the CAGE or CAGE-AID in older adults because the questions in these tools are less likely to apply to older adults.

We should not ignore other substances, however. In one study of older adults in Florida, prescription drug misuse was more prevalent than alcohol abuse (Schonfeld et al. 2010). This population is certainly not immune to the opioid epidemic, and opioid use disorder is also of significant concern in older adults. In fact, one study of nationwide Medicaid data in the United States showed that the largest population undergoing methadone maintenance treatment was individuals ages 50–59 years—our soon-to-be older adults (Cotton et al. 2018). Cannabis use is also growing in older adults and should be considered when assessing for psychiatric illness in this population, although certainly the evidence tying use of cannabis to depression or anxiety is not as robust as that for alcohol, opioids, and other substances (Levy et al. 2020).

Table 3–2. Instruments for assessing substance use in older adults

Instrument	Substances covered	Description	Use in older adults	Our recommendation
AUDIT and AUDIT-C	Alcohol	AUDIT-C asks three questions: How often the patient drinks, how many drinks he or she has on a typical day, and how often he or she has had six or more drinks on one occasion in the past year. It is scored on a 12-point scale.	A score of 3 or more is considered positive, with 7 or more being highly sensitive for AUD in older adults (Dawson et al. 2005; Towers et al. 2011).	We like the AUDIT-C but find that the question of six drinks or more is less applicable to older adults.
MAST-G and SMAST-G	Alcohol	SMAST-G consists of 10 yes or no questions, scored as +1 for "yes" responses and 0 for "no" responses. A cutoff of 2 or more warrants further investigation.	The MAST-G has a sensitivity of 0.94 and specificity of 0.78, with a cutoff of 5+ (Blow et al. 1992).	This is our favorite, given that it's well validated in older adult populations and is easy to administer and understand.
SDS	Any substance	SDS asks five questions: Does the patient think his or her use is out of control? Does the thought of missing use make the patient anxious or worried? Does the patient worry about use of the drug? Does the patient wish to stop use? How difficult would it be for the patient to stop? Items are rated on a 0–3 scale.	SDS has been validated in a sample of 246 older adults, with optimal cut-off of 6+, sensitivity 0.76, and specificity 0.86 (Cheng et al. 2019).	We like this tool as well and find it's the best tool for older adults to screen for more than just alcohol use.

Note. AUDIT=Alcohol Use Disorders Identification Test; AUDIT-C=Alcohol Use Disorders Identification Test-Concise; MAST-G=Michigan Alcohol Screening Test—Geriatric Version; SMAST-G=Short Michigan Alcohol Screening Test—Geriatric Version; SDS=Severity of Dependence Scale.

Older adults are at the greatest risk of prescription drug interactions; adverse effects; and prescription drug misuse, which may be intentional or unintentional. Almost any prescription medication can be misused. This includes nonadherence, taking more or less than prescribed, sharing with others, obtaining the drug from a nonmedical source, taking the drug for psychoactive effects, or using the drug in combination with substances of abuse for desired effects other than those that are intended. Older adults are also especially at risk of exploitation for their prescribed substances—for example, a caregiver, relative, or friend may abuse the older adult's prescribed opioids.

Many prescription medications can precipitate anxiety, depression, or other psychiatric symptoms. These medications are listed (not exhaustively) in Table 3–3 (Alexopoulos 2005; Grossberg et al. 2017; Kotlyar et al. 2005).

PSYCHOLOGICAL, PSYCHOSOCIAL, AND PERSONALITY FACTORS

Personality Traits and Disorders

Personality traits and disorders are important considerations in late-life depression and anxiety, and there are a number of studies examining their connections to late-life disorders. Higher extroversion as a personality trait correlates with improved prognosis for recovery from a depressive episode (Hayward et al. 2013). Neuroticism, described by Aziz and Steffens (2013, p. 10) as "an enduring tendency to experience negative emotional states," is associated with poor distress tolerance, hopelessness, increased risk of developing depressive and anxiety disorders (including in late-life), and poorer treatment outcomes (Aziz and Steffens 2013; Davison et al. 2012; Hayward et al. 2013; Steffens et al. 2013; Steunenberg et al. 2006). High levels of neuroticism and low self-rated mastery have also been linked to greater risk of relapse of depression for older adults (Steunenberg et al. 2010). Having high levels of obsessional personality traits is also linked with increased risk for late-life depression and anxiety, worse treatment outcomes, and higher risk of suicide (Aziz and Steffens 2013). The personality trait of external locus of control predicts development and persistence of depression and anxiety disorders (Beekman et al. 2001). Frank diagnosable personality disorders also have been linked to worse outcomes overall, greater likelihood of development of an anxiety or depressive disorder, and greater likelihood of chronicity or recurrence of anxiety or depression (Abrams and Bromberg 2006; Morse and Lynch 2004).

Table 3–3. Medications and substances that may contribute to depression and anxiety in older adults

Medication/ substance	Clinical indication	Psychiatric side effect(s)
ACE inhibitors	Hypertension	Depressive symptoms
Benzodiazepines	Anxiety, alcohol withdrawal treatment, muscle spasm	Depressive symptoms, sedation
Calcium channel blockers	Hypertension	Depressive symptoms
Carbidopa/levodopa and other anti-parkinsonian agents	Parkinson's disease, tremor, restless leg syndrome, EPSE from antipsychotics	Insomnia, depressive symptoms, anxiety symptoms, agitation, mania, psychosis
Cimetidine and other H_2 antihistamines	Gastroesophageal reflux disease, peptic ulcer disease	Altered mental status, depressive symptoms
Clonidine	Hypertension, tic disorder	Depressive symptoms
Estrogens	Vulvar or vaginal atrophy in menopause, menopausal vasomotor symptoms	Depressive symptoms
Hydralazine	Hypertension, hypertensive crisis, congestive heart failure	Psychosis, anxiety, and depressive symptoms
Interferon alpha	Cancer, condyloma acuminata, hepatitis C and B	Depressive symptoms including suicidal ideation, anxiety
Methyldopa	Hypertension	Depressive symptoms
Opioids	Pain	Depressive symptoms
Progesterone	Menopausal vasomotor symptoms	Depressive symptoms
Propranolol and other β-blockers	Hypertension, congestive heart failure and cardiovascular disease, tremor, anxiety	Depressive symptoms
Reserpine	Hypertension, tardive dyskinesia	Depressive symptoms

Table 3–3. Medications and substances that may contribute to depression and anxiety in older adults *(continued)*

Medication/ substance	Clinical indication	Psychiatric side effect(s)
Steroids (systemic glucocorticoids)	Asthma, COPD exacerbation, systemic inflammatory response, rheumatological conditions, autoimmune conditions	Insomnia, depressive symptoms, mood lability, mania, psychosis, anxiety symptoms including panic
Tamoxifen	Breast cancer	Depressive symptoms
VMAT-2 inhibitors	Tardive dyskinesia	Depressive symptoms

Note. ACE=angiotensin-converting enzyme; COPD=chronic obstructive pulmonary disease; EPSE=extrapyramidal side effects; H_2=histamine-2 receptor; VMAT-2=vesicular monoamine transporter type 2.

The best way to assess for personality traits and diagnosable personality disorders remains the psychiatric diagnostic interview. In older adults this must be coupled with historical and collateral information, given the enduring nature of these traits and patterns. Structured clinical interviews and general personality inventories can aid in better understanding of these traits, but in general, diagnosis and understanding take time. For the purposes of this book, we do not focus on the nuances and use of particular tools.

We do want to be sure to point out that it is also crucial to consider the role of acquired illness in changing overall personality by coarsening or dampening various traits and aspects. For example, someone who has an underlying tendency to be more rigid but was historically able to compensate and is generally able to be flexible may experience an intensifying of his or her rigidity due to acquired medical illness in later life. This newly acquired pathological rigidity does not qualify for a personality disorder, which must be present across the life span—rather, the DSM-5 diagnosis of personality change due to another medical condition is most appropriate to describe these cases (American Psychiatric Association 2013). Neurocognitive disorders are the best example of late-life medical illness leading to personality change, especially frontotemporal dementia; stroke and traumatic brain injury also commonly have this effect in later life (Oxman 2015).

Trauma

When we speak of trauma and traumatic events, we are talking about events that meet criterion A for posttraumatic stress disorder (PTSD) per DSM-5, which requires that the person have experienced actual or threatened death, serious injury, or sexual violence through direct experience or direct witnessing of the event, by learning of an event occurring to a close loved one, or by experiencing repeated or extreme exposure to such events (as would a first responder or someone in a similar role). (For the DSM-5 criteria for PTSD, see Box 2–4 in Chapter 2, "Introduction to Late-Life Anxiety and Related Disorders.") In a study using surveys of adults in 24 countries spanning all continents save Antarctica, more than 70% reported exposure to at least one such event in their lifetimes. Thus, trauma is nearly ubiquitous, although older adults surveyed were more likely to report experience of collective trauma such as war or natural disasters rather than interpersonal violence such as muggings, accidental injury or death, or sexual violence (Benjet et al. 2016). Older adults are less likely to meet full criteria for PTSD but may still have significant symptoms that can affect their quality of life (Cook and Simiola 2018).

Symptoms of anxiety and depressive disorders can certainly overlap with PTSD. Criterion D for PTSD specifically discusses negative mood and cognitive symptoms, and the hyperarousal associated with PTSD can be confused with somatic anxiety symptoms. Trauma- and stressor-related disorders are another "do not miss" diagnostic category that should be on the differential when assessing older adults for anxiety or depression. Clinicians must screen for criterion A traumatic events with gentle care so as not to trigger worsening of trauma symptoms without having the time or focus of the session to address them. While keeping in mind that these topics are sensitive, it is also important to ask with comfort and confidence so as not to trigger stigma responses. For my patients of any age, I always preface such questions with an explanation of why I am asking about these difficult experiences:

> It's important to me as a psychiatrist to understand whether my patients have experienced traumatic events in their lives, but I want to do so without delving into potentially triggering details in this first session. May I ask if you've experienced a traumatic event in your lifetime, such as being seriously injured, assaulted, or abused emotionally, physically, or sexually, or witnessing or hearing of the violent death or injury of a loved one?

Find a standard phrasing that works best for you, and try to ask every time you are first assessing someone.

Grief, Loss, and Bereavement

The longer we live, the more loss we accumulate. Bereavement in later life is most commonly thought of as the loss of loved ones through death. The loss of a spouse is one such grief that has been better studied in older adults. That said, there are other losses to grieve in later life, and losses include difficult transitions that older adults may experience such as loss of functionality or independence or having to move from independent living to varying levels of long-term care. Additionally, the loss of the sense of smell (often studied as a harbinger of neurological illness, although not so much in terms of how it can affect quality of life) may be significant. If career or employment was an important part of the person's earlier life, the transition to retirement via either choice or necessity also brings with it grief and loss. We should consider all potential losses when evaluating elders for depression or anxiety. It is important to consider that every loss, including the loss of spouse or other loved one, is unique to the individual: Was the loss sudden or unexpected? Or was the loss anticipated for months or years of a long illness, such that some of the grieving was done before the death? Is there a (generally healthy) sense of relief, perhaps that the loved one is no longer suffering or that heavy caregiving duties are at an end? There is no calculator that can predict how an elder will process individual losses (Bruce 2002).

We recommend taking a meaning-centered approach to exploring grief and loss with older adult patients, including as it may relate to depression and anxiety in late life. Asking our patients what a loss means to them may yield helpful information, but I often find that this is too vague, and elders with depressive disorders may find it especially difficult to answer such a broad question. Often, a general sense of the meaning of the loss to the patient emerges out of asking for more details about how the loss has affected him or her.

A discussion of distinguishing grief from MDD and a discussion of complicated grief, a severe form of acute grief that lasts longer than expected and results in functional impairment, can be found in Chapter 1, subsection "Depression and Grief" and Table 1–2.

Social Support

It is critical to assess social support of elders with anxiety or depression. It is a complex factor and includes the elder's perception of his or her social support as well as more objective measures and aspects. The negative impacts of social isolation have been well demonstrated in older adults, and they have been associated with depressive and anxiety symptoms. Low perceived social support also predicts poorer prognosis for older adults with depression (Blazer 2005; Bruce 2002). The most important aspect to assess for in our elders is their perception of their levels of social support. As we discuss the difficulties of their presenting problem, I will often ask my older patients, "Who do you have to support you in all this?" or "Who do you have in your life for support?" If an older adult appears to have strong support from, for example, adult children or neighbors, a response of "No one" or "I don't have anyone to support me" will give you important information about the patient's perception of his or her support. In situations such as this one in which older adult patients lack insight or their perceptions are colored by their depression, you may need to obtain collateral information about the details of supports available to them.

Socioeconomic Status and Financial Stressors

Lower socioeconomic status and lower household income are associated with increased risk for late-life depression around the world (Barua et al. 2010; Glaesmer et al. 2011). It should come as no surprise that older adults facing financial stressors are at greater risk for both anxiety and depressive disorders. Indeed, the Geriatric Anxiety Scale measures anxiety specifically related to finances, recognizing the importance of financial considerations for older adults (Segal et al. 2010). In the United States, 23% of older adults living in two-elder households and half of older adults living alone lack the financial resources to meet their basic needs (Mutchler et al. 2019). Therefore, we recommend that the social history portion of any evaluation of an older adult with depression or anxiety include questions about financial stressors.

Educational Attainment and Health Literacy

Social determinants of health are intricately interwoven. By examining one aspect of an older adult's history as it relates to health, we may be capturing the effects of many upstream and downstream factors. One area where this applies is in educational background and health literacy. Childhood experiences and opportunities afforded when older adults were young and receiving their primary, secondary, and potential postsecondary educations were influenced by a variety of factors, including potential structural racism and socioeconomic inequalities. Studies looking at health and health outcomes, including those focused on older adults, have measured how these factors relate to educational attainment and health literacy. Lower educational attainment has been linked with increased risk of late-life depression (Abrams and Mehta 2019). We recommend that a full social history taken at time of assessment for late-life depression or anxiety include educational attainment and occupational history.

Health literacy reflects the ability to process and understand health information to make informed decisions for care. It can be helpful to understand your older adult patient's level of health literacy because studies have demonstrated that targeting interventions to the patient's health literacy level leads to better outcomes (Schapira et al. 2017). A variety of tools have been designed to measure health literacy, including some in languages other than English. We recommend using the Rapid Estimate of Adult Literacy in Medicine—Short Form (REALM-SF), which has been studied across health care settings (Arozullah et al. 2007). The REALM-SF consists of a list of seven medical terms (behavior, exercise, menopause, rectal, antibiotics, anemia, jaundice) and directs the administrator to request that the patient read each word. If the word is mispronounced or if the patient takes more than 5 seconds to say the word, no point is given. The score is equal to the number of words read correctly, and a corresponding level is assigned, with suggested written materials that may be most helpful to a patient at that level: 0, third grade and below; 1–3, fourth to sixth grade; 4–6, seventh to eighth grade; 7, high school. The U.S. National Library of Medicine, in collaboration with Boston University, funds a Health Literacy Tool Shed (for a link, see "Resources for Clinicians" at the end of this chapter).

CULTURAL AND SPIRITUAL FACTORS

Although cultural and spiritual factors are covered in greater detail in Chapter 6, "Comprehensive Cultural Assessment of the Older Adult With Depression and Anxiety," we wish to briefly address the implications for assessment here. A tool such as the DSM-5 Cultural Formulation Interview, also discussed in Chapter 6, can help the clinician better understand the role of culture in an elder with depression.

Gender and Sexual Identity

Here we briefly discuss gender and sexual identity along spectra and how these identities relate to late-life anxiety and depression. When we discuss gender and sexual identity diversity, we are generally talking about older adult members of the LGBTQ+ (lesbian, gay, bisexual, transgender, and queer, with the plus representing additional identities such as intersex, nonbinary, and asexual) community, of which there are approximately one million in the United States (Yarns et al. 2016). According to the Williams Institute (2019), 7% of adults older than age 65 in the United States identify as LGBTQ+.We do want to touch broadly on how depression and anxiety may affect LGBTQ+ older adult men and women differently from heterosexual cisgender (identifying as the gender assigned at birth) elders and the differences in how LGBTQ+ patients present with these symptoms. These areas are important to consider and to ask our patients about for many reasons, including differences in risk and prevalence of mental health concerns among older adults identifying as LGBTQ+. These identities can be particularly relevant when considering our elder patients and their care from culturally informed and meaning-centered perspectives.

Recognizing that traditional research has been conducted in a gender binary, it has been well established that women have demonstrated higher rates of depression and anxiety throughout the life span, including in older age (Abrams and Mehta 2019). Likewise, LGBTQ+ elders are more likely than heterosexual cisgender elders to experience anxiety and depressive disorders in later life (Fredriksen-Goldsen et al. 2011). In spite of significant recent advances in codifying into law the inherent human rights of the LGBTQ+ community, our LGBTQ+ elders have lived the vast majority of their lives under oppression, discrimination, and threat of violence and death. In spite of advances, these threats continue to some extent into the present day. Living under this type of minority stress contributes to the greater rates of mental illness in this population, and to have survived all these years under oppression demonstrates resilience (Yarns et al. 2016).

One phenomenon that's important to mention is that of older adults facing a move to long-term care and finding themselves having to go "back into the closet" to avoid discrimination. Sometimes, discriminatory long-term care facilities are the only options available in the elder's area, and even if a facility bills itself as LGBTQ+ accepting or even affirming, not all staff may uphold those values. Older LGBTQ+ adults facing a move into long-term care are especially vulnerable (Johnson et al. 2005).

It's important to not assume that all older adults are cisgender and heterosexual unless they tell you otherwise. You should ask your older patients respectfully about their sexual and gender identities and about their experiences with and fears about discrimination. Further details on the mental health of LGBTQ+ older adults are covered in Chapter 6.

Race, Ethnicity, and Migration

As mentioned earlier, socioeconomic status, opportunity, and psychosocial stressors are unequally distributed across the older adult population worldwide on the basis of race and ethnicity (Abrams and Mehta 2019). The degree of inequalities differs by country; for the purposes of this book, we focus on the United States. This inequality is due in part to the effects of racism, which centers whiteness, in all its forms: structural, institutional, historical, cultural, and interpersonal. Migration, and status as an immigrant, is also of consideration here. The stress of being Black, indigenous, or a person of color, or to present as anything other than white in the United States, is a key part of what leads to adverse health outcomes for these populations. Racism is indeed a public health crisis. Details of how mental health and race and ethnicity interact are reviewed in Chapter 1 and discussed further in Chapter 6, but in general, Black Americans may experience higher rates of depression (Barry et al. 2014). Therefore, it is important to consider race and ethnicity and immigrant status as they pertain to personal experience and stress, and these things should be explored with elders who are presenting for evaluation of anxiety and depression.

Religion and Spirituality

Religion and spirituality are covered in more detail in Chapter 6, but here we would like to discuss assessment of religious and spiritual practices and beliefs among older adults as they relate to depression and anxiety. In general, higher levels of spirituality and religiosity are associated with decreased prevalence of anxiety and depression. In a cross-sectional study of Brazilian adults, Vitorino et al. (2018) measured levels of spirituality and religiosity among older adults and divided them into four groups on the basis of their level of spirituality (high or low) and their level of religiosity (high or low). They then compared these groups in terms of quality of life, depressive symptoms, anxiety, optimism, and happiness. Elders in the high spirituality and high religiosity group fared the best in all factors; those in the low spirituality and high religiosity group had the next best ratings, followed by the high spirituality and low religiosity group. The low spirituality and low religiosity group had the lowest ratings.

Asking our older adult patients about religious and spiritual beliefs is an important part of a comprehensive assessment and should be considered an essential aspect of the assessment of elders with late-life depression or anxiety. For example, the FICA Spiritual History Tool (Borneman et al. 2010) was developed to allow clinicians to incorporate open-ended questions into obtaining a history:

- Faith: Do you consider yourself spiritual or religious? Do you have spiritual beliefs that help you cope with stress? What gives your life meaning?

- Importance and influence: What importance does your faith or belief have in your life? On a scale of 0 (not important) to 5 (very important), how would you rate the importance of faith or belief in your life? Have your beliefs influenced you in how you handle stress? What role do your beliefs play in your health care decision-making?
- Community: Are you part of a spiritual or religious community? Is this of support to you, and how? Is there a group of people you really love or who are important to you?
- Address in care: How would you like your health care provider to use this information about your spirituality as he or she cares for you?

ORGANIZATIONAL FRAMEWORKS FOR A COMPREHENSIVE ASSESSMENT

How do we capture, summarize, and convey all aspects of our comprehensive assessment of the older adult presenting with depression or anxiety? Here we discuss some helpful frameworks to guide clinicians.

The *biopsychosocial model* was first proposed by psychiatrist George Engel at the University of Rochester in the 1970s (Engel 1977). It ushered in a new wave of holistic medicine—treating patients as whole, complex people, considering biological, psychological, and social aspects—rather than the previous reductionism of the purely biomedical model. The biopsychosocial model has its critics (Ghaemi 2009), but it remains a worthwhile way to conscientiously approach the assessment of our patients (Tripathi et al. 2019). Other researchers have advocated for adopting an additional spiritual dimension, such that we consider biopsychosocial-spiritual factors for our patients (Sulmasy 2002). Table 3–4 presents considerations that may come into play in evaluating an anxious or depressed elder using this framework.

Another potential framework to use is the Wisconsin Star Method. Developed by Timothy Howell, a geriatric psychiatrist at the University of Wisconsin, as a method for approaching complex problems in geriatrics, this method employs a comprehensive, meaning-centered approach to mapping out these complex problems. The person and his or her medical problem (in this case, late-life anxiety or depression) goes at the center of the star, and the arms represent 1) medical factors, 2) medications, 3) behavioral factors, 4) personal factors, and 5) social factors. These factors are mapped out around the star to demonstrate their complex interplay and to allow for an organized assessment and development of recommendations for further diagnosis and treatment. The Wisconsin

Table 3–4.　The biopsychosocial-spiritual framework

	Historical factors	Current factors	Treatment implications
Biological factors	• Genetics • Previous illness from recent times back to childhood • Biological development	• Current illness • Current medications • Current substance use • Physical examination, including mental status examination	• Laboratory studies • Diagnostic imaging • Biological treatments, including medications and therapies such as bright light, electroconvulsive therapy, and transcranial magnetic stimulation
Psychological factors	• Trauma • Grief and loss • Relationships • Psychological development	• Psychological stressors • Personality traits, structure, and disorder(s) • Coping skills, defenses, and cognitive distortions • Psychological impact of illness	• Psychological testing and diagnostics • Psychotherapy
Social factors	• Social development • Educational attainment and occupational history • Socioeconomic status and developmental hardships	• Support system and relationships • Occupation, roles, and stressors • Cultural identities	• Referrals to community programs and case management • Social engagement, healthy diet and exercise, relationship building, and hobbies

Table 3–4. The biopsychosocial-spiritual framework (*continued*)

	Historical factors	Current factors	Treatment implications
Spiritual factors	• Historical role of spirituality and religion in life, including specific behaviors (e.g., prayer)	• Current spiritual and religious identities, affiliations, beliefs, behaviors, religious support (resources of the religious community), and religious coping	• Explore whether and how the patient would like possible modalities involved in treatment (e.g., mindfulness practice, which may be purely psychological for some but often has spiritual elements)

Note. A clinician may organize the information obtained when assessing an older adult with depression or anxiety using a biopsychosocial-spiritual framework. See text for additional details.

Star can be especially helpful for team-based discussions of diagnostically challenging situations. Figure 3–1 illustrates this method (Howell 2015).

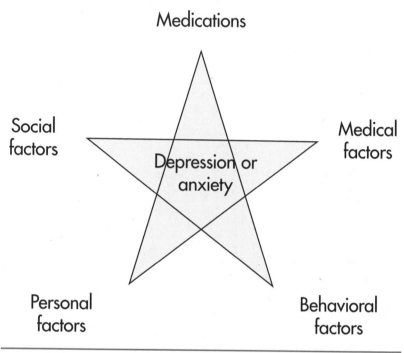

Figure 3–1.   Wisconsin Star Method.

See text for a description and the case example for an illustration of using the Wisconsin Star Method. The Madison Veterans Administration Hospital, the University of Wisconsin School of Medicine and Public Health, the Division of Mental Health and Substance Abuse Services of the Wisconsin Department of Health Services, NAMI Wisconsin, and members of the Wisconsin Geriatric Psychiatry Initiative provided in-kind support for the development of the Wisconsin Star Method.

In the following case, we apply each of these frameworks to help organize the assessment of an older adult with depression and anxiety.

CASE EXAMPLE: "WHY WON'T SHE ACCEPT HELP WE'RE TRYING TO GIVE HER?"

Ms. Miller is a 73-year-old divorced woman who had intermittently experienced depression and anxiety over the course of her life, but nothing as bad as the previous year. She has not been taking care of herself, resulting in alarmed phone calls from neighbors, including one to the local adult protective services agency, which assigned a social worker to her case. Ms. Miller, however, has refused all entreaties. Her depression and anxiety have worsened, and self-care has declined. She now presents for her sixth primary care visit in as many months, this time for a follow-up of a recent emergency department evaluation.

Ms. Miller's history was compiled over several visits with primary care clinicians and social workers. She initially developed depression and anxiety as a teen following the unexpected death of her mother in a motor vehicle accident. Her grades faltered, but she completed high school, although just barely. She married her high school sweetheart when she became pregnant with their first child. She experienced post-partum depression following the birth of each of her three children. Her third child, Peter, died from leukemia at age 7; she was quite angry at his doctors for missing the diagnosis and blamed the local hospital for his death. Ms. Miller went into a "deep depression" following Peter's death, essentially staying in bed for several months. She did not receive treatment for this depression or for the postpartum depressive episodes, but she noted that her strong Catholic faith helped her get through these times. Her husband traveled extensively for work and became increasingly emotionally distant. About 5 years after Peter's death, the Millers divorced, and Ms. Miller finished raising their two other children essentially on her own. Once both children left the house, she took her first job—driving a school bus for the local school district—at age 43. She loved this job, especially all the interactions with the children. She had brief periods of depression and anxiety, but these did not significantly interfere with her work, and she managed them through prayer and going to church more often. She was never psychiatrically hospitalized and had never had a suicide attempt. She had one brief trial of an antidepressant (she did not recall which one) but stopped it because of gastrointestinal side effects. She reports no history of trauma or abuse. There is no known family psychiatric history. She quit smoking 20 years ago, and she does not drink alcohol. She identifies as heterosexual and cisgender; her last romantic relationship ended about 5 years ago.

Everything changed 1 year ago. Ms. Miller developed glaucoma and cataracts, leading to problems with her vision, which did not resolve completely after cataract surgery. This, in turn, led to concerns about her driving the school bus. She also found herself feeling increasingly irritable and snapped at the school children several times, leading to a complaint from a parent. She was asked to retire, which she did grudgingly. Afterward, she became more sullen and less interested in activities such as going to church and socializing with her neighbors. Her children, who both live out of town, noticed that she called them less frequently and that she rarely picked up the phone. Her neighbors noticed that she rarely left the house.

At her first primary care visit 6 months ago, Ms. Miller's physical examination was notable for a 15-pound weight loss over the past year, evidence of peripheral neuropathy in legs, and a slightly unsteady gait—but otherwise was normal. Her Patient Health Questionnaire nine-item rating scale (PHQ-9) score was elevated at 18, and her Generalized Anxiety Disorder-7 (GAD-7) score was elevated at 15. Bedside cognitive testing was normal (Saint Louis University Mental Status [SLUMS] examination score of 28/30). Ms. Miller was taking hydrocholorothiazide for hypertension, and she was found to be slightly hypertensive, so her dosage was adjusted. She was also taking simvastatin (for history of hyperlipidemia), glucosamine-chondroitin (for joint aches), and timolol eye drops (for glaucoma). Laboratory test results were normal. Sertraline was ordered, and it was recommended she see a therapist. Ms. Miller stopped sertraline after three doses because of nausea and did not call to schedule an appointment with a therapist.

Over the next 6 months, the situation deteriorated. Ms. Miller lost additional weight, started falling behind on paying her bills, refused assistance from family and neighbors, stopped going to church, and stopped returning phone calls. She allowed the adult protective services case manager into her home, despite being ashamed at the state of the house, and the case worker found that Ms. Miller was not following any of the recommendations of the primary care provider (e.g., to start taking art classes at the local community center). One week ago, she was evaluated in the emergency department following a fall in which she struck her head. She was alert and fully oriented but appeared unkempt. Neurological examination and neuroimaging were normal, but she had lost another 10 pounds and was found to have orthostatic hypotension and hyponatremia due to dehydration, for which she received a liter of intravenous fluids. A hospital social worker gave her pamphlets about depression support groups. She was prescribed bupropion, but she stopped it after 3 days because of nausea. Her children and neighbors are worried about her, and the social services staff and clinicians involved in her case are frustrated, not sure what to do next.

Table 3–5 and Figure 3–2 depict a biopsychosocial-spiritual formulation and Wisconsin Star Method assessment, respectively, for Ms. Miller.

Bedside Assessment

SUICIDE RISK ASSESSMENT

We cover suicide risk in detail in Chapter 4, "Suicide Risk Reduction in Older Adults," so we present an overview here. Suicide is a critical concern in older adults because the risk for suicide increases dramatically with age (Conwell et al. 2002; Grossberg et al. 2017). Older adult men are at the greatest risk, and the rate of completed suicide compared with attempts is also much higher in older adults. Older adults, both men and women, are more likely to use highly lethal means, with the most common means being a firearm (Bessey et al. 2018). Older adults who kill themselves are highly likely to have had a health care encounter in the months prior (Heisel 2006). Anxiety disorders substantially increase the risk for suicide in older adults, as do depressive disorders (Khan et

Table 3–5. Biopsychosocial-spiritual formulation for Ms. Miller

	Past	Present
Biological factors	• Gastrointestinal side effects from psychiatric medications • Former tobacco smoker • History of postpartum depression and depression following death of son	• Depression and anxiety • Vision loss due to glaucoma • Chronic pain • Weight loss • Dehydration and hypotension • Recent fall • Hyponatremia
Psychological factors	• Death of mother in car accident when patient was a teen • Death of son from leukemia at age 7 • Divorce after death of son and after husband became emotionally distant • Going back to work and raising children on her own after divorce	• Mistrust of doctors • Very independent, ashamed about seeking help from others • Lack of structure following forced retirement
Social factors	• Had been financially independent, managing own household	• Financial impact of retirement unknown • Socially isolated, less contact with children
Spiritual factors	• Going to church and prayer very important	• Has not been going to church lately

al. 200?; Wulsin et al.1999). All of this means that it is crucial that we screen for and address suicide in our older adult patients, especially those with anxiety and depressive disorders.

Assessing suicide risk should start with screening. My personal recommendation for screening tools is the Columbia Suicide Severity Rating Scale (C-SSRS), but the Patient Health Questionnaire two-item rating scale plus the ninth question from the nine-item scale (PHQ-2+9) followed by the nine-item rating scale (PHQ-9) if positive is also a validated screening method. The C-SSRS first asks about passive ideation, such as a wish to be dead or wish to go to sleep and not wake up. It then moves gradually into asking about having any thoughts about actually killing oneself and, if this is positive, moves into asking about ideation of possible methods, thoughts of methods with some intent to act, and finally having a plan for suicide. The C-SSRS is a well-validated tool (Posner et al. 2011), but neither the C-SSRS nor the PHQ-2+9 methods

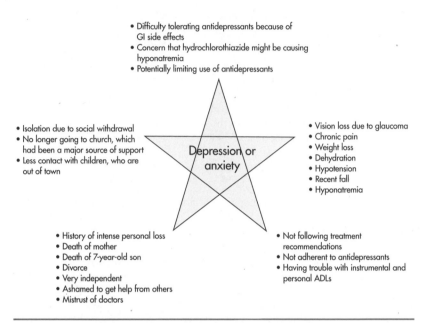

Figure 3–2. **Wisconsin Star Method assessment for Ms. Miller.**

See text for a description and the case example for an illustration of using the Wisconsin Star Method. The Madison Veterans Administration Hospital, the University of Wisconsin School of Medicine and Public Health, the Division of Mental Health and Substance Abuse Services of the Wisconsin Department of Health Services, NAMI Wisconsin, and members of the Wisconsin Geriatric Psychiatry Initiative provided in-kind support for development of the Wisconsin Star Method.

Abbreviations. ADLs=activities of daily life; GI=gastrointestinal.

have been studied specifically in older adults. For access to the C-SSRS, see the link to the Columbia Lighthouse Project in the "Resources for Clinicians."

Once an older adult screens positive with one of the above tools, we recommend further assessment. It is critical to assess a suicidal older adult's ideation about methods and access to means in more detail. You should start with an open-ended question about methods, such as "Have you thought about ways you would try to kill yourself?" and follow up with specific questions about other common methods even if they have not been mentioned. The means that I typically ask about are 1) access to firearms and ideation about using them for suicide, 2) stockpiling of medications and thoughts of overdose, 3) thoughts of hanging oneself (perhaps with preparation such as finding a rope for a noose), 4) thoughts of jumping from a high place, 5) thoughts of cutting as a means for suicide, and 6) thoughts of carbon monoxide poisoning. Patients may also have considered stopping eating and drinking or refusing medical interventions as ways of ending their lives.

Another aspect of risk assessment is a detailed history of suicidal ideation and behavior, including dates of prior attempts, methods used, and how the attempt resolved. For example, did the patient self-abort the attempt, and did he or she then seek help? Did someone else abort the attempt? Was the attempt unsuccessful and the patient never told anyone until now? Also important to ask about is family history of suicidal behavior, suicide in other loved ones, or recent suicide of someone with whom the patient identifies, which can all increase risk. The following psychological factors are associated with risk of suicide and should be assessed: depression, anxiety, insomnia, hopelessness, feeling that one is a burden, recent diagnosis of dementia, and recent loss. Chronic pain and other medical conditions should also be noted because they can increase the risk of suicide.

Suicide risk assessment involves more than just screening and should be comprehensive, meaning that your risk assessment must also include weighing the full complement of risk and protective factors present for each older adult patient as an individual. As you can see in Chapter 4, there is a useful tool called the Suicide Assessment Five-Step Evaluation and Triage (SAFE-T), which comes as a pocket card and is available freely from the Substance Abuse and Mental Health Services Administration (see "Resources for Clinicians" for a link).

Finally, treating depression reduces the risk of suicide. For example, a pooled analysis of three treatment studies of late-life depression (totaling nearly 400 subjects) found that whereas 77.5% of participants reported suicidal ideation at the start of treatment, none did after 12 weeks of treatment (Szanto et al. 2003). In short, please screen for suicide and further assess suicide risk in older adults being assessed for depression or anxiety, and know that treatment reduces risk. We discuss evidence-based interventions for addressing underlying psychiatric conditions and reducing suicide risk in greater detail in Chapter 4, subsections "Psychiatric Medications and Other Biological Treatments" and "Psychotherapy."

SCREENING FOR COGNITIVE IMPAIRMENT

Depression and cognitive impairment are intricately linked. Depression has clear effects on cognition, and late-life depression is connected to the presence or development of dementia. Patients with depression or anxiety can present with behavioral and psychological symptoms of dementia as well. Depression in older adults has long been known to lead to a phenomenon described as *pseudodementia*, whereby individuals suffering from depression will have decreased cognitive function, predominantly in the attention domain, which may give the appearance of deficits in the memory domain. If an elder cannot pay attention and encode information, he or she certainly can't remember that information, and this mimics an amnestic dementia. Likewise, anxiety disorders can affect attention and also lead to a similar phenomenon. In contrast with pseudodementia, there is also evidence that some older adults who first present with depression or anxiety with cognitive impairments in multiple domains (described by Alexopoulos et al. [1993] as the *dementia syndrome of depression* [DSD]) will have persistent cognitive deficits, and a portion of these individuals will progress to frank dementia. This is the concept of late-onset depression and/or anxiety as being prodromal for the development of dementia, as discussed in greater detail in Chapter 1. This has been documented in several studies; Alexopoulos et al. (1993) examined depressed elders over 3 years and noted that those with DSD were more than 4.5 times as likely to develop dementia than were elders with depression free of DSD.

In addition to using tools for broad bedside assessment of cognitive function, it may be especially important to screen in particular for executive dysfunction in older adults with depression. This is evidenced by available data, including a study of 468 older adults with DSM-IV-defined major depressive episode in which researchers measured participants' executive functioning via neuropsychological testing. The study demonstrated that executive dysfunction predicted failure to complete treatment. The authors suggested that identifying patients with poor executive function may allow for intervention to improve treatment completion (Cristancho et al. 2018). Indeed, Alexopoulos and others have described a form of depression seen in older adults, termed *depression executive dysfunction syndrome* (Alexopoulos 2003; Alexopoulos et al. 2002). As the name suggests, individuals with this type of depression meet MDD criteria but also have significant frontostriatal dysfunction, described as reduced verbal fluency, impaired naming, profound apathy, paranoia, and psychomotor retardation with additional vegetative symptoms.

We recommend screening all older adults presenting for assessment of anxiety or depression with a brief validated cognitive instrument. In general, if an elder has been tested before using one instrument, it would be prudent to retest with the same instrument in order to be able to compare apples to apples. However, elders who are tested multiple times with the same instrument may "learn" the test, thus making retest results less reliable. For example, I once started to test an elder who had been tested multiple times with the SLUMS examination, and she essentially quoted from this instrument, saying, "Oh yes, this one, Jill the very successful stockbroker!" In some ways, if this occurs, it suggests that the patient's memory domain at least is relatively intact.

If, after testing and full evaluation for depression and anxiety, questions remain about cognitive status and there is evidence of impairment, it may be reasonable to pursue formal neuropsychological testing. The tools used during neuropsychological testing vary on the basis of the patient's age and the concerns precipitating testing; therefore, we recommend that you provide as much information about the specific cognitive concerns as possible in your referral to the neuropsychologist. There are several brief validated cognitive instruments to choose from, and we summarize the details of the most commonly used tools in Table 3–6.

The diagnosis of *major neurocognitive disorder* (also known as dementia) requires both cognitive impairment and functional impairment (assessment of functional status is discussed later in the section "Functional Assessment"). If only cognitive impairment is present, without functional impairment, then the diagnosis is *mild neurocognitive disorder* (or mild cognitive impairment). It is also important to specify potential or possible suspected etiology of the impairment, but details of this are beyond the scope of this book. Suffice it to say that when assessing late-life depression or anxiety, clinicians should at minimum be screening for cognitive impairment.

DEPRESSION RATING SCALES

Many conventional depression screening tools or rating scales designed for a general adult population include a number of items focused on somatic symptoms of depression, and this can make them less useful for older adults for whom physical disability or functional impairment is less likely to be due to depression and may serve as confounders. We summarize commonly used depression rating scales and their evidence for use in older adults in Table 3–7 (informed by the studies cited therein, but also by Balsamo et al. (2018b). In general, it is our recommendation that the Geriatric Depression Scale (GDS) is the best tool for depression screening in cognitively typical older adults. In older adults with mild cognitive impairment, or even those with mild dementia, the GDS may still be useful. The cutoff point in terms of cognitive impairment and usefulness of the GDS is not hard and fast, but for older adults with significant cognitive impairment, we find that the gold standard remains the Cornell Scale for Depression in Dementia (CSDD).

Regarding the data supporting the use of the GDS, an early study examining the sensitivity and specificity of the original 30-question GDS form demonstrated a sensitivity of 84% and specificity of 95%

Table 3–6.   Instruments for identifying cognitive impairment in older adults

Instrument	Availability	Details	Our comments
Saint Louis University Mental Status (SLUMS) examination (Tariq et al. 2006)	Free to use	Time: 7–10 minutes Administered by clinician to elder	With the MoCA becoming essentially proprietary, this may become our go-to instrument. It does not have measures specific to executive function. In practice, we find this tool is "easier" than the MoCA such that scores will be higher than on the MoCA.
Montreal Cognitive Assessment (MoCA; Nasreddine et al. 2005)	Must pay for training to use the tool as of 2020	Time: 10–15 minutes Administered by clinician to elder	The MoCA tests multiple domains and is available in multiple versions and languages. Previously, it was our preferred test for detecting milder impairment. It is now proprietary, with required (and not free) training for those who administer the test.
Mini-Mental State Examination (MMSE; Folstein et al. 1975)	Copyrighted; must pay to use	Time: 7–10 minutes Administered by clinician to elder	The MMSE is proprietary and of limited sensitivity in detecting mild cognitive impairments. It is predominantly used in research and institutional settings. Gone are the days when medical students would have to memorize the MMSE.
Mini-Cog (Borson et al. 2000)	Free to use	Time: 2–5 minutes Administered by clinician to elder	The Mini-Cog is free and is an excellent, well-validated test to utilize when time is of the essence.

Table 3–6. Instruments for identifying cognitive impairment in older adults *(continued)*

Instrument	Availability	Details	Our comments
AD8 (Galvin et al. 2005)	Free to use	Time: 3 minutes or less Self-administered by informant (preferably someone who knows the patient well) or elder	The AD8 has lower sensitivity and specificity in milder impairments, but it is excellent when an informant is available. The test can be given in a packet to the elder to be completed prior to the actual assessment visit, or it can be completed in the waiting room.
Frontal Assessment Battery (FAB; Dubois et al. 2000)	Free to use	Time: 10–15 minutes Administered by clinician to elder	The FAB is the best test for differentiating mild frontotemporal dementia from mild Alzheimer's disease.

Table 3–7. Instruments for assessing depression in older adults

Instrument	Availability	Details	Use in older adults	Our recommendation
Patient Health Questionnaire (PHQ)	Free to use	Time: 1–5 minutes Administration: self-report Items: 2- and 9-item forms; responses are on a 0–3 scale of frequency; available in multiple languages	Validated in older adult primary care populations (Phelan et al. 2010)	The PHQ is an acceptable tool for use in older adults and is quick and easy to use; it has less utility in cognitive impairment.
Geriatric Depression Scale (GDS)	Free to use	Time: 2–7 minutes Administration: self-report Items: 5-, 15- (short form), and 30-item forms; responses are in yes/no format Available in multiple languages	Designed specifically for and well validated for use in older adults (Sheikh and Yesavage 1986; Yesavage et al. 1982–1983)	We recommend the GDS first for everyday use in cognitively intact and mildly impaired older adults.
Hospital Anxiety and Depression Scale (HADS)	Copyrighted; must pay to use	Time: 2–5 minutes per subscale Administration: self-report Items: separate anxiety and depression scales may be combined; responses are on a 0–3 scale of frequency or severity Available in multiple languages	Some studies support use in older adults (Djukanovic et al. 2017), but other studies call its use into question (Samaras et al. 2013)	We don't recommend using the HADS as a first-line tool for depression assessment; the GDS has clinical utility in geriatric inpatients and acutely ill older adults.

Table 3–7. Instruments for assessing depression in older adults *(continued)*

Instrument	Availability	Details	Use in older adults	Our recommendation
Center for Epidemiologic Studies Depression Scale (CES-D)	Free to use	Time: 2–5 minutes Administration: self-report Items: 20-, 10-, and 8-item forms; responses are on a 0–4 scale of frequency Available in multiple languages	Some studies support use in older adults (Dozeman et al. 2011), but other studies call its use into question (Saracino et al. 2017)	We don't recommend using the CDS-D as a first-line tool for depression assessment because it may be more confusing to use, even for cognitively typical older adults. The GDS would be preferable.
Beck Depression Inventory-II (BDI-II)	Copyrighted; must pay to use	Time: 5–10 minutes Administration: self-report Items: 21 items; responses are on a 0–3 scale of severity Available in multiple languages	Some studies support use in older adults (Segal et al. 2008; Steer et al. 2000)	The BDI-II is useful for better and more qualitatively capturing depression severity, but having to pay for use limits its accessibility.
Cornell Scale for Depression in Dementia (CSDD)	Free to use	Time: 30+ minutes Administration: two parts both completed by the clinician based on interview of caregiver and elder Items: each symptom rated as NA or 0–2 severity Available in English only	Designed specifically for and well validated for use in older adults with dementia (Alexopoulos et al. 1988a) and also validated in older adults without dementia (Alexopoulos et al. 1988b)	We recommend the CSDD as the gold standard for assessing depression in older adults with mild to moderate dementia.

Table 3–7. Instruments for assessing depression in older adults *(continued)*

Instrument	Availability	Details	Use in older adults	Our recommendation
Neuropsychiatric Inventory Questionnaire (NPI-Q)	Free to use	Time: 5–10 minutes Administration: two-part caregiver self-report Items: responses are on a 1–3 scale of severity for how they affect the elder and a 0–5 scale for how they affect the caregiver Available in multiple languages	Designed specifically for and well validated for use in older adults with dementia (Kaufer et al. 2000)	We recommend use of the NPI-Q for assessment of neuropsychiatric or behavioral and psychological symptoms of dementia, which may include depression. It can be used with any level of cognitive impairment; many elders with mild cognitive impairment will have BPSD.

Note. See text for further discussion.
Abbreviations. BPSD=behavioral and psychological symptoms of dementia; NA=not applicable.

when using 11/30 as a cutoff in a mixed population of community-dwelling older adults and psychiatrically hospitalized older adults (Brink et al. 1982). In another study, in a sample of 257 adults ages 75 years and older, the sensitivity and specificity for the GDS in detecting depression with a cutoff point of 3±15 were 100% and 72%, respectively (Arthur et al. 1999). In a 2003 systematic review of 18 studies examining the performance of depression screening instruments in an older adult population in primary care, the authors found the GDS 15-item short form (GDS-15) to be highly sensitive and specific, with a sensitivity ranging from 79% to 100% and specificity ranging from 67% to 80% for cutoffs from 3 to 5 out of 15 (Watson and Pignone 2003). An important question to consider when weighing the merits of various rating scales is whether they can detect one condition in the presence of another. An examination of the Beck Depression Inventory (BDI) and full GDS in a sample of anxious older adults with and without depression (as clinically diagnosed) showed that both of these scales performed well at detecting depression in these anxious elders (Snyder et al. 2000).

ANXIETY RATING SCALES

Many anxiety rating scales have been developed for use in older adults, or, if they were not specifically developed for older adults, they have been examined in this population. Table 3–8 summarizes the properties of various commonly used instruments for assessing anxiety in older adults, along with our recommendations, informed by the studies cited therein, but also by Balsamo et al. (2018a).

Older adults are not as accurate as younger adults at identifying symptoms of depression and anxiety (Wetherell et al. 2009). There has been some research devoted to whether self-report measures for anxiety are appropriate for older adults. One such study examined use of the Beck Anxiety Inventory (BAI), State-Trait Anxiety Inventory (STAI), Hospital Anxiety and Depression Scale (HADS), and another scale not commonly used (Dennis et al. 2007). The authors reported that the BAI, STAI, and HADS were all adequate for screening for and assessing severity of anxiety, but the STAI was more error prone, so their recommendation of the three measures was for the BAI or HADS. They further reported, after reassessing the cohort of older adults, that none of the measures was effective for assessing change in anxiety severity over time.

Another question that has been raised is whether clinician assessment of anxiety severity based on a diagnostic interview aligns well with patient self-report on rating scales. Hopko et al. (2000) examined

Table 3–8. Instruments for assessing anxiety in older adults

Instrument	Availability	Details	Use in older adults	Our recommendation
Generalized Anxiety Disorder-7 (GAD-7)	Free to use	Time: 1–5 minutes Administration: self-report Items: 7 items rated on a 0–3 scale of frequency Available in multiple languages	One study supports use in older adults (Vasiliadis et al. 2015)	The GAD-7 is our second recommendation if time does not allow for scoring of the GAS, but there is less evidence supporting use in older adults.
Geriatric Anxiety Scale (GAS)	Free to use in its original version; if the short form or LTC form is desired, must contact Dr. Segal	Time: 2–10 minutes Administration: self-report Items: original version is 30 items on a 0–3 severity scale, with first 25 items representing three domains (cognitive, somatic, and affective anxiety) and last 5 items exploring content areas of worry; short form is 10 items; LTC version recently developed with yes/no responses Available in multiple languages	Designed specifically for and well validated for use in older adults (Gould et al. 2014; Mueller et al. 2015; Pifer and Segal 2020; Segal et al. 2010)	If time allows, the GAS is our preferred instrument given that it was designed specifically for older adults and is readily available; the self-report is fairly quick, but the scoring takes more time.

Table 3–8. Instruments for assessing anxiety in older adults *(continued)*

Instrument	Availability	Details	Use in older adults	Our recommendation
Geriatric Anxiety Inventory (GAI)	Available free for research and academic use on the GAI website but must apply for a license	Time: 2–7 minutes Administration: self-report Items: 20 items rated as agree/disagree, 5-item short-form version available Available in multiple languages	Designed specifically for and well validated for use in older adults, including those with cognitive impairment (Byrne and Pachana 2011; Pachana et al. 2007)	Given that one must apply for a license to use the GAI, this tool is a bit harder to access and therefore is not our preferred option, but it is well-validated and its agree/disagree response system may be easier for older adults with cognitive impairment to use.
Hospital Anxiety and Depression Scale (HADS)	Copyrighted; must pay to use	Time: 2–5 minutes per subscale Administration: self-report Items: separate anxiety and depression scales may be combined; responses are on a 0–3 scale of frequency or severity Available in multiple languages	Some studies support use in older adults (Creighton et al. 2019; Haworth et al. 2007)	The HADS anxiety subscale appears to have more clinical utility in elders than the depression subscale, but copyright restrictions limit availability.
Beck Anxiety Inventory (BAI)	Copyrighted; must pay for use	Time: 5–10 minutes Administration: self-report Items: 21 items rated from 0–3 severity Available in multiple languages	Some studies support use in older adults (Therrien and Hunsley 2012)	The BAI is useful for better and more qualitatively capturing anxiety symptom severity, but having to pay for use limits its accessibility.

Table 3–8. Instruments for assessing anxiety in older adults *(continued)*

Instrument	Availability	Details	Use in older adults	Our recommendation
Rating Anxiety in Dementia (RAID)	Free to use (accessible as an appendix to the 1999 validation article)	Time: 30+ minutes Administration: clinician-rated based on interview with elder and caregiver Items: 20 items, with the first 18 scored 0–3 on severity level and the last 2 items assessing presence of panic or phobias Available in English only	Designed specifically for and well validated for use in older adults with dementia (Shankar et al. 1999)	We have not used the RAID tool regularly, but the available evidence supports its use for diagnosing anxiety disorders in dementia.
Neuropsychiatric Inventory Questionnaire (NPI-Q)	Free to use	Time: 5–10 minutes Administration: two-part caregiver self-report Items: responses are on 1–3 scale of severity for how they affect the elder and a 0–5 scale for how they affect the caregiver Available in multiple languages	Designed specifically for and well validated for use in older adults with dementia (Kaufer et al. 2000)	We recommend use of the NPI-Q for assessment of neuropsychiatric symptoms or BPSD, which may include anxiety; it can be used with any level of cognitive impairment because many patients with mild cognitive impairment will have BPSD.

Note. See text for further discussion.
Abbreviations. BPSD=behavioral and psychological symptoms of dementia; LTC= long-term care.

this issue using the DSM-IV Anxiety Disorders Interview Schedule (ADIS-IV), a structured interview by clinicians, and self-report of older adult patients with generalized anxiety disorder via four measures (the Penn State Worry Questionnaire [PSWQ], Worry Scale [WS], STAI, and BDI). The authors found that there were significant correlations between patient and clinician ratings of severity, but presence of a comorbid mood disorder correlated with higher clinician rating of severity compared with patient rating.

Screening for Depression and Anxiety in Special Populations

CULTURALLY DIVERSE ELDERS

One important question to consider when examining the evidence base for all rating scales among older adults is whether they perform adequately across diverse cultural, ethnic, and international groups. Although our audience and the literature examined for this book come predominantly from the United States, Canada, and Europe, the implications of the evidence base for diverse populations and international audiences must not be ignored.

For late-life anxiety disorders, the instrument that appears to have been most widely adapted cross-culturally and linguistically is the Geriatric Anxiety Inventory (GAI). Versions have been validated in Chinese (Yan et al. 2014), Italian (Ferrari et al. 2017), French Canadian (Champagne et al. 2018), Portuguese (Ribeiro et al. 2011), Brazilian Portuguese (Massena et al. 2015), Spanish (Márquez-González et al. 2012), and Iranian (Bandari et al. 2019) populations. Performance of the GAI has been validated in a large multisite cross-national analysis (Molde et al. 2020). The newer Geriatric Anxiety Scale (GAS) has also been studied internationally and in diverse populations, and it has been validated in community-dwelling older Italian adult populations (Gatti et al. 2018).

Within the United States, anxiety rating scales for older adult populations have also been studied in a lower socioeconomic and predominantly African American group. Shrestha et al. (2020) examined the Penn State Worry Questionnaire-Abbreviated (PSWQ-A), GAD-7, and Geriatric Anxiety Inventory-Short Form (GAI-SF) in a community-based, low-income sample of African American and white older adults. The authors found that the PSWQ-A and GAD-7 performed best in both African American and white groups, whereas the GAI-SF performed well only in the African American subgroup. They suggested that the PSWQ-A and GAD-7 had the greatest utility in their low-income group of elders.

ELDERS WITH COGNITIVE IMPAIRMENT

As noted in the subsection "Depression Rating Scales," we recommend using the CSDD to screen for depression in older adults with cognitive impairment. With respect to screening for anxiety, Boddice et al. (2008) found that the ability of the GAI to distinguish anxious older adults from nonanxious older adults was not affected by cognitive status in any setting. Further study of the GAI has confirmed its utility in capturing anxiety symptoms in older adults with cognitive impairment (Diefenbach et al. 2014).

ELDERS RESIDING IN LONG-TERM CARE

Another important consideration is how rating scales perform across settings and, for our population, whether they have utility in long-term care settings. The GAI and GAI-SF have been validated in long-term care settings (Gerolimatos et al. 2013). In a study by Gould et al. (2016), the GAI was used successfully along with the 15-item GDS in a geriatric primary care clinic within the U.S. Department of Veterans Affairs system, although the authors noted that the GAI did not perform as well in distinguishing clinically diagnosed depressive disorders from anxiety disorders as they had hoped.

In one study looking at older long-term care residents (Dozeman et al. 2011), the Center for Epidemiologic Studies Depression Scale (CES-D) was studied in terms of its utility to screen for both anxiety and depression as compared with a diagnostic instrument (the Mini-International Neuropsychiatric Instrument [MINI]). They found that the CES-D performed well and had a sensitivity of at least 80% across the board, with optimal cutoff scores between 18 and 22 on a scale of 0–60. The CES-D was best able to predict major depression and persistent depressive disorder, with similarly good performance for detecting any combination of depressive and/or anxiety disorders.

Another study examining the performance of multiple anxiety rating scales in older adults in long-term care settings looked at the GAI, Hospital Anxiety and Depression Scale–Anxiety subscale (HADS-A), and Rating Anxiety in Dementia (RAID), along with a structured diagnostic interview to serve as the standard (Creighton et al. 2019). The authors found that the GAI with a cutoff of 9+ yielded a sensitivity of 90% and specificity of 86%, the HADS-A with a cutoff of 6+ yielded sensitivity of 90% and specificity of 81%, and the RAID with a cutoff of 11+ yielded sensitivity of 85% and specificity of 73%. Creighton et al. (2019) determined that although all three measures were adequate in their performance, the GAI performed the best.

ACUTELY ILL ELDERS AND THOSE WITH SPECIFIC MEDICAL CONDITIONS

The HADS was designed to detect depression and anxiety in inpatient medical settings but was not designed specifically for older adults, and its performance in hospitalized elders has been called into question. In a study of hospitalized older adults with and without dementia (with dementia severity rated via the Clinical Dementia Rating), the depression subscale of the HADS was not able to reliably detect depression compared with diagnosis by a psychiatrist after a clinical diagnostic interview, regardless of the presence of dementia or of dementia severity (Samaras et al. 2013). Both the HADS and the GDS-15 have been studied in outpatients with chronic heart failure. A cohort of 88 older adults with congestive heart failure were interviewed and completed the GDS-15 and both the anxiety and depression subscales of the HADS. The GDS-15 performed well at a standard cutoff of 5±15, with a sensitivity of 82% and specificity of 83%. The HADS for anxiety also performed fairly well, with a standard cutoff of 7±21, sensitivity of 94%, and specificity of 85%. The HADS for depression required a reduced cutoff for acceptable performance, with a cutoff of 4± t21 yielding a sensitivity of 86% and specificity of 79%. The authors noted that the HADS Depression subscale (HADD) required this reduced cutoff to ensure that elders with depression were not missed (Haworth et al. 2007).

It is also important to consider how these rating scales perform in patients with specific diseases. The GAI has been demonstrated to be useful in assessing for generalized anxiety disorder among patients with Parkinson's disease but without dementia (Matheson et al. 2012). The GAI and HADS have has also been studied and found effective for this purpose in older adults with COPD (Cheung et al. 2012) and among older adults on inpatient stroke services, in which case the GAI was superior to the HADS in terms of sensitivity in detecting clinically significant anxiety (Kneebone et al. 2016). A systematic review of anxiety rating scales in Parkinson's disease (Mele et al. 2018) looked at the BAI, GAI, Hamilton Anxiety Rating Scale, HADS Anxiety subscale, and the Parkinson's Anxiety Scale (PAS). The GAI had the best sensitivity (86%) and a specificity of 88%. The PAS has both a self-rating portion and an observer-rating portion, and the observer-rated portion had a sensitivity of 71% and the highest specificity of all tools at 91%. The authors recommended the GAI as perhaps the best all-around scale.

In older adults with Parkinson's disease, the GDS appears to perform well at detecting depression but does best with detecting depression when symptoms of apathy, low energy, and anxious distress are present (Lopez et al. 2018). Lopez and colleagues noted that this may be due to these particular symptoms being predominant in depressed elders with Parkinson's disease.

There is also a question of how standard geriatric depression rating scales perform in older adults with cancer. In a study of 201 cancer patients ages 70 and older who were undergoing active treatment, Saracino et al. (2017) compared their scores on the GDS-15, HADS, and CES-D with diagnosis of depression via the depression module of the Structured Clinical Interview for DSM Disorders (SCID). Unfortunately, the published standard cutoffs for all three measures failed to achieve an appropriate sensitivity in detecting clinically significant depression in this population, missing up to 83% of depressed older adult cancer patients. The CES-D performed the best but still not acceptably. The authors cautioned that these commonly used screens for geriatric depression may be inadequate for older adults with cancer.

Functional Assessment

Universal, comprehensive functional assessment of older adults should be adopted in health care. Our recommendation is to assess both activities of daily living and instrumental activities of daily living, and our preferred tools for this are the Katz Index of Independence in Activities of Daily Living and the Lawton-Brody Scale of Instrumental Activities of Daily Living. Our adapted versions of these scales can be found in Tables 3–9 and 3–10 (Katz 1983; Lawton and Brody 1969).

Assessing Decision-Making Capacity

Medical decision-making capacity refers to the ability of a patient to understand and appreciate the risks, benefits, and alternatives of a proposed treatment, apply this understanding to his or her own situation, and clearly and consistently express a choice. This is a topic of particular concern in older adults, given the increasing prevalence of cognitive impairment with increasing age. It's also particularly relevant as we con-

Table 3–9.   Katz Index of Independence in Activities of Daily Living

Activity	Description of independence in each activity
Bathing	Bathes self completely or needs help with only one area of the body
Dressing	Gets appropriate clothes out and puts them on independently; still independent if needs help only with tying shoes
Toileting	Uses the toilet and provides appropriate postvoid cleaning without assistance
Transferring	Moves in and out of bed or a chair without assistance from another person (use of mechanical aides still qualifies for independence)
Continence	Exercises complete control over urination and defecation
Feeding	Gets food from plate to mouth without assistance from another person (still qualifies for independence if another prepares the food, including cutting or blending to appropriate consistency for dietary needs)

Note.   The clinician assesses the person's ability to perform activities of daily living as independent, requires assistance, or dependent. The total score is equal to the number of activities in which the person is independent, from 0 to 6.

Source.   Adapted from Katz 1983.

sider late-life depression, and perhaps also late-life anxiety, because these conditions can affect cognition and insight and may render usually capable older adults incapable of weighing risks and benefits of a proposed treatment as it pertains to themselves.

Often, the answer to a question of capacity in an ill older adult is very clear, but other times there is more ambiguity. When there is uncertainty, we recommend formal evaluation of capacity. This can be done by any physician of any specialty and does not require psychiatric consultation, even if the elder in question has a psychiatric diagnosis. We recommend use of one of two tools: the Aid to Capacity Evaluation (ACE; Etchells et al. 1996) or the Assessment of Capacity for Everyday Decision-Making (ACED; Lai et al. 2008). These tools are in the public domain and can be accessed online free of charge.

Screening for Elder Abuse

About 11% of older adults are victims of elder abuse (Dong et al. 2014). Older adults are considered a vulnerable population in the United States, with health care professionals qualifying as mandated reporters.

Table 3–10. Lawton-Brody Scale of Instrumental Activities of Daily Living

Activity	Functional levels and corresponding score	
	Intact functioning	Impaired functioning
Use of telephone	1 = Operates telephone independently; looks up and dials numbers 1 = Dials only a few well-known numbers 1 = Answers telephone only	0 = Unable to use telephone without assistance
Shopping	1 = Manages all shopping independently	0 = Shops only for small items 0 = Needs to be accompanied but still shops 0 = Unable to shop
Food preparation	1 = Plans, prepares, and serves meals independently	0 = Prepares meals if supplied with ingredients 0 = Heats and serves prepared meals 0 = Needs to have meals prepared and served
Housekeeping	1 = Maintains home alone or with minor assistance 1 = Performs light daily tasks only 1 = Performs light daily tasks but cannot maintain level of cleanliness 1 = Needs help with all home maintenance tasks	0 = Does not participate in any home maintenance tasks
Laundry	1 = Does personal laundry completely 1 = Launders small items	0 = All laundry done by others

Table 3–10. Lawton–Brody Scale of Instrumental Activities of Daily Living *(continued)*

Activity	Functional levels and corresponding score	
	Intact functioning	Impaired functioning
Transportation	1 = Travels independently on public transit or drives own vehicle 1 = Arranges own travel via taxi or ride share but does not use public transportation 1 = Uses public transit when accompanied by others	0 = Travels only as arranged by others 0 = Does not travel at all
Medication management	1 = Able to organize and take medications at correct time in correct dosages	0 = Able to take medications appropriately if arranged by others 0 = Not capable of dispensing own medications
Management of finances	1 = Manages all financial matters independently 1 = Manages day-to-day purchases but may need help with banking or major purchases	0 = Unable to manage money

Note.   The clinician tallies the number of activities in which the person has intact functioning, resulting in a score of 0–8.

Source.   Lawton and Brody 1969.

Elder abuse can come in the form of physical abuse, psychological and verbal abuse, sexual abuse, financial abuse and exploitation, and neglect. Self-neglect is actually the most common form of elder abuse—because of cognitive or other impairments, elders can neglect their own needs and safety. Risk factors include cognitive impairment, female sex, younger old age, lower income, and a shared living environment. Perpetrators other than the elders themselves are most likely family members, usually adult children or spouses, and are more likely to have health problems, including substance abuse, and to have additional legal and financial problems (Lachs and Pillemer 2015).

The assessment of an elder for possible abuse is especially challenging—often, elders lack insight or are dependent on their abuser, leading them to be reluctant to report abuse. A number of screening tools are available, such as the Elder Abuse Suspicion Index (EASI; Yaffe et al. 2008). Elders suspected to be victims of abuse by another should always be interviewed separately and alone about possible abuse.

Local authorities, typically adult protective services or a similar agency with or without law enforcement, should be involved if there is a suspicion of abuse. To ensure the safety of the elder, confrontation of the suspected abuser is not recommended until local authorities are involved because such confrontation may risk making the elder a focus of increased abuse (Lachs and Pillemer 2015). For further discussion, see Chapter 6, section "Elder Abuse."

Laboratory, Imaging, and Other Assessments

A basic physical and neurological examination is indicated in a depressed older adult. This should include measurement of vital signs. We recommend laboratory examination in all cases of late-life depression or anxiety, especially during the initial assessment. Standard tests that we recommend are listed in Table 3–11, along with recommendations for additional testing when indicated. Certainly, clinicians can use their own judgment, and if some of the recommended tests have been performed recently, they may not need to be repeated.

Depending on the situation, an electrocardiogram (ECG) may be warranted. If evaluating for anxiety and palpitations are reported or if there is clinical suspicion of arrhythmia, an ECG is a good first step, but longer-term monitoring (e.g., Holter monitor) may be required for full evaluation. Clinicians may also want to obtain a baseline ECG to mea-

Table 3–11. Laboratory testing in the assessment of late-life depression and anxiety

Recommendation	Laboratory test(s)	Rationale
Standard (for all elders)	CBC with differential	Anemia can lead to depressive or anxiety symptoms. MCV may provide evidence of excessive alcohol use.
Standard (for all elders)	Basic metabolic panel	Metabolic testing may reveal renal disease, hyponatremia (possibly caused by antidepressant), hyperglycemia, and other electrolyte abnormalities.
Standard (for all elders)	Calcium and magnesium levels	Hypercalcemia and other disturbances have been associated with psychiatric disease.
Standard (for all elders)	TSH with reflex T4	Thyroid disease can mimic or cause depression or anxiety.
Standard (for all elders)	Vitamin B_{12}, folate ± other B vitamins	Pernicious anemia and vitamin B_{12} deficiency, as well as deficiencies in folate and other B vitamins, increase in prevalence with age and have been linked with psychiatric and neurological disease.
May be indicated	Vitamin D	Vitamin D deficiency may be a treatable cause of depression.
May be indicated	Liver function	Hepatic impairment and disease have been associated with psychiatric illness and may also have implications for medication treatment choice.
May be indicated	Albumin	Testing albumin may help approximate nutritional status.
May be indicated	Urinalysis	Testing may be useful depending on setting and presence of acute mental status change coupled with appropriate clinical suspicion; urinary tract infection has been associated with acute mental status changes in older adults.

Table 3–11. Laboratory testing in the assessment of late-life depression and anxiety *(continued)*

Recommendation	Laboratory test(s)	Rationale
May be indicated	Syphilis testing (see Gatchel et al. 2015 for more details of specific tests)	Untreated tertiary syphilis has been associated with psychiatric and neurological disease.
May be indicated	Lyme disease	Untreated Lyme disease has been associated with psychiatric and neurological disease.
May be indicated	Additional endocrine laboratory testing (e.g., sex hormones, dexamethasone suppression test)	See subsection "Medical Conditions."

Abbreviations. CBC=complete blood count; MCV=mean corpuscular volume; T4=thyroxine; TSH=thyroid stimulating hormone.

sure the QT interval if prescribing a medication that can prolong the QT interval (e.g., citalopram).

Neuroimaging may be recommended, depending on the circumstances, but it is not a standard part of assessment for late-life depression or anxiety. If there are focal neurological signs or cognitive impairment affecting more than just the attention domain, neuroimaging is warranted. In general, a computed tomography (CT) scan without contrast is best for evaluating suspected subdural hematoma or other intracranial bleeding. MRI is the preferred study for examining structural changes or abnormalities, but if there are contraindications for your patient, CT with and without contrast would be acceptable. If OSA is suspected (for example, if the STOP-BANG screening tool is positive), then polysomnography should be considered.

Communicating With Family and Others

It may be useful to gather collateral information from loved ones and support persons, with consent from the patient. We also need to consider our older adults' family histories. Even in late-onset depression or anxiety there can be genetic or epigenetic contributions, as well as intergenerational trauma and other considerations that may play a role in our patients' depressive illness. This extends to family history of suicide, substance abuse, and also family history of mental illness treatment and treatment response. A full family psychiatric history should be taken for each older adult patient. This should include not just parents, grandparents, and siblings but also children. Older adults may have a variety of other in-home supports, or they may be living in a long-term care facility. These supports, such as case managers, home health workers, long-term care workers, and other partners, should be contacted for collateral information.

Making the Diagnosis

Although rating scales can play a role in the assessment of late-life depression and anxiety, they are, of course not, sufficient. As with any medical assessment, we must first take a good history (here, rating scales may serve as a jumping-off point for discussion); follow with indicated physical examination, including neurological and mental status examinations; and consider laboratory or neuroimaging assessments that may be indicated, as discussed previously in the subsection "Laboratory, Imaging, and Other Assessment." It is only once we have collected and considered all the relevant factors that we can make a diagnosis of a depressive or an anxiety disorder in an older adult.

DEPRESSIVE DISORDERS

One critical point to consider is whether an older adult in a current major depressive episode has unipolar or bipolar illness. It is important to screen for past mania, including obtaining a collateral report, if possible. Another important diagnostic break point is whether the major depressive episode and illness are primary or whether they are instead secondary to substance use, a medication, or a general medical condition. We also want to emphasize the *other specified depressive disorder* category in DSM-5 because it is much more common in later life to have clinically significant depression that does not meet full criteria for MDD but that nonetheless may merit treatment. *Minor depression* is often clinically significant in older adults, and in this population it can have similar effects to those of MDD in terms of impairment in functioning, increased utilization of medical services, and increased disability and morbidity as well as increased mortality; see Chapter 1, subsection "Minor Depression," for further discussion (Beekman et al. 1997; Lavretsky and Kumar 2002).

If a depressive disorder is suspected, it is critical to consider whether the older adult has had prior depressive episodes. These may or may not have been identified and treated at the time they occurred for various reasons, including greater burden of stigma in different time periods in history. If a patient has had prior episodes, you need to know if the symptom profile, severity, and overall "feel" of the depression has changed across episodes. You should detail prior treatment—were medications, psychotherapy, neuromodulation, or other therapeutics used, and what was the response? It is important to detail prior medication trials and, if possible, the dose ranges and duration of use for each agent. Often, patients will have had inadequate trials, and a "failed" medication may still be an option. Any allergic or adverse reactions should be identified anjd documented.

The diagnosis of a major depressive episode depends on the diagnostic criteria. See Box 1–2 in Chapter 1 for the diagnostic criteria for MDD and Table 3–12 for the good old SIGECAPS mnemonic and the WWARTS mnemonic. It is important to note that older adults with depression may present with predominantly somatic concerns (e.g., nausea) and are more prone than younger adults to experience alexithymia (difficulty describing their mood). Other depressive disorders include persistent depressive disorder (dysthymia), substance/medication-induced depressive disorder, depressive disorder due to another medical condition, other specified depressive disorder (including subthreshold or minor depression), and unspecified depressive disorder.

We should also consider severity, course, and additional specifiers. When diagnosing MDD, the clinician should specify whether there has been a single episode or whether the disease has been recurrent. The severity should also be specified: mild, moderate, or severe, with or without psychotic features. If an older adult is experiencing psychotic features with a major depressive episode, the severity is automatically classed as severe. Additional specifiers that may be relevant to consider include *seasonal pattern* (previously seasonal affective disorder), *melancholic features* (profound unshakable anhedonia, symptoms worst in the mornings with early morning awakening, loss of appetite), *atypical features* (sensitivity to interpersonal rejection, leaden paralysis, overeating, oversleeping), and *anxious distress* (accompanying anxiety that is not present outside major depressive episodes) (American Psychiatric Association 2013).

It is also important to mention bereavement as it pertains to MDD. DSM-5 did away with the bereavement exception that prevented diagnosis of MDD during acute grief, and although this was controversial with some people who say that it pathologizes grief, what it allows clinicians to do is to treat grieving elders who are really suffering with symptoms over and above a typical grief that would meet criteria for MDD. For further discussion, see Chapter 1, subsection "Depression and Grief."

Table 3–12. Mnemonics for symptoms of depression and anxiety

Major depression

S	Sleep disturbance—insomnia or hypersomnia
I	Interest—lack of interest or enjoyment (anhedonia)
G	Guilt—pathological feelings of guilt, shame, or worthlessness
E	Energy—decreased energy levels
C	Concentration—difficulty concentrating
A	Appetite—changes in appetite
P	Psychomotor—either slowing or agitation/restlessness
S	Suicide—thoughts of suicide

Anxiety

W	Wound up—feeling keyed up or on edge
W	Worn-out—being easily fatigued
A	Absent-minded—difficulty concentrating or mind going blank
R	Restless—restlessness
T	Touchy—irritability
S	Sleepless—difficulty falling or staying asleep

Source. Caplan and Stern 2008; Coupland 2002.

Persistent depressive disorder, previously referred to as dysthymia, is defined as significant depressive symptoms lasting for 2 years or more. Elders with this condition may also have concurrent major depressive episodes—formerly known as double depression, but now subsumed into the diagnosis of persistent depressive disorder. Depressive disorders may also be secondary, due to substance use, medications, or a general medical condition, as we have described.

ANXIETY DISORDERS

A key diagnostic issue is distinguishing nonpathological worry or anxiety that is situationally appropriate and not causing functional impairment from an anxiety disorder. It should also be noted that PTSD has been reconceptualized as a trauma- and stressor-related disorder, and obsessive-compulsive disorder (OCD) has been reconceptualized as an obsessive-compulsive and related disorder—that is, neither is listed among the anxiety disorders. However, the emotional core of both conditions remains anxiety. As with depressive disorders, there is also the question of whether the anxiety disorder is primary or secondary to substance use, medication(s), or a general medical condition. We recommend also considering adults with previously undiagnosed mild autism spectrum disorder. For an overview of specific anxiety disorders, see Table 2–4 in Chapter 2.

Generalized anxiety disorder (GAD) is the most common anxiety disorder across age groups (diagnostic criteria are listed in Box 2–1 in Chapter 2). It involves feelings of nervousness, anxiousness, or edginess; pathological worry about many different subjects; muscle tension and trouble relaxing; and often irritability. Symptoms must be present more often than not for at least 6 months. *Panic disorder* consists of panic attacks and a fear of recurrence of panic that results in avoidance and may be accompanied by *agoraphobia* (fear of entering situations from which escape is not possible, often characterized by an unwillingness to leave home). See Chapter 2, Box 2–2 for diagnostic criteria for panic disorder and Box 2–3 for diagnostic criteria for agoraphobia. *Social phobia* is somewhat self-explanatory, with fear of judgment or embarrassment in social situations leading to avoidance and stress. It may be generalized or performance only (such that it is an issue only with public speaking or music or theater performances, for example). *Specific phobias* may be present and of concern in older adults, and the specific *fear of falling* is especially prevalent among older populations. Anxiety disorders also may be secondary to substance use, medication(s), or a general medical condition. For a more detailed discussion of all of these conditions, as well as PTSD and OCD, we refer you to Chapter 2, section "Clinical Presentation."

Summary: Comprehensively Assessing the Older Adult With Depression or Anxiety

The assessment of late-life depression and anxiety should include considerations of medical comorbidities and possible medical condition confounders, possible contributions from medications or substances, and contributions from psychosocial factors as well. Assessment of the depressed or anxious elder should include a comprehensive history that includes family and social histories, suicide risk assessment, screening for cognitive impairment, use of validated instruments to measure symptom severity and frequency, functional assessment, considerations of decision-making capacity and the potential for elder abuse, physical examination with laboratory assessment, and possibly additional diagnostic testing. Clinicians can use such frameworks as the biopsychosocial or biopsychosocial-spiritual model or Wisconsin Star

Method to organize the assessment. A thorough assessment will ensure the best possible treatment and chance at meaningful recovery for our older adult patients. See Figure 3–3 for a summary of the assessment of late-life depression and anxiety.

KEY POINTS

- Older adults have higher levels of medical and other comorbidity.
  - Medical conditions can influence, mimic, and precipitate anxiety and depression in older adults. Careful consideration and comprehensive assessment should reveal the potential presence or impact of medical contributions to depression or anxiety in older adults.
  - Older adults are less likely to be screened for substance use disorders but are just as likely, if not more likely, to benefit from treatment. A variety of validated instruments can be used to aid in evaluation for problematic substance use in older adults. We recommend the Short Michigan Alcohol Screening Test—Geriatric Version (SMAST-G) for alcohol and the Severity of Dependence Scale (SDS) for screening more broadly for substance use disorders.
  - Older adults are at risk for medication misuse, and many medications can precipitate depressive or anxiety symptoms. Older adults may be especially sensitive to adverse effects or drug-drug interactions that may cause or worsen symptoms.
  - Trauma screening should be done for all older adults presenting for assessment of late-life anxiety or depression. Bereavement, grief, and loss are especially pertinent in older adult populations and should be considered. Perceived social support and adequacy of actual social support should be assessed also.
  - Screening for cognitive impairment is an essential part of assessment of the depressed or anxious older adult. A variety of brief validated cognitive instruments are available, including the Saint Louis University Mental Status (SLUMS) examination, the Mini-Cog, and the AD8, all three of which can be accessed free of charge and are well validated.

- A number of other factors may contribute to depression and anxiety and should be included in any assessment.
  - Personality traits and personality disorders may influence the risk for, presentation of, and course of anxiety and depressive disorders in older adults.
  - Socioeconomic status, financial stressors, educational attainment, occupational history, and health literacy level are all important considerations in the comprehensive evaluation of older

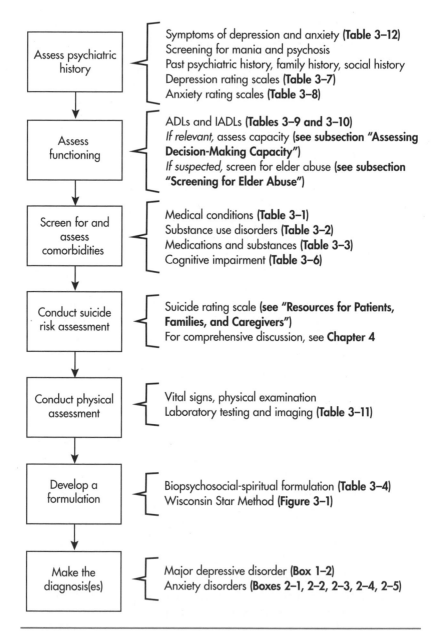

Figure 3–3. Summary of assessment of depression and anxiety in older adults.

Abbreviations. ADLs=activities of daily living; IADLs=instrumental activities of daily living.

adults for anxiety or depression. The Rapid Estimate of Adult Literacy in Medicine—Short Form (REALM-SF) is a fast and easy way to approximate health literacy level in older adult patients

- Women have greater risk for and higher prevalence of anxiety and depression across age groups, including in later life. LGBTQ+ and racial and ethnic minority elders have experienced and continue to experience unequal stressors compared with heterosexual, cisgender, and white elders.

- Religious and spiritual beliefs and practices should be assessed as part of a comprehensive evaluation for late-life anxiety and depression. Consider using the FICA Spiritual History Tool.

• Suicide risk assessment is especially critical in older adult assessment for depression or anxiety. It should be comprehensive. The Columbia Suicide Severity Rating Scale (C-SSRS) is our preferred tool for screening. Suicide Assessment Five-Step Evaluation and Triage (SAFE-T) is a method for comprehensive risk assessment and can be downloaded free of charge as a pocket card from the Substance Abuse and Mental Health Services Administration (see "Resources for Patients, Families, and Caregivers").

• We recommend using rating scales to aid in diagnosis and assist in monitoring treatment outcomes.

- Depression rating scales are available for assessing depressive symptoms in older adults. We recommend the Geriatric Depression Scale (GDS) for cognitively typical older adults, and it may be used in older adults with mild cognitive impairments or possibly even mild dementia. The Cornell Scale for Depression in Dementia (CSDD) is the gold standard for assessing depressive symptoms in dementia, but the Neuropsychiatric Inventory Questionnaire (NPI-Q) may also be used.

- Anxiety rating scales are available for assessing anxiety symptoms in older adults. Our recommendations are not quite as strong for one over another in this case, but we typically use the Generalized Anxiety Disorder-7 (GAD-7) for fast screening and the GAS if more time is available for scoring for a more comprehensive picture. The Rating Anxiety in Dementia (RAID) or NPI-Q may be used for assessing anxiety symptoms in older adults with dementia.

- Rating scales for depression and anxiety have also been studied in special populations of older adults, such as those with cognitive impairment, those in long-term care, and those with acute illness or special medical conditions. We have summarized this evidence for you but have no additional recommendations for special scales in these populations.

- Other important assessments include functioning, decision-making capacity, and elder abuse.
  - Functional assessment of activities of daily living and instrumental activities of daily living) should be performed when evaluating older adults. We recommend the Katz and Lawton-Brody tools for this assessment.
  - Older adults may lose the capacity to make medical decisions, usually due to cognitive impairment. In order to evaluate medical decision-making capacity, we recommend the Aid to Capacity Evaluation (ACE) or Assessment of Capacity for Everyday Decision Making (ACE-D) tools.
  - Older adults are at risk of elder abuse, so clinicians should maintain a high index of suspicion and consider using a screening tool such as the Elder Abuse Suspicion Index.
- Physical examination, laboratory examination, and possibly other diagnostic testing are also part of the assessment of late-life depression and anxiety.
- It is important to communicate with families and supports and potentially with long-term care facilities, home health agencies, or other community supports. Collateral information can be especially helpful in assessment of late-life anxiety and depression.
- Biopsychosocial or biopsychosocial-spiritual models and the Wisconsin Star Method can serve as a useful framework for organizing assessments.
- Making a diagnosis of a depressive or an anxiety disorder in an older adult requires comprehensive assessment as we have outlined above. Diagnostic criteria should be consulted such that the clinician is providing the clearest and most appropriate diagnosis to guide treatment and recovery.

Resources for Patients, Families, and Caregivers

Hazelden Betty Ford Foundation

"How Do You Talk to Older Adults Who May be Addicted?"

www.hazeldenbettyford.org/articles/how-to-talk-to-an-older-person-who-has-a-problem-with-alcohol-or-medications

- Article with helpful tips on how to talk to an older person who has problems with alcohol or drugs

National Resource Center on LGBT Aging

www.lgbtagingcenter.org

- Technical assistance resource center aimed at improving the quality of services and supports offered to lesbian, gay, bisexual, and/or transgender older adults

American Society on Aging

"Aging, Social Relationships, and Health Among Older Immigrants"

www.jstor.org/stable/26556029

- Blog post with helpful information on older adult immigrant health

Resources for Clinicians

Alcohol Use Disorders Identification Test (AUDIT)

https://auditscreen.org

- Access the full AUDIT
- Learn more about the AUDIT with easy access to helpful information

Health Literacy Tool Shed

http://healthliteracy.bu.edu

- Collaboration between the U.S. National Library of Medicine and Boston University that provides a searchable database of peer-reviewed tools to measure individual health literacy in a variety of languages; it has been validated in a variety of care settings

American Medical Association

"Creating an LGBTQ-Friendly Practice"

www.ama-assn.org/delivering-care/population-care/creating-lgbtq-friendly-practice

- Helpful tips on how to make your practice welcoming and affirming for LGBTQ+ patients, including older adults

Stanford Ethnogeriatrics Curriculum

https://geriatrics.stanford.edu

- Brief but comprehensive curricula organized into modules on the basis of ethnicity/identity
- Highly recommended

Columbia Lighthouse Project

http://cssrs.columbia.edu

- Identification of risk and suicide prevention

- Access the Columbia Suicide Severity Rating Scale (C-SSRS)
- Learn how family, friends, and health care professionals can use the C-SSRS

Substance Abuse and Mental Health Services Administration Suicide Assessment Five-Step Evaluation and Triage (SAFE-T)

https://store.samhsa.gov/product/SAFE-T-Pocket-Card-Suicide-Assessment-Five-Step-Evaluation-and-Triage-for-Clinicians/sma09-4432

- Access and download the SAFE-T pocket card

Saint Louis University Mental Status (SLUMS) Examination

www.slu.edu/medicine/internal-medicine/geriatric-medicine/aging-successfully/assessment-tools/mental-status-exam.php

- Access the SLUMS
- Learn more about the test
- Watch the training video on how to administer the test

Mini-Cog

https://mini-cog.com

- Access the Mini-Cog
- Learn more about the examination

Montreal Cognitive Assessment (MoCA)

www.mocatest.org

- Access the training required to administer the MoCA (cost involved)
- Once trained, you may access the various versions of the test

Alzheimer's Association AD8 Dementia Screening Interview

www.alz.org/media/Documents/ad8-dementia-screening.pdf

- Access the AD8
- Access additional information on the AD8 test

Geriatric Anxiety Inventory (GAI)

http://gai.net.au

- Access the GAI
- Access additional information on the GAI

References

Abrams LR, Mehta NK: Changes in depressive symptoms over age among older Americans: differences by gender, race/ethnicity, education, and birth cohort. SSM Popul Health 7:100399 2019 31024986

Abrams RC, Bromberg CE: Personality disorders in the elderly: a flagging field of inquiry. Int J Geriatr Psychiatry 21(11):1013–1017, 2006 17061248

Alexopoulos GS: Role of executive function in late-life depression. J Clin Psychiatry 64(suppl 14):18–23, 2003 14658931

Alexopoulos GS: Depression in the elderly. Lancet 365(9475):1961–1970, 2005 15936426

Alexopoulos GS, Abrams RC, Young RC, et al: Cornell Scale for Depression in dementia. Biol Psychiatry 23(3):271–284, 1988a 3337862

Alexopoulos GS, Abrams RC, Young RC, et al: Use of the Cornell scale in nondemented patients. J Am Geriatr Soc 36(3):230–236, 1988b 3339232

Alexopoulos GS, Meyers BS, Young RC, et al: The course of geriatric depression with "reversible dementia": a controlled study. Am J Psychiatry 150(11):1693–1699, 1993 8105707

Alexopoulos GS, Meyers BS, Young RC, et al: 'Vascular depression' hypothesis. Arch Gen Psychiatry 54(10):915–922, 1997 9337771

Alexopoulos GS, Kiosses DN, Klimstra S, et al: Clinical presentation of the "depression-executive dysfunction syndrome" of late life. Am J Geriatr Psychiatry 10(1):98–106, 2002 11790640

Alguire C, Chbat J, Forest I, et al: Unusual presentation of pheochromocytoma: thirteen years of anxiety requiring psychiatric treatment. Endocrinol Diabetes Metab Case Rep 2018:17–0176, 2018 29644077

American Psychiatric Association: Diagnostic and Statistical Manual of Mental Disorders, 5th Edition. Arlington, VA, American Psychiatric Association, 2013

Anglin RE, Rosebush PI, Mazurek MF: The neuropsychiatric profile of Addison's disease: revisiting a forgotten phenomenon. J Neuropsychiatry Clin Neurosci 18(4):450–459, 2006 17135373

Arozullah AM, Yarnold PR, Bennett CL, et al: Development and validation of a short-form, rapid estimate of adult literacy in medicine. Med Care 45(11):1026–1033, 2007 18049342

Arthur A, Jagger C, Lindesay J, et al: Using an annual over-75 health check to screen for depression: validation of the short Geriatric Depression Scale (GDS15) within general practice. Int J Geriatr Psychiatry 14(6):431–439 1999 10398352

Aziz R, Steffens DC: What are the causes of late-life depression? Psychiatr Clin North Am 36(4):497–516, 2013 24229653

Balsamo M, Cataldi F, Carlucci L, et al: Assessment of anxiety in older adults: a review of self-report measures. Clin Interv Aging 13:573–593, 2018a 29670342

Balsamo M, Cataldi F, Carlucci L, et al: Assessment of late-life depression via self-report measures: a review. Clin Interv Aging 13:2021–2044, 2018b 30410319

Bandari R, Heravi-Karimooi M, Miremadi M, et al: The Iranian version of Geriatric Anxiety Inventory (GAI-P): a validation study. Health Qual Life Outcomes 17(1):118, 2019 31296228

Barry KL, Blow FC: Drinking over the lifespan: focus on older adults. Alcohol Res 38(1):115–120, 2016 27159818

Barry LC, Thorpe RJ Jr, Penninx BW, et al: Race-related differences in depression onset and recovery in older persons over time: the health, aging, and body composition study. Am J Geriatr Psychiatry 22(7):682–691, 2014 24125816

Barua A, Ghosh MK, Kar N, et al: Socio-demographic factors of geriatric depression. Indian J Psychol Med 32(2):87–92, 2010 21716860

Beekman AT, Deeg DJ, Braam AW, et al: Consequences of major and minor depression in later life: a study of disability, well-being and service utilization. Psychol Med 27(6):1397–1409, 1997 9403911

Beekman AT, Deeg DJ, Geerlings SW, et al: Emergence and persistence of late life depression: a 3-year follow-up of the Longitudinal Aging Study Amsterdam. J Affect Disord 65(2):131–138, 2001 11356236

Benjet C, Bromet E, Karam EG, et al: The epidemiology of traumatic event exposure worldwide: results from the World Mental Health Survey Consortium. Psychol Med 46(2):327–343, 2016 26511595

Bessey LJ, Radue RM, Chapman EN, et al: Behavioral health needs of older adults in the emergency department. Clin Geriatr Med 34(3):469–489, 2018 30031428

Bharwani IL, Hershey CO: The elderly psychiatric patient with positive syphilis serology: the problem of neurosyphilis. Int J Psychiatry Med 28(3):333–339, 1998 9844837

Blazer DG: Depression and social support in late life: a clear but not obvious relationship. Aging Ment Health 9(6):497–499, 2005 16214696

Blazer DG, Moody-Ayers S, Craft-Morgan J, et al: Depression in diabetes and obesity: racial/ethnic/gender issues in older adults. J Psychosom Res 53(4):913–916, 2002 12377303

Blow FC, Brower KJ, Schulenberg JE, et al: The Michigan Alcoholism Screening Test—Geriatric Version (MAST-G): a new elderly specific screening instrument. Alcohol Clin Exp Res 16:372, 1992

Boddice G, Pachana NA, Byrne GJ: The clinical utility of the Geriatric Anxiety Inventory in older adults with cognitive impairment. Nurs Older People 20(8):36–39, quiz 40, 2008 18982897

Borneman T, Ferrell B, Puchalski CM: Evaluation of the FICA Tool for Spiritual Assessment. J Pain Symptom Manage 40(2):163–173, 2010 20619602

Borson S, Scanlan J, Brush M, et al: The Mini-Cog: a cognitive 'vital signs' measure for dementia screening in multi-lingual elderly. Int J Geriatr Psychiatry 15(11):1021–1027, 2000 11113982

Breslow RA, Castle IP, Chen CM, et al: Trends in alcohol consumption among older Americans: National Health Interview Surveys, 1997 to 2014. Alcohol Clin Exp Res 41(5):976–986, 2017 28340502

Brink TL, Yesavage JA, Lum O, et al: Screening tests for geriatric depression. Clin Gerontol 1(1):37–43, 1982

Bruce ML: Psychosocial risk factors for depressive disorders in late life. Biol Psychiatry 52(3):175–184, 2002 12182924

Bunevicius R, Prange AJ Jr: Thyroid disease and mental disorders: cause and effect or only comorbidity? Curr Opin Psychiatry 23(4):363–368, 2010 20404728

Byrne GJ, Pachana NA: Development and validation of a short form of the Geriatric Anxiety Inventory—the GAI-SF. Int Psychogeriatr 23(1):125–131, 2011 20561386

Caplan JP, Stern TA: Mnemonics in a mnutshell: 32 aids to psychiatric diagnosis. Curr Psychiatry 7(10):27–33, 2008

Carney RM, Freedland KE: Depression, mortality, and medical morbidity in patients with coronary heart disease. Biol Psychiatry 54(3):241–247, 2003 12893100

Champagne A, Landreville P, Gosselin P, et al: Psychometric properties of the French Canadian version of the Geriatric Anxiety Inventory. Aging Ment Health 22(1):40–45, 2018 27656951

Cheng S, Siddiqui TG, Gossop M, et al: The Severity of Dependence Scale detects medication misuse and dependence among hospitalized older patients. BMC Geriatr 19(1):174, 2019 31234786

Cheung G, Patrick C, Sullivan G, et al: Sensitivity and specificity of the Geriatric Anxiety Inventory and the Hospital Anxiety and Depression Scale in the detection of anxiety disorders in older people with chronic obstructive pulmonary disease. Int Psychogeriatr 24(1):128–136, 2012 21794199

Conwell Y, Duberstein PR, Caine ED: Risk factors for suicide in later life. Biol Psychiatry 52(3):193–204, 2002 12182926

Cook JM, Simiola V: Trauma and aging. Curr Psychiatry Rep 20(10):93, 2018 30194546

Cordella M, Poiani A: Behavioral Oncology: Psychological, Communicative, and Social Dimensions. New York, Springer-Verlag, 2014

Cotton BP, Bryson WC, Lohman MC, et al: Characteristics of Medicaid recipients in methadone maintenance treatment: a comparison across the lifespan. J Subst Abuse Treat 92:40–45, 2018 30032943

Coupland NJ: Worry WARTS have generalized anxiety disorder. Can J Psychiatry 47(2):197, 2002 11926087

Creighton AS, Davison TE, Kissane DW: The psychometric properties, sensitivity and specificity of the Geriatric Anxiety Inventory, hospital anxiety and depression scale, and rating anxiety in dementia scale in aged care residents. Aging Ment Health 23(5):633–642, 2019 29470096

Cristancho P, Lenze EJ, Dixon D, et al: Executive function predicts antidepressant treatment noncompletion in late-life depression. J Clin Psychiatry 79(3):16m11371, 2018 29659205

Davison TE, McCabe MP, Knight T, et al: Biopsychosocial factors related to depression in aged care residents. J Affect Disord 142(1–3):290–296, 2012 22901400

Dawson DA, Grant BF, Stinson FS, Zhou Y: Effectiveness of the derived Alcohol Use Disorders Identification Test (AUDIT-C) in screening for alcohol use disorders and risk drinking in the US general population. Alcohol Clin Exp Res 29(5):844–854, 2005 15897730

Dennis RE, Boddington SJ, Funnell NJ: Self-report measures of anxiety: are they suitable for older adults? Aging Ment Health 11(6):668–677, 2007 18074254

Diefenbach GJ, Bragdon LB, Blank K: Geriatric anxiety inventory: factor structure and associations with cognitive status. Am J Geriatr Psychiatry 22(12):1418 1426, 2014 23954040

Dissanayaka NN, White E, O'Sullivan JD, et al: The clinical spectrum of anxiety in Parkinson's disease. Mov Disord 29(8):967–975, 2014 25043800

Djukanovic I, Carlsson J, Årestedt K: Is the Hospital Anxiety and Depression Scale (HADS) a valid measure in a general population 65–80 years old? A psychometric evaluation study. Health Qual Life Outcomes 15(1):193, 2017 28978356

Dozeman E, van Schaik DJ, van Marwijk HW, et al: The Center for Epidemiological Studies Depression scale (CES-D) is an adequate screening instrument for depressive and anxiety disorders in a very old population living in residential homes. Int J Geriatr Psychiatry 26(3):239–246, 2011 20623777

Dong X, Chen R, Simon MA: Elder abuse and dementia: a review of the research and health policy. Health Aff (Millwood) 33(4):642–649, 2014 24711326

Dubois B, Slachevsky A, Litvan I, Pillon B: The FAB: a Frontal Assessment Battery at bedside. Neurology 55(11):1621–1626, 2000 11113214

Duru OK, Xu H, Tseng CH, et al: Correlates of alcohol-related discussions between older adults and their physicians. J Am Geriatr Soc 58(12):2369–2374, 2010 21087224

Economou NT, Ilias I, Velentza L, et al: Sleepiness, fatigue, anxiety and depression in chronic obstructive pulmonary disease and obstructive sleep apnea—overlap—syndrome, before and after continuous positive airways pressure therapy. PLoS One 13(6):e0197342, 2018 29889828

Engel GL: The need for a new medical model: a challenge for biomedicine. Science 196(4286):129–136, 1977 847460

Etchells E, Sharpe G, Elliott C, et al: Bioethics for clinicians 3: capacity. CMAJ 155(6):657–661, 1996 8823211

Fiest KM, Dykeman J, Patten SB, et al: Depression in epilepsy: a systematic review and meta-analysis. Neurology 80(6):590–599, 2013 23175727

Ferrari S, Signorelli MS, Cerrato F, et al: Never too late to be anxious: validation of the Geriatric Anxiety Inventory, Italian version. Clin Ter 168(2):e120–e127, 2017 28383623

Folstein MF, Folstein SE, McHugh PR: "Mini-mental state": a practical method for grading the cognitive state of patients for the clinician. J Psychiatr Res 12(3):189–198, 1975 1202204

Folstein M, Liu T, Peter I, et al: The homocysteine hypothesis of depression. Am J Psychiatry 164(6):861–867, 2007 17541043

Fredriksen-Goldsen KI, Kim HJ, Emlet CA, et al: The Aging and Health Report: Disparities and Resilience Among Lesbian, Gay, Bisexual, and Transgender Older Adults. Seattle, WA, Institute for Multigenerational Health, 2011

Galvin JE, Roe CM, Powlishta KK, et al: The AD8: a brief informant interview to detect dementia. Neurology 65(4):559–564, 2005 16116116

Gatchel J, Legesse B, Tayeb S, et al: Neurosyphilis in psychiatric practice: a case-based discussion of clinical evaluation and diagnosis. Gen Hosp Psychiatry 37(5):459–463, 2015 26022384

Gatti A, Gottschling J, Brugnera A, et al: An investigation of the psychometric properties of the Geriatric Anxiety Scale (GAS) in an Italian sample of community-dwelling older adults. Aging Ment Health 22(9):1170–1178, 2018 28675312

Gerolimatos LA, Gregg JJ, Edelstein BA: Assessment of anxiety in long-term care: examination of the Geriatric Anxiety Inventory (GAI) and its short form. Int Psychogeriatr 25(9):1533–1542, 2013 23782768

Gerstenblith TA, Stern TA: Lyme disease: a review of its epidemiology, evaluation, and treatment. Psychosomatics 55(5):421–429, 2014 25016354

Ghaemi SN: The rise and fall of the biopsychosocial model. Br J Psychiatry 195(1):3–4, 2009 19567886

Glaesmer H, Riedel-Heller S, Braehler E, et al: Age- and gender-specific prevalence and risk factors for depressive symptoms in the elderly: a population-based study. Int Psychogeriatr 23(8):1294–1300, 2011 21729425

Gleason OC, Pierce AM, Walker AE, et al: The two-way relationship between medical illness and late-life depression. Psychiatr Clin North Am 36(4):533–544, 2013 24229655

Gould CE, Segal DL, Yochim BP, et al: Measuring anxiety in late life: a psychometric examination of the geriatric anxiety inventory and geriatric anxiety scale. J Anxiety Disord 28(8):804–811, 2014 25271176

Gould CE, Beaudreau SA, Gullickson G, et al: Implementation of a brief anxiety assessment and evaluation in a Department of Veterans Affairs geriatric primary care clinic. J Rehabil Res Dev 53(3):335–344, 2016 27273145

Grossberg GT, Beck D, Zaidi SNY: Rapid depression assessment in geriatric patients. Clin Geriatr Med 33(3):383–391, 2017 28689570

Haworth JE, Moniz-Cook E, Clark AL, et al: An evaluation of two self-report screening measures for mood in an out-patient chronic heart failure population. Int J Geriatr Psychiatry 22(11):1147–1153, 2007 17457953

Hayward RD, Taylor WD, Smoski MJ, et al: Association of five-factor model personality domains and facets with presence, onset, and treatment outcomes of major depression in older adults. Am J Geriatr Psychiatry 21(1):88–96, 2013 23290206

Heisel MJ: Suicide and its prevention among older adults. Can J Psychiatry 51(3):143–154, 2006 16618005

Hopko DR, Bourland SL, Stanley MA, et al: Generalized anxiety disorder in older adults: examining the relation between clinician severity ratings and patient self-report measures. Depress Anxiety 12(4):217–225, 2000 11195758

Howell T: The Wisconsin Star Method: understanding and addressing complexity in geriatrics, in Geriatrics Models of Care: Bringing "Best Practice" to an Aging America. Edited by Malone ML, Capezuti E, Palmer RM. New York, Springer International, 2015, pp 87–94

Johnson MJ, Jackson NC, Arnette JK, et al: Gay and lesbian perceptions of discrimination in retirement care facilities. J Homosex 49(2):83–102, 2005 16048895

Katz S: Assessing self-maintenance: activities of daily living, mobility, and instrumental activities of daily living. J Am Geriatr Soc 31(12):721–727, 1983 6418786

Kaufer DI, Cummings JL, Ketchel P, et al: Validation of the NPI-Q, a brief clinical form of the Neuropsychiatric Inventory. J Neuropsychiatry Clin Neurosci 12(2):233–239, 2000 11001602

Khan A, Leventhal RM, Khan S, et al: Suicide risk in patients with anxiety disorders: a meta-analysis of the FDA database. J Affect Disord 68(2–3):183–190, 2002 12063146

Kneebone II, Fife-Schaw C, Lincoln NB, et al: A study of the validity and the reliability of the Geriatric Anxiety Inventory in screening for anxiety after stroke in older inpatients. Clin Rehabil 30(12):1220–1228, 2016 26647422

Kotlyar M, Dysken M, Adson DE: Update on drug-induced depression in the elderly. Am J Geriatr Pharmacother 3(4):288–300, 2005 16503326

Krishnan KR, Hays JC, Blazer DG: MRI-defined vascular depression. Am J Psychiatry 154(4):497–501, 1997 9090336

Lachs MS, Pillemer KA: Elder abuse. N Engl J Med 373(20):1947–1956, 2015 26559573

Lai JM, Gill TM, Cooney LM, et al: Everyday decision-making ability in older persons with cognitive impairment. Am J Geriatr Psychiatry 16(8):693–696, 2008 18669948

Lawton MP, Brody EM: Assessment of older people: self-maintaining and instrumental activities of daily living. Gerontologist 9(3):179–186, 1969 5349366

Lavretsky H, Kumar A: Clinically significant non-major depression: old concepts, new insights. Am J Geriatr Psychiatry 10(3):239–255, 2002 11994211

Lehmann SW, Fingerhood M: Substance-use disorders in later life. N Engl J Med 379(24):2351–2360, 2018 30575463

Le Roux C, Tang Y, Drexler K: Alcohol and opioid use disorder in older adults: neglected and treatable illnesses. Curr Psychiatry Rep 18(9):87, 2016 27488204

Levy C, Galenbeck E, Magid K: Cannabis for symptom management in older adults. Med Clin North Am 104(3):471–489, 2020 32312410

Lopez FV, Split M, Filoteo JV, et al: Does the Geriatric Depression Scale measure depression in Parkinson's disease? Int J Geriatr Psychiatry 33(12):1662–1670, 2018 30251374

Márquez-González M, Losada A, Fernández-Fernández V, et al: Psychometric properties of the Spanish version of the Geriatric Anxiety Inventory. Int Psychogeriatr 24(1):137–144, 2012 21813040

Massena PN, de Araújo NB, Pachana N, et al: Validation of the Brazilian Portuguese version of Geriatric Anxiety Inventory—GAI-BR. Int Psychogeriatr 27(7):1113–1119, 2015 24946782

Matheson SF, Byrne GJ, Dissanayaka NN, et al: Validity and reliability of the Geriatric Anxiety Inventory in Parkinson's disease. Australas J Ageing 31(1):13–16, 2012 22417148

Mele B, Holroyd-Leduc J, Smith EE, et al: Detecting anxiety in individuals with Parkinson disease: a systematic review. Neurology 90(1):e39–e47, 2018 29212828

Molde H, Nordhus IH, Torsheim T, et al: A cross-national analysis of the psychometric properties of the Geriatric Anxiety Inventory. J Gerontol B Psychol Sci Soc Sci 75(7):1475–1483, 2020 30624724

Morse JQ, Lynch TR: A preliminary investigation of self-reported personality disorders in late life: prevalence, predictors of depressive severity, and clinical correlates. Aging Ment Health 8(4):307–315, 2004 15370047

Mueller AE, Segal DL, Gavett B, et al: Geriatric Anxiety Scale: item response theory analysis, differential item functioning, and creation of a ten-item short form (GAS-10). Int Psychogeriatr 27(7):1099–1111, 2015 24576589

Mutchler J, Li Y, Roldán NV: Living Below the Line: Economic Insecurity and Older Americans, Insecurity in the States 2019. Boston, MA, Center for Social and Demographic Research on Aging, November 2019. Available at: https://scholarworks.umb.edu/demographyofaging/40. Accessed May 18, 2021.

Nagappa M, Liao P, Wong J, et al: Validation of the STOP-BANG questionnaire as a screening tool for obstructive sleep apnea among different populations: a systematic review and meta-analysis. PLoS One 10(12):e0143697, 2015 26658438

Nanni MG, Caruso R, Mitchell AJ, et al: Depression in HIV infected patients: a review. Curr Psychiatry Rep 17(1):530, 2015 25413636

Nasreddine ZS, Phillips NA, Bédirian V, et al: The Montreal Cognitive Assessment, MoCA: a brief screening tool for mild cognitive impairment. J Am Geriatr Soc 53(4):695–699, 2005 15817019

Oxman TE: Personality disorders, in The American Psychiatric Publishing Textbook of Geriatric Psychiatry, 5th Edition. Edited by Steffens DC, Blazer DG, Thakur ME. Arlington, VA, American Psychiatric Publishing, 2015, pp 491–506

Pachana NA, Byrne GJ, Siddle H, et al: Development and validation of the Geriatric Anxiety Inventory. Int Psychogeriatr 19(1):103–114, 2007 16805925

Park JH, Jeon BH, Lee JS, et al: CADASIL as a useful medical model and genetic form of vascular depression. Am J Geriatr Psychiatry 25(7):719–727, 2017 28434675

Parks KA, Parks CG, Onwuameze OE, et al: Psychiatric complications of primary hyperparathyroidism and mild hypercalcemia. Am J Psychiatry 174(7):620–622, 2017 28669204

Patten SB, Marrie RA, Carta MG: Depression in multiple sclerosis. Int Rev Psychiatry 29(5):463–472, 2017 28681616

Phelan E, Williams B, Meeker K, et al: A study of the diagnostic accuracy of the PHQ-9 in primary care elderly. BMC Fam Pract 11:63, 2010 20807445

Pifer MA, Segal DL: Geriatric Anxiety Scale: development and preliminary validation of a long-term care anxiety assessment measure. Clin Gerontol 43(3):295–307, 2020 32036777

Posner K, Brown GK, Stanley B, et al: The Columbia-Suicide Severity Rating Scale: initial validity and internal consistency findings from three multisite studies with adolescents and adults. Am J Psychiatry 168(12):1266–1277, 2011 22193671

Rasmussen SA, Rosebush PI, Smyth HS, et al: Cushing disease presenting as primary psychiatric illness: a case report and literature review. J Psychiatr Pract 21(6):449–457, 2015 26554329

Reijnders JS, Ehrt U, Weber WE, et al: A systematic review of prevalence studies of depression in Parkinson's disease. Mov Disord 23(2):183–189, quiz 313, 2008 17987654

Ribeiro O, Paúl C, Simões MR, et al: Portuguese version of the Geriatric Anxiety Inventory: transcultural adaptation and psychometric validation. Aging Ment Health 15(6):742–748, 2011 21656405

Robinson RG: Poststroke depression: prevalence, diagnosis, treatment, and disease progression. Biol Psychiatry 54(3):376–387, 2003 12893112

Samaras N, Herrmann FR, Samaras D, et al: The Hospital Anxiety and Depression Scale: low sensitivity for depression screening in demented and nondemented hospitalized elderly. Int Psychogeriatr 25(1):82–87, 2013 22971288

Saracino RM, Weinberger MI, Roth AJ, et al: Assessing depression in a geriatric cancer population. Psychooncology 26(10):1484–1490, 2017 27195436

Schapira MM, Swartz S, Ganschow PS, et al: Tailoring educational and behavioral interventions to level of health literacy: a systematic review. MDM Policy Pract 2(1):2381468317714474, 2017 30288424

Segal DL, Coolidge FL, Cahill BS, et al: Psychometric properties of the Beck Depression Inventory II (BDI-II) among community-dwelling older adults. Behav Modif 32(1):3–20, 2008 18096969

Segal DL, June A, Payne M, et al: Development and initial validation of a self-report assessment tool for anxiety among older adults: the Geriatric Anxiety Scale. J Anxiety Disord 24(7):709–714, 2010 20558032

Schonfeld L, King-Kallimanis BL, Duchene DM, et al: Screening and brief intervention for substance misuse among older adults: the Florida BRITE project. Am J Public Health 100(1):108–114, 2010 19443821

Shankar KK, Walker M, Frost D, et al: The development of a valid and reliable scale for rating anxiety in dementia (RAID). Aging and Mental Health 3:39–49, 1999

Sheikh J, Yesavage J: Geriatric Depression Scale (GDS): recent evidence and development of a shorter version. Clin Gerontol 5:165–172, 1986

Shrestha S, Ramos K, Fletcher TL, et al: Psychometric properties of worry and anxiety measures in a sample of African American and Caucasian older adults. Aging Ment Health 24(2):315–321, 2020 30810345

Sneed JR, Rindskopf D, Steffens DC, et al: The vascular depression subtype: evidence of internal validity. Biol Psychiatry 64(6):491–497, 2008 18490003

Snyder AG, Stanley MA, Novy DM, et al: Measures of depression in older adults with generalized anxiety disorder: a psychometric evaluation. Depress Anxiety 11(3):114–120, 2000 10875052

Steer RA, Rissmiller DJ, Beck AT: Use of the Beck Depression Inventory-II with depressed geriatric inpatients. Behav Res Ther 38(3):311–318, 2000 10665163

Steffens DC, McQuoid DR, Smoski MJ, et al: Clinical outcomes of older depressed patients with and without comorbid neuroticism. Int Psychogeriatr 25(12):1985–1990, 2013 23941723

Steunenberg B, Beekman AT, Deeg DJ, et al: Personality and the onset of depression in late life. J Affect Disord 92(2–3):243–251, 2006 16545466

Steunenberg B, Beekman AT, Deeg DJ, et al: Personality predicts recurrence of late-life depression. J Affect Disord 123(1–3):164–172, 2010 19758704

Sulmasy DP: A biopsychosocial-spiritual model for the care of patients at the end of life. Gerontologist 42(Spec No 3):24–33, 2002 12415130

Szanto K, Mulsant BH, Houck P, et al: Occurrence and course of suicidality during short-term treatment of late-life depression. Arch Gen Psychiatry 60(6):610–617, 2003 12796224

Tariq SH, Tumosa N, Chibnall JT, et al: Comparison of the Saint Louis University Mental Status examination and the Mini-Mental State Examination for detecting dementia and mild neurocognitive disorder—a pilot study. Am J Geriatr Psychiatry 14(11):900–910, 2006 17068312

Taylor MA, Doody GA: CADASIL: a guide to a comparatively unrecognised condition in psychiatry. Advances in Psychiatric Treatment 14(5):350–357, 2008

Taylor WD, Aizenstein HJ, Alexopoulos GS: The vascular depression hypothesis: mechanisms linking vascular disease with depression. Mol Psychiatry 18(9):963–974, 2013 23439482

Therrien Z, Hunsley J: Assessment of anxiety in older adults: a systematic review of commonly used measures. Aging Ment Health 16(1):1–16, 2012 21838650

Towers A, Stephens C, Dulin P, et al: Estimating older hazardous and binge drinking prevalence using AUDIT-C and AUDIT-3 thresholds specific to older adults. Drug Alcohol Depend 117(2–3):211–218, 2011 21402452

Tripathi A, Das A, Kar SK: Biopsychosocial model in contemporary psychiatry: current validity and future prospects. Indian J Psychol Med 41(6):582–585, 2019 31772447

Vaishnavi S, Rao V, Fann JR: Neuropsychiatric problems after traumatic brain injury: unraveling the silent epidemic. Psychosomatics 50(3):198–205, 2009 19567758

Vasiliadis HM, Chudzinski V, Gontijo-Guerra S, et al: Screening instruments for a population of older adults: the 10-item Kessler Psychological Distress Scale (K10) and the 7-item Generalized Anxiety Disorder Scale (GAD-7). Psychiatry Res 228(1):89–94, 2015 25956759

Vitorino LM, Lucchetti G, Leão FC, et al: The association between spirituality and religiousness and mental health. Sci Rep 8(1):17233, 2018 30467362

Wan L, Li Y, Zhang Z, et al: Methylenetetrahydrofolate reductase and psychiatric diseases. Transl Psychiatry 8(1):242, 2018 30397195

Waterman L, Stahl ST, Buysse DJ, et al: Self-reported obstructive sleep apnea is associated with nonresponse to antidepressant pharmacotherapy in late-life depression. Depress Anxiety 33(12):1107–1113, 2016 27636232

Watson LC, Pignone MP: Screening accuracy for late-life depression in primary care: a systematic review. J Fam Pract 52(12):956–964, 2003 14653982

Wetherell JL, Petkus AJ, McChesney K, et al: Older adults are less accurate than younger adults at identifying symptoms of anxiety and depression. J Nerv Ment Dis 197(8):623–626, 2009 19684501

Wiglusz MS, Landowski J, Cubała WJ: Prevalence of anxiety disorders in epilepsy. Epilepsy Behav 79:1–3, 2018 29223931

Williams Institute: LGBT Data & Demographics. Los Angeles, CA, UCLA School of Law, January 2019. Available at: https://williamsinstitute.law.ucla.edu/visualization/lgbt-stats/?topic=LGBT#density. Accessed October 13, 2021.

Wulsin LR, Vaillant GE, Wells VE: A systematic review of the mortality of depression. Psychosom Med 61(1):6–17, 1999 10024062

Yaffe MJ, Wolfson C, Lithwick M, et al: Development and validation of a tool to improve physician identification of elder abuse: the Elder Abuse Suspicion Index (EASI). J Elder Abuse Negl 20(3):276–300, 2008 18928055

Yan Y, Xin T, Wang D, et al: Application of the Geriatric Anxiety Inventory-Chinese Version (GAI-CV) to older people in Beijing communities. Int Psychogeriatr 26(3):517–523, 2014 24252312

Yarnell S, Li L, MacGrory B, et al: Substance use disorders in later life: a review and synthesis of the literature of an emerging public health concern. Am J Geriatr Psychiatry 28(2):226–236, 2020 31340887

Yarns BC, Abrams JM, Meeks TW, et al: The mental health of older LGBT adults. Curr Psychiatry Rep 18(6):60, 2016 27142205

Yesavage JA, Brink TL, Rose TL, et al: Development and validation of a geriatric depression screening scale: a preliminary report. J Psychiatr Res 17(1):37–49, 1982–1983 7183759

CHAPTER 4

Suicide Risk Reduction in Older Adults

Lucy Y. Wang, M.D.

PRÉCIS

Suicide is a tragic outcome for patients and their loved ones, and it is increasingly being recognized as a public health priority. Psychiatric illnesses that contribute to suicide risk are treatable, which provides an opportunity to relieve suffering and prevent suicide in many elders. In this chapter, we first review the scope and seriousness of suicide in older adults, highlighting how older adults, and older men in particular, are a high-risk group. This is followed by a discussion of how we, as individual mental health or medical providers, can screen, assess, and intervene to reduce suicide risk in our patients. Because of the importance of systems-level interventions, we also review opportunities at the wider clinic or facility level, as well as available public health resources. We also address situations that are seen more often in older than younger adults, such as suicide risk in dementia, suicide in skilled nursing facilities, and end-of-life considerations.

Scope

The United States is experiencing an alarming increase in the rate of suicide: from 2000 to 2016, the age-adjusted suicide rate increased 30% overall (Hedegaard et al. 2018b). Although increases were highest among middle-age adults, suicide rates have historically been high in older men, and they have remained so. The group with the highest suicide rate in 2016 was, indeed, men ages 75 and older, with 39.2 deaths per 100,000. This number is markedly higher than that of the next-highest risk group, men ages 45–64, at 29.1 deaths per 100,000. And the rate in older men dwarfs that of women in their highest-risk age category (ages 45–64), which was 9.9 deaths per 100,000. Another concerning trend is that the younger old, ages 65–74, saw suicide rates increase from 2000 to 2016 in both men and women. Figures 4–1 and 4–2 present suicide rates in the United States for females and males, respectively. There are also significant differences in suicide risk among elders of different ethnic and racial groups, as presented in Figure 4–3. Suicide rates are also higher in rural areas than urban and suburban areas (Hedegaard et al. 2018a).

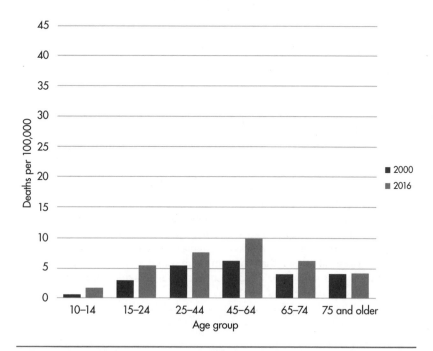

Figure 4–1.   Suicide rates for females by age group in 2000 and 2016.
Source.   Adapted from Hedegaard et al. 2018b.

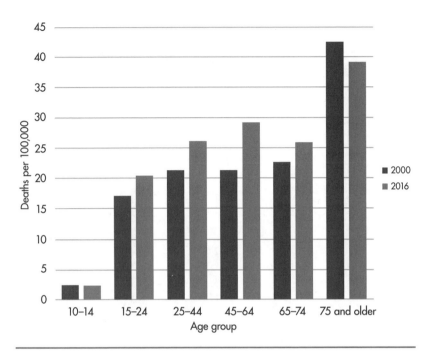

Figure 4–2. **Suicide rates for males by age group in 2000 and 2016.**
Source. Adapted from Hedegaard et al. 2018b.

Suicide is also a global health problem. Approximately 800,000 people die from suicide yearly worldwide (World Health Organization 2019). Although most of the world's suicides occur in low- and middle-income countries (79%), high-income countries have the highest age-standardized suicide rate (11.5 per 100,000); in high-income countries, rates of suicide are highest among middle-age and older adults (World Health Organization 2019).

The ratio of suicide attempts to completed suicides differs notably between younger people and older adults. In adolescents, for each death from suicide, there are estimated to be as many as 200 attempts, whereas in older adults, for each death from suicide it is estimated that there are only 2–4 attempts (Yeates 2014). The higher lethality in older adults is explained in part by the choosing of more lethal means; for example, older men, in particular, die from suicide predominantly by firearms. Many older adults own one or more firearms—in one study, 38.6% of older adults reported having a firearm in the home (Morgan et al. 2019). In addition, the purchase of a firearm is associated with a marked increase in suicide risk, especially within the first 30 days of purchase (Studdert et al. 2020). Remarkably, 91% of firearm deaths

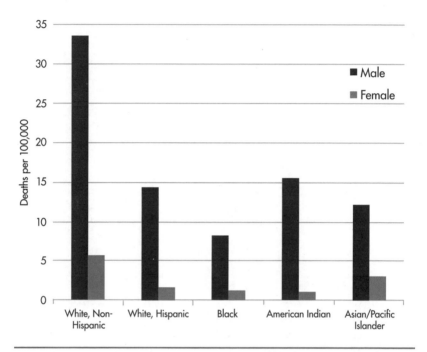

Figure 4–3.   Suicide rates in the United States among adults 65 years and older by ethnicity and gender in 2018.

Rates are per 100,000. Note that the counts for Black Hispanic, American Indian Hispanic, and Asian/Pacific Islander Hispanic elders were very low (three or fewer total deaths in each category) and therefore are not included.
Source.   CDC WISQARS. Accessed January 2021.

among elders in the United States are self-inflicted (Morgan et al. 2019). In addition, frailty or other health factors may make it less likely that older adults will recover from physical trauma or critical illness (e.g., following an overdose) compared with younger people. In Figure 4–4, we present the frequency of means of suicide used by older adults.

Given high suicide rates in men ages 75 and older and growing rates in both men and women ages 65–74, suicide is considered a major area of concern for any health care professional working with older adults. These numbers also highlight that we as clinicians are positioned to intervene in a meaningful way. By being aware of the elevated risk and the means by which our patients can die from suicide, we are better equipped to screen, assess, and implement risk reduction approaches for our patients.

Asking about suicidal ideation in older adults seeking mental health care is critical. Psychological autopsy studies have found that only 8% of elders who ultimately died from suicide denied having ideation

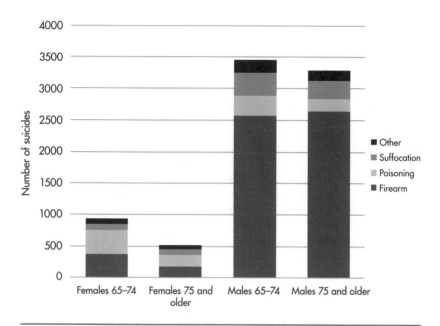

Figure 4–4.   Means of suicide in older adults in the United States in 2016.

Source.   Adapted from Hedegaard et al. 2018b.

when asked directly (Heisel 2006). In addition, in the last year of their life, 40% had reported suicidal ideation to a health care professional and 75% had reported it to a family member. In the next section, we review screening for suicidality in older adults in detail.

Screening for Suicidality

The traditional medical model for prevention is screening for an illness, usually through inquiry, a test, or a procedure, implemented by a nurse or other medical provider. When the screening is positive, it triggers a more thorough evaluation from a physician or specialist, with confirmation of the illness followed by appropriate treatment. Suicide prevention and risk reduction have taken on a similar model, starting with screening, often by a triage nurse or physician, followed by evaluation by a physician and referral to a psychiatrist in many cases. This should result in an appropriate treatment disposition, such as psychiatric hospitalization, intensive outpatient treatment, or a more routine referral to outpatient mental health care. We present a model of screening for, assessing, and addressing suicidality in older adults in Figure 4–5.

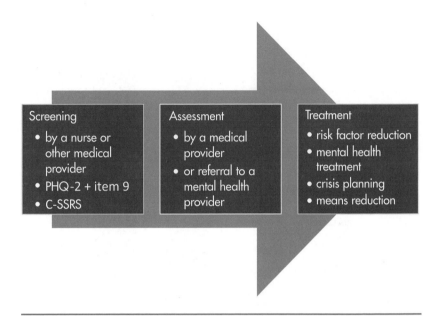

Figure 4–5.   Model of screening for, assessing, and addressing suicidality in older adults.

See text for further details.

Abbreviations.   C-SSRS=Columbia Suicide Severity Rating Scale; PHQ-2 t+item 9=Patient Health Questionnaire, two-item version plus item 9 from the nine-item version.

ROLE OF SCREENING

The role of screening for suicide risk is still being defined. Screening for any illness is considered appropriate when a treatment is available for that illness. Suicide risk interventions do exist and work, but many of them depend on access to mental health care. Because mental health care access is lacking in many places, it is reasonable to ask whether screening for suicide risk provides sufficient benefit to implement universally. The U.S. Preventive Services Task Force (USPSTF) 2014 recommendation states that "The current evidence is insufficient to assess the balance of benefits and harms of screening for suicide risk in adolescents, adults, and older adults in primary care" (LeFevre and U.S. Preventive Services Task Force 2014). The USPSTF does recommend depression screening in the general adult population, including older adults, although it adds that screening should be implemented with adequate systems in place to ensure accurate diagnosis, effective treatment, and appropriate follow-up (Siu et al. 2016). For hospital systems, the Joint Commission's National Patient Safety Goal 15.01.01 clearly recommends screening for suicidal ideation in those who are being seen for a behavioral health condition (The Joint Commission 2019). Although it stops short of requiring suicide risk screening in individuals being evaluated or treated for other medical conditions, the report clarifies that many patients being evaluated for medical conditions are at risk for comorbid mental health conditions and that providers should consider suicide risk as part of a clinical assessment if indicated. The authors of the guidelines also comment that "some organizations that care for vulnerable populations with a high prevalence of suicidal ideation have successfully implemented universal screening" (The Joint Commission 2019, p. 4). Although these guidelines stop short of recommending universal screening at this time, health systems that do have adequate mental health resources should implement, and many have implemented, universal screening. My experience with primary care providers is not that they question the importance of screening suicide risk but rather that they have difficulty figuring out what to do with a positive screen, including challenges finding adequate mental health treatment for the older patient.

SCREENING TOOLS

No suicide screening tools have been specifically validated for older adults, but in practice they are the same tools as those we use for all adults. Two common suicide screening instruments are the Patient Health Questionnaire two-item rating scale supplemented by the ninth question from the nine-item scale (PHQ-2+9) and the Columbia Suicide Severity Rating Scale (C-SSRS) screening tool. Both have been made freely available by their developers and have been widely used.

The PHQ-2 consists of the first two questions of the PHQ-9 and includes inquiries about the presence of depressed mood and loss of enjoyment (items 1 and 2). Many primary care offices screen for depression with the PHQ-2 and if positive proceed to the full PHQ-9. However, we recommend including item 9 (which asks about thoughts of dying or suicide) in addition to the PHQ-2 at the outset so as not to miss older adults with thoughts of suicide who do not screen positive for depression (Raue et al. 2014). Two large retrospective studies correlate PHQ-9 item 9 with suicide attempts and completed suicide, further supporting the inclusion of item 9 as a screening instrument (Louzon et al. 2016; Simon et al. 2013).

The C-SSRS screening tool is an abbreviated form of a longer research-validated suicide risk rating scale (Posner et al. 2011). The screening version asks questions in a stepwise manner, first inquiring about desire to die, followed by thoughts of taking one's own life, and then inquiring about suicide plan and intent. It includes a last question about past suicide attempts because a history of suicide attempts markedly increases suicide risk. Therefore, it not only acts as a screening measure but also begins one of the key steps in risk assessment: an inquiry into suicide plan, intent, and risk factors. The C-SSRS is applicable to different populations, ranging from children to older adults, and there are trainings available for individuals who are not medical providers, including teachers, coaches, first responders, and family members. One consideration, however, is that although the full C-SSRS is validated, the C-SSRS screening tool as yet has fewer studies than the PHQ-9 demonstrating a correlation with suicide.

Please refer to the "Resources for Clinicians" at the end of the chapter for more information on screening tools.

Older adults are less likely than younger adults to be screened for suicidality in emergency departments, and even when they screen positive, older adults are less likely to receive mental health evaluations and to be offered referral resources (Arias et al. 2017; Betz et al. 2016). The reasons behind this are unclear; clinicians may assume that older adults are at lower risk of suicide or, alternatively, may believe that suicide is "normal" for older adults' life stage or situation. I have had many patients ask me, "Wouldn't anyone with my health problems want to die?" A medical student once said to me, "If I were in a nursing home, I would probably be suicidal, too." In fact, ageism—negative attitudes toward and stereotypes about aging and older adults, including among older adults themselves—may pose barriers to identifying and addressing suicidality in older adults (Van Orden and Deming 2018). Admittedly, there may be other complicating conditions that limit screening or referrals for treatment, such as dementia or delirium. That being said, we should be aware of our own biases, and we should be vigilant about screening for and assessing suicide risk in older adults.

Suicide Risk Assessment

The goal of the *suicide risk assessment* is to determine the severity and level of risk a patient is at for suicide, with a view to implementing interventions to reduce this risk level and facilitating the level of care needed. This assessment weighs the balance between risk factors and protective factors, incorporating the severity of suicidal thoughts, behaviors, and intent. In this chapter we review these steps in detail (summarized in Figure 4–6).

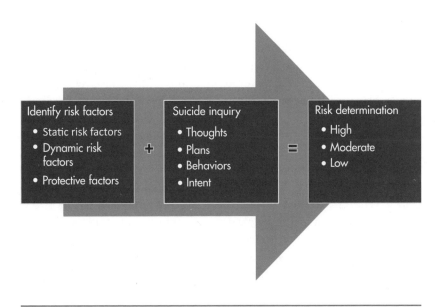

Figure 4–6. Suicide risk assessment.
See text and Tables 4–1 and Table 4–2 for further details.

Readers should also be aware of a useful pocket reference called the Suicide Assessment Five-Step Evaluation and Triage (SAFE-T) pocket card that summarizes the suicide risk assessment in five steps. This pocket card is based on the American Psychiatric Association *Practice Guideline for the Assessment and Treatment of Patients With Suicidal Behaviors* (American Psychiatric Association 2010) and is available free at the Substance Abuse and Mental Health Services Administration (SAMHSA) website. (See "Resources for Clinicians" for more details.)

IDENTIFYING RISK FACTORS

We identify suicide risk factors for two reasons:

- To determine a patient's risk level, thereby informing what level of care is safest and most appropriate. We cover this topic in this subsection.
- To aid in treatment planning because the interventions one chooses for reducing risk are tailored to the dynamic, or modifiable, risk factors and protective factors that have been identified. We discuss this topic in the section "Suicide Risk Reduction Interventions."

Suicide researchers have identified a number of static risk factors, dynamic risk factors, and protective factors in all populations, including older adults. Some risk factors have been identified as being more prevalent or salient in older adults, as highlighted in Table 4–1 (Steele et al. 2018). Older age, in and of itself, is a notable risk factor, particularly in males. Other static risk factors in older adults include race (white being higher risk), history of prior suicide attempts, personal history of abuse, family history of suicide, and chronic mental illness; this list is much like that seen in younger adults. Dynamic risk factors pertinent to geriatric populations include current psychiatric illness (depression in particular), psychological symptoms (perceived burdensomeness, guilt, hopelessness, impulsivity, poor perception of health), acute medical illness, current substance use, access to lethal means, financial stress, and social isolation. It is not uncommon in geriatric psychiatry to see this patient profile, such as individuals with depression and multiple medical problems, living on a limited fixed income, whose spouse and other family and friends have passed away and who feel like a burden on their families or on society. In fact, older adults who die from suicide are characterized by some combination of psychiatric illness, physical illness, pain, social isolation, and/or functional impairment (Van Orden and Deming 2018).

Because we are writing this book in the midst of the SARS-CoV-2 disease (COVID-19) pandemic, we would be remiss if we did not comment on the impact of the pandemic on suicide risk in older adults. The severe acute respiratory syndrome (SARS) epidemic in 2003 was associated with an increase in elder suicide in Hong Kong, perhaps due to disruptions in social networks and in access to health care (Chan et al. 2006). Interestingly, thus far in the COVID-19 pandemic, older adults seem to have less suicidal ideation than do younger adults (Vahia et al. 2020).

We can view protective factors in older adults as the opposite of some risk factors. Protective factors include a strong sense of social connectedness, fewer medical comorbidities, no history of prior suicide attempts, being active in the community, not being socially isolated, and strong family support in geographical proximity. This list highlights the role of social connectedness, both actual and perceived, in suicide risk reduction (Steele et al. 2018).

SUICIDE INQUIRY

A *suicide inquiry* involves eliciting a patient's thoughts about suicide and determining the imminence of suicide behaviors. The C-SSRS screening tool, as previously described in the subsection "Screening Tools," includes questions that provide some of this information. Beyond

Table 4–1.　Suicide risk and protective factors

Static risk factors	Dynamic risk factors	Protective factors
Older age	Acute medical illness	Access to and engagement with health care
Male sex	**Poor perception of health**	
Race (white)		Access to and engagement with mental health care
Mental health history	**Social isolation**	
• **History of mental illness**	Psychosocial stressors	Fewer medical comorbidities
• **History of suicide attempts**	• Homelessness	
• History of mental health hospitalizations	• Legal problems	Family relationships
	• Financial problems	• **Family support in geographic proximity**
	• Relationship problems	• Meaningful family relationships
• History of nonsuicidal self-directed violence (e.g., cutting)	Psychological symptoms	
	• **Impulsivity**	• Has a significant other
	• **Hopelessness**	• Responsibilities for someone else (e.g., children, elder)
	• Insomnia	
Losses	• Agitation	
• Loss of a loved one	• Problem-solving difficulties	
• Loss of a relationship	• Anger	Protective personal traits or beliefs
• Unstable housing	• Rumination	• Strong desire to live
• Job loss	• **Perceived burden-someness**	• Motivation for treatment
Medical conditions	• **Guilt**	• Hope for the future
• Traumatic brain injury	• Intoxication	• Pattern of help seeking
• HIV/AIDS	Current psychiatric conditions	• Beliefs against suicide
• Chronic pain	• **Depression**	• Cognitive flexibility
Membership in a minority group at increased risk (e.g., LGBTQ+)	• Anxiety	**Social connectedness**
	• Personality disorder	• Ethnic groups
	• Psychotic disorder	• Religious groups
	• Eating disorder	• Friends
	• **Substance use**	• Community support
Personal history of trauma or abuse	**Access to lethal means**	Religious or spiritual beliefs
	• Firearms	
Family history of suicide	• Large quantities of medications	
Widowed, divorced, or single marital status		

Note.　Included are risk factors for any age group that are applicable to older adults. Factors that have been specifically identified in studies of older adults are in boldface type.
Source.　American Psychiatric Association 2010; Department of Veterans Affairs 2019; Steele et al. 2018.

the C-SSRS, a suicide inquiry includes questions about severity and about how often and how long thoughts about suicide have been occurring. This inquiry also involves whether these thoughts include plans to take one's own life and details about such plans, including timing, means, and whether the patient has initiated any preparatory actions. Finally, suicide intent can be assessed by gauging to what degree patients expect to carry out a plan and their belief that they will die from the attempt, as opposed to being self-injurious but with nonlethal intent.

Many providers naturally feel uncomfortable initiating this line of questioning. I find it helpful to put the questioning into context both for myself and for the patient: "I noticed the answers you wrote on the questionnaire the nurse gave you earlier. I would like to spend a few moments to talk about those answers." Or you might say, "We just discussed how you are going through a difficult time (with your health, financial situation, etc.). Sometimes, when people are going through difficult situations, they can have thoughts about giving up or not wanting to live any more. Is this something that you experience as well?" If the response is affirmative, you can increase the level of detail in your questions in a natural progression: "How long have you been feeling this way?" "Have these thoughts progressed to a point where you are thinking of taking your own life?" "Have you considered how you would take your life?" "Have you taken steps to move forward with this plan?" "How close are you to following through with this plan?"

RISK DETERMINATION

A critical next step is estimating the risk of suicide, which is based on the risk factors involved and the results of a suicide inquiry. The suicide risk level in turn helps determine next steps in treatment, including the appropriate setting and referrals. If a patient has many risk factors and a high degree of suicidality (e.g., strong intent, high lethality plan, preparatory behaviors), the risk level is considered high, and psychiatric hospitalization is recommended. On the other end of the spectrum, if there are few risk factors, there are more protective factors, and suicidality is low (e.g., no plan, no intent), then outpatient treatment and working on a safety plan are appropriate. The decision on the setting also incorporates an assessment of what is needed to maintain safety (e.g., locked unit, supervision, means reduction) and which interventions are needed to reverse the trajectory of worsening suicidal ideation (e.g., family involvement, psychotherapy, medication changes). Availability of resources may influence treatment recommendations: such options as same-day and next-day emergency mental health appointments or partial hospitalization and intensive outpatient can be safe alternatives to an inpatient admission but are not available in all areas. Table 4–2 summarizes risk determination and associated interventions.

Table 4–2. Estimating suicide risk level and determining appropriate interventions

Risk and protective factors	Results of suicide inquiry	Risk level	Interventions to consider
Severe psychiatric illness or multiple risk factors; protective factors not relevant	Persistent suicidal ideation, suicide plan, suicide intent, suicide rehearsal	High	Voluntary or involuntary admission
Multiple risk factors, few protective factors	Suicidal ideation with plan; no intent or behavior	Moderate	Voluntary admission, intensive outpatient or partial hospitalization programs, crisis planning
Few risk factors, strong protective factors	Suicidal ideation or thoughts of death; no plan, intent, or behavior	Low	Intensive outpatient or partial hospitalization programs, outpatient mental health treatment, crisis planning

Note. See text and "Resources for Clinicians" for more information.

Source. Adapted from the Suicide Assessment Five-Step Evaluation and Triage (SAFE-T) pocket card (Substance Abuse and Mental Health Services Administration 2009).

Finally, documentation is important. Documenting the risk determination, rationale, and initial treatment planning is key not only from a medicolegal perspective but also to communicate this information to future providers because a transfer of care is often involved, such as from an emergency department to an outpatient provider. It is also helpful to document the patient's presentation at the time because risk factors and suicidal ideation are fluid, and a risk level at one point in time may improve or worsen at a later time point (American Psychiatric Association 2010).

Suicide Risk Reduction Interventions

Reducing suicide risk involves tailoring treatment to address modifiable risk factors while bolstering protective factors. This is the case regardless of the setting—a psychiatric inpatient unit, an intensive outpatient program, or a general outpatient clinic. Treatment of psychiatric illness is a major component in risk factor reduction; other key interventions include *safety planning* and *means reduction*. Table 4–3 summarizes these steps.

Table 4–3. Suicide risk reduction strategies

Reduce risk factors

• Treat psychiatric disorders and address psychological factors

  - Psychiatric medication and other biological treatments

  - Psychotherapy

• Discuss means reduction

Enhance protective factors

• Encourage social connectedness

• Engage family or friends if appropriate

Discuss safety

• Review emergency resources

• Construct a suicide safety plan

PSYCHIATRIC MEDICATIONS AND OTHER BIOLOGICAL TREATMENTS

Pharmacological approaches for addressing psychiatric illness are a mainstay of treatment. Medications are certainly warranted when the illness is so severe that it includes suicidal ideation. We consider any medication for psychiatric illness that has greater benefits than risks—including antidepressants, mood stabilizers, and antipsychotics—to be appropriate, bearing in mind that some medications may be harmful or even lethal in overdose. We cover medications and other biological treatments of depression and anxiety in Chapter 5, "Management of Late-Life Depression and Anxiety," so they will not be fully detailed here. However, a few of them have been studied specifically with respect to suicide risk reduction and are worth mentioning.

Two large collaborative care studies, which specifically targeted older adults with depression in primary care settings, evaluated thoughts of dying or thoughts of suicide in response to a collaborative care intervention: the Prevention of Suicide in Primary Care Elderly: Collaborative Trial (PROSPECT; Alexopoulos et al. 2009) and Improved

Mood—Promoting Access to Collaborative Care Treatment (IMPACT; Unützer et al. 2006). These interventions included a psychotherapy intervention plus an antidepressant, usually a selective serotonin reuptake inhibitor (IMPACT), and citalopram specifically in PROSPECT. For additional information about collaborative care models in the treatment of late-life depression and anxiety, see Chapter 5, subsection "Collaborative Care."

Both IMPACT and PROSPECT were successful in decreasing the percentage of patients expressing thoughts of dying and thoughts of suicide. Because medication trials were one piece of larger collaborative care interventions, it is not entirely accurate to conclude that antidepressants were specifically helpful in reducing suicidal ideation and depression. However, the trials reinforce the role pharmacological treatments can play in a broader intervention that includes multifaceted approaches toward screening and treatment.

Furthermore, a meta-analysis of 372 placebo-controlled, randomized trials of antidepressants (99,231 subjects, 8.6% of whom were at least 65 years old) found a reduction in suicidality (ideation or worse) in older adults assigned to antidepressant treatment (Stone et al. 2009). The odds ratio of suicidality for antidepressant versus placebo was 0.37 (95% CI of 0.18–0.76) for subjects at least 65 years old and 0.22 (95% CI 0.06–0.78) for those at least 75 years old. In fact, the odds ratio declined at a rate of 2.6% per year—that is, the older the patient, the stronger the protective effect of antidepressants appears to be.

Two medications in younger adults have also been identified as being particularly helpful in reducing suicidal ideation and even suicide rates: lithium, for treatment of bipolar disorder or as an augmentation strategy in depression (Smith and Cipriani 2017), and clozapine, for treatment of schizophrenia (Meltzer et al. 2003); in fact, clozapine is FDA approved for reducing suicidal behavior in patients with schizophrenia or schizoaffective disorder. Although we have very little information on the antisuicide effects of lithium and clozapine specifically in older adults (Lepkifker et al. 2007), it is reasonable to consider these medications in older patients with an appropriate indication and for whom suicide is a concern. Lithium, specifically, has been studied for treatment-resistant depression in older adults, with demonstrated benefit with regard to symptom response rates (Cooper et al. 2011). Side effects and strict monitoring requirements, especially for clozapine, will limit tolerability in geriatric populations. But given the severity of illness, these medications may be appropriate and worthy of consideration.

Ketamine and esketamine have also gained visibility as treatment options in severe depression involving suicide risk. Ketamine can reduce suicidal ideation rapidly and has been recognized as having a role in cases of severe depression in which urgent treatment to reduce risk is needed (Wilkinson et al. 2018). Information on ketamine in older adults remains limited, but Ochs-Ross et al. (2020) performed a study of esketamine in older adults. Although this study did not demonstrate superiority for esketamine over a more usual antidepressant treatment, subgroup analyses suggested that "younger" older adults ages 65–74 years may have had more benefit. The study could not examine effects on suicide because most participants did not have thoughts of suicide when entering the study. For a more detailed discussion of ketamine and esketamine in older adults, see Chapter 5, subsections "Sedative-Hypnotics and Other Medications for Insomnia" and "Treating Psychotic Depression."

Electroconvulsive therapy (ECT) has a long-standing track record of efficacy in late-life depression and is therefore considered a gold standard by many (Meyer et al. 2020). It results in a rapid and highly effective response, with reports of remission rates consistently better in older adults than in younger adults. It is considered a generally safe procedure even in patients with medical comorbidities. In a study that included older adults, ECT was found to be highly effective for addressing suicidal ideation: 76% of subjects with "high expressed suicidal intent" had resolution of suicidal ideation within nine ECT sessions conducted over 3 weeks (Kellner et al. 2005). We would thus consider ECT a treatment of choice in older adults with treatment-resistant depression, particularly in severe illness where there is a high suicide risk, grave disability, or psychosis. For a more detailed discussion of the risks and benefits of ECT in older adults, see Chapter 5, subsection "Electroconvulsive Therapy."

Repetitive transcranial magnetic stimulation (rTMS) is another neuromodulation approach that has gained traction because it is better tolerated than ECT (McDonald 2016). Response rates for depression are far lower than with ECT, but the side-effect burden is also notably lower because no anesthesia is involved and there are no cognitive adverse effects. The effect of rTMS on suicide risk is not yet clear (Bozzay et al. 2020). An initial treatment course typically lasts 4–6 weeks, so rTMS is not thought to be appropriate in urgent situations where a rapid response is desired, as it would in ECT. To learn more about rTMS in older adults, see Chapter 5, subsection "Repetitive Transcranial Magnetic Stimulation."

PSYCHOTHERAPY

Psychotherapy is another key approach to suicide risk reduction. Psychological risk factors salient in older adults include perceived burdensomeness, guilt, hopelessness, impulsivity, and poor perception of health; many if not all of these can be helped through psychotherapy. As with medications, any psychotherapeutic approach that can reduce psychiatric illness severity would be appropriate; those that improve late-life depression, anxiety, and insomnia are described in greater detail in Chapter 5, section "Psychotherapy." In this subsection, we discuss two types of therapy that were included in the IMPACT and PROSPECT studies (mentioned in the previous subsection) and resulted in reductions in thoughts of dying and suicidal ideation in study participants. These two therapies are interpersonal psychotherapy (IPT) and problem-solving therapy (PST).

In IPT, interpersonal problems are considered key factors in contributing to the genesis and maintenance of depression and therefore are focused targets for treatment (Weissman et al. 2000). This approach has the therapist identify one of four possible interpersonal problem areas that may be contributing to depression: grief, interpersonal role disputes, role transition, or interpersonal deficits. Specific therapeutic approaches are then implemented depending on the area of focus identified. IPT is considered well suited to older adults because grief and role transitions are common in this population. In addition to the IMPACT trial (Unützer et al. 2006), a small uncontrolled trial also found IPT helpful in addressing suicidal ideation in elders at risk for suicide (Heisel et al. 2015). For further discussion, see Chapter 5, subsection "Interpersonal Psychotherapy."

PST focuses on the development of skills to address difficult life situations (Nezu et al. 2013). The therapist practices a stepwise approach: first help the patient identify and define a problem the patient wishes to address, then help set appropriate goals, generate solutions, implement a solution, and reevaluate the solution. Because executive functioning impairment is common in older adults with depression, this approach may be well suited to improving both function and depressive symptoms in older adults—in fact, PST has been found to reduce suicidal ideation in older adults with executive dysfunction (Gustavson et al. 2016). A modification of PST, problem adaptation therapy (PATH), was found to be helpful for depression and suicidality in elders with major depressive disorder and dementia (Kiosses et al. 2015). For further discussion, see Chapter 5, subsection "Problem-Solving Therapy."

Alas, finding therapists who are skilled in these approaches and are comfortable and willing to work with older adults can be a challenge.

It is worth mentioning that cognitive-behavioral therapy (CBT), which can be more accessible than PST and IPT, may be of benefit with regard to reduction of suicide risk. CBT has been demonstrated to be feasible and effective in older adults for depression in general. In clinical trials of younger adults, CBT showed greater improvement in measures of suicidal thoughts and behaviors than did treatment as usual (Leavey and Hawkins 2017). Although studies of CBT specifically evaluating suicide risk in older adults are limited, the efficacy seen in younger adults as well as CBT's ability to reduce depression severity in older adults suggest that this modality is an appropriate consideration in a suicide risk reduction plan. For more detail, see Chapter 5, subsection "Cognitive-Behavioral Therapy."

MEANS REDUCTION

Means reduction is also an important intervention (Jin et al. 2016). As noted earlier, nearly 40% of older adults have a firearm in the home. However, although access to firearms and stockpiles of medications dangerous in overdose are frequently involved in these discussions, other means may also be important to address depending on the patient's past suicide attempts or plans.

A means reduction strategy is best done with input from the patient, incorporating his or her values and ideas, because in most cases the patient is the one who will take the initiative to implement the means reduction strategies discussed. Removing access entirely, such as disposing of stockpiled medications or having a firearm removed from the home, is ideal. When patients prefer not to pursue this route, it is helpful to ask them to generate ideas to add extra steps between themselves and the medication, firearms, or other means. Adding these steps allows an impulsive or emotionally driven action extra time to resolve or allows time for another intervention to take place. Examples include locking medications in a lock box or a gun in a gun safe, using gun locks, separating firearms from ammunition, or asking a friend or family member to take possession of these items temporarily until the crisis resolves. Sometimes, a concerned friend or family member will offer to help the patient remove means from the home. More rarely but possibly in some jurisdictions depending on the laws for that area, law enforcement may remove firearms from the home.

PSYCHOSOCIAL INTERVENTIONS

A dynamic risk factor for suicide is social isolation, and protective factors include having a strong sense of social connectedness and being active in the community. Therefore, bolstering social connectedness can go a long way toward reducing suicide risk in a patient. A good starting place is to ask patients whom they consider to be their support network. Family members, faith-based organizations, and other community groups tend to be common answers to this question. Encourage the patient's efforts to maintain or improve existing relationships

For some patients, family relationships may be strained because depression can negatively affect their interpersonal skills and their ability to interact with others in a healthy way. In some cases, family therapy or couples therapy may be helpful. Regardless of whether or not family therapy is indicated, psychoeducation for the family in and of itself can be highly effective, and it can be done through a family meeting or by referring the family to advocacy organizations such as the National Alliance on Mental Illness (NAMI). NAMI not only provides conferences and educational materials but also offers a robust family peer support program and opportunities for patients and family members to engage in advocacy themselves.

Many communities have opportunities available that are geared toward supporting older adults, providing them places in which to engage in social and fulfilling activities. Senior centers tend to be useful referrals because they often have reduced-cost meals where attendees eat in a community setting, hobby- or interest-focused gatherings, and exercise and other classes. Faith-based organizations provide similar opportunities as well. Many community colleges or parks and recreation departments offer retiree classes with reduced tuition. In a related fashion, fostering volunteerism in patients also meets this need because volunteering promotes well-being not just through the activity itself but also by providing connection to an organization and fostering altruism. The opportunities for volunteering are varied and too broad to describe here, but a good starting point is to inquire with the patient about his or her skills and interests. Recreational therapists can provide directions toward this aim as well.

SUICIDE SAFETY PLANNING

When there is more than minimal suicide risk, health care professionals can help the patient construct a suicide safety plan both in outpatient settings and on discharge from an inpatient unit or the emergency department. Table 4–4 details the elements of a suicide safety plan. Patients can also easily find templates online and develop their own safety plans independently. One well-recommended format was developed by Stanley and Brown (2012) and includes five components: warning signs, internal coping strategies, people or social settings that provide distraction, people who can be called to help, and professionals who can be called during a crisis. There is also a section in which ways to make the environment safer (i.e., means reduction) are documented.

Table 4–4.   Elements of a suicide safety plan

Safety plan	Prompts	Examples
1. Warning signs	What are your warning signs that thoughts of suicide could get worse? When would be a good time to use this safety plan?	*Thoughts:* "I cannot take it anymore." "I don't see any hope." *Emotions:* depression, hopelessness, irritability *Behaviors:* withdrawing from friends and family, drinking more than usual *Physical signs:* pain, not sleeping
2. Internal coping strategies	What are things you can do on your own to help?	Go for a walk, listen to music, exercise, play with a pet, read a book, work on a hobby
3. People and social settings that provide distraction	Sometimes being in certain places or being with certain people helps. What places, groups, or people help you feel better?	Coffee shops, places of worship, 12-step meetings, friends and family members
4. People to call for help	Who are friends or family members you can talk to about what you are going through?	
5. Professionals or agencies to call for help	If you need to go to an urgent care or emergency room, where will you go? *If the patient is receiving mental health treatment:* Who are the people on your mental health team?	In addition to the patient's ideas, include the National Suicide Lifeline: 1-800-273-TALK (8255)
6. Making the environment safe	What are items in your home that you have thought about using to hurt yourself? What can you do to make the environment around you safer? Do you own a firearm?	Give firearms to family or friends for safekeeping, use gun locks or a gun safe, dispose of stock-piled medications

Source.   Adapted from Stanley and Brown 2012.

Each section of the suicide safety plan includes prompting questions that help individuals write down the strategies they can implement on the spot when thoughts of suicide begin to worsen (Stanley and Brown 2012). I explain to my patients that the plan is a tool they develop beforehand, similar to a fire escape plan, so they have something they can easily reference when in a crisis situation. The safety plan has a graduated approach, which involves first being aware of one's own warning signs, then using strategies one can implement on one's own (e.g., coping strategies, engaging in social contact), and then reaching out for help (trusted family and friends, health care professionals). An advantage of a safety plan such as this is that the primary author is the patient, not the clinician (although the plan can be completed with a clinician's assistance), so the plan is tailored to what the patient believes would be helpful and therefore can be implemented more easily when needed. The safety plan also contains a section to document how to make the environment safer; this is a helpful prompt for addressing whether or not a patient has easy access to lethal means and how to reduce that access both at the time of the safety planning discussion and in the future when warning signs or suicidal thoughts occur.

One additional resource to offer all patients is the National Suicide Prevention Lifeline, 1-800-273-TALK (8255), and this phone number should be included in any safety plan. This resource was established in 2005 by SAMHSA and Vibrant Emotional Health. Trained counselors are available 24 hours a day, 7 days a week, and they field calls from people in crisis or distress nationwide. The system is made up of a large network of local crisis centers, with national oversight and guidance from a team of leaders in the field of suicide prevention. If a caller is a U.S. veteran, an additional benefit is that a log of the call is transmitted to providers at the caller's VA medical center, which facilitates prompt local follow-up.

Systems-Level Approaches to Suicide Risk Reduction

Suicide risk assessment and reduction strategies are vital skills in a mental health provider's skill set, and, in addition, suicide is well recognized as a public health problem. Interventions that are systematized to larger-scale settings are necessary because many patients do not choose to engage with their individual health care providers with regard to thoughts of suicide. These larger-scale approaches are varied and broad, and examples include innovations in health care delivery, community care, and policy.

HEALTH CARE DELIVERY: COLLABORATIVE CARE MODEL

As noted previously, IMPACT and PROSPECT were two pioneering studies that examined a collaborative care model for late-life depression (Alexopoulos et al. 2009; Unützer et al. 2006). This model involves using evidence-based screening measures for all older adults in a primary care clinic and, if the screening is positive, referring the patient to a care manager who provides short-term psychotherapy and acts as a liaison between the primary care provider and a mental health team. A psychiatric prescriber is part of the mental health team and provides medication recommendations to the primary care provider. This comprehensive approach offers the benefits of universal depression screening, evidence-based psychotherapy, care coordination, and access to specialty consultants.

Both studies showed benefit of collaborative care over usual care in measures assessing suicide risk. IMPACT assessed whether participants had 1) any thoughts of death and dying and 2) thoughts of suicide. At baseline, more than half of the participants endorsed thoughts of death and dying, and approximately 15% endorsed thoughts of suicide. Over a follow-up period of 24 months, the numbers of participants who endorsed both thoughts of death and dying and thoughts of suicide decreased in those engaged in the intervention but remained at baseline numbers in the usual care group. PROSPECT used the Scale for Suicide Ideation and reported results based on answers to questions on the scale that were considered to be reflective of active ideation. At baseline, 35% in the intervention group and 24% of those in the usual care group were considered positive for suicidal ideation. These percentages decreased in both groups, and follow-up at 24 months did not show a difference between the groups. However, subgroup analysis suggested that the intervention was more effective in reducing suicidal ideation among patients with major depression than those with minor depression.

The collaborative care model has gained traction in the United States; for example, it has been recognized as an evidence-based practice by SAMHSA and has been recommended as a best practice, including by the Surgeon General's Report on Mental Health and the President's New Freedom Commission on Mental Health. The U.S. Centers for Medicare and Medicaid Services (CMS) added Medicare billing codes in 2018 specifically to provide reimbursement for collaborative care. For mental health professionals seeking to implement collaborative care in their clinic, trainings and toolkits are freely available from the American Psychiatric Association and the University of Washington Advancing Integrated Mental Health Solutions (AIMS) Center (see "Resources for Clinicians"). For additional discussion regarding collaborative care, see Chapter 5, subsections "Collaborative Care" and "Community-Based Interventions."

PUBLIC SERVICES FOR THE HEALTH AND WELL-BEING OF OLDER ADULTS

In the United States, the 1965 Older Americans Act established a National Aging Network, whose mission is to help vulnerable older adults maintain independence and dignity within their communities. This network begins at the federal level with the Administration on Aging, which provides funding to state units on aging with the purpose of providing services to older adults and their caregivers. State units on aging allocate these funds to area agencies on aging (AAAs) at the local level to implement programs and collaborate with other agencies. AAAs have five core services: elder rights, caregiver support, nutrition, health and wellness, and supportive services. Examples of service areas supported by AAAs include home-delivered meals (e.g., "Meals on Wheels"), adult day services, senior centers, caregiver support programs, and transportation services.

Connecting patients to a local AAA can provide a means to address suicide risk factors related to social isolation and to promote both physical and mental health. Alleviating food and financial instability and providing means for social connection through senior centers or through the aid of transportation services, as well as transportation assistance in getting to medical and mental health appointments, are a few examples of how these agencies provide practical help to older adults. Many also offer case management services or outreach services to vulnerable older adults and can screen for depression, anxiety, substance use, and suicide risk.

NATIONAL STRATEGY FOR SUICIDE PREVENTION

The National Strategy for Suicide Prevention was first released in 2001 by the U.S. Surgeon General, with a subsequent revision in 2012 (Office of the Surgeon General 2012). It provides nationwide goals, objectives, and strategies for suicide reduction; achievements include the creation of the National Suicide Prevention Lifeline and the establishment of the

Suicide Prevention Resource Center (SPRC). The SPRC now in turn supports the National Action Alliance for Suicide Prevention and the Zero Suicide initiative. These organizations and initiatives provide tools for health care systems, as well as for community organizations such as faith-based communities, workplaces, and sports groups. They also provide expert guidelines around such topics as research priorities or media messaging. Although these efforts are not directly related to suicide risk in older adults, it is helpful to acknowledge that public health initiatives at the national level are considered key to reducing suicide risk on a larger scale. On the more practical side, the Zero Suicide initiative provides tools for clinics and health care facilities, which can be found easily on their website or obtained for free by request.

Suicide in Special Populations

DEMENTIA AND SUICIDE RISK

The question of whether dementia contributes to suicide risk is a challenging one. Cognitive impairment can increase risk because it makes it more difficult to problem solve stressors, decreases social awareness, and contributes to impulsivity. On the other hand, cognitive impairment may decrease risk in that it reduces one's ability to formulate and carry out a suicide plan. Many older adults with dementia also are closely supervised by caregivers at home or have moved to a long-term care facility, which reduces opportunities to access lethal means.

Studies indicate that suicide behaviors are lower in persons with dementia than in the general population as a whole. That being said, of those with dementia who do die from suicide, the majority are newly diagnosed with dementia (Seyfried et al. 2011). A recent diagnosis of mild cognitive impairment or dementia increases the risk of suicide attempt (Günak et al. 2021). Other factors associated with suicide in patients with dementia are a history of depression and history of depression treatment. The period right after diagnosis in elders with a history of depression is a high-risk period because they may lack full cognitive resources to problem solve or cope with this difficult diagnosis, but their cognitive impairment is mild enough that they have the capability to carry out a suicide plan. The implication for providers who give patients the bad news of a dementia diagnosis is that they need to be aware of suicide risks; monitor the patient's reactions and other risk factors; and, as with any severe diagnosis, ensure that the patient receives appropriate follow-up treatment. The case example provides an illustration of this scenario.

CASE EXAMPLE: "IF I GET ALZHEIMER'S, JUST SHOOT ME"

Mr. Armstrong is a 78-year-old divorced white man with no prior neuropsychiatric history who presented to his primary care provider 1 week earlier with concerns about his memory. At that time, he reported misplacing objects and having had trouble with remembering people's names and keeping up with his bills for about a year. He got lost driving twice. His children commented to him that he was getting repetitive in his stories. He had watched his sister's decline as a result of Alzheimer's disease and told his doctor, "I don't want to die like that; if I get Alzheimer's disease, just shoot me." Mr. Armstrong denied any other symptoms of depression, and his PHQ-9 score was 3 (one point each for low energy, trouble falling asleep, and trouble concentrating). His physical examination was unremarkable. At the primary care appointment, he said he did not intend to hurt himself, but he was anxious to learn why he was having memory problems. The doctor referred Mr. Armstrong to a neurologist to evaluate his memory problems and to a psychiatrist to further assess his suicidality.

Mr. Armstrong now presents for a psychiatric diagnostic evaluation. He reports that he has never seen a psychiatrist or therapist before. He has found himself ruminating about the possibility he has Alzheimer's disease, and he reiterates that he would rather die than "suffer like my sister did." He has had difficulty falling asleep because of this difficult-to-control worry, and he sometimes feels tense and restless; he has also found himself more irritable in his phone calls with his children. He does not feel hopeless—in fact, he hopes that he does not have Alzheimer's disease so he can pursue his retirement plans. He is easily fatigued, and he often naps during the daytime. He denies that he is depressed or anhedonic. He reports no past history of mania, psychosis, or other psychiatric disorders.

Mr. Armstrong is carefully screened for suicidal ideation. He denies any current passive or active suicidal ideation. He denies having a plan to harm himself. He does not have a gun at home and has no stockpiles of medications, no noose, and no other means of harming himself; he is not aware of the concept of voluntarily stopping eating and drinking. He divulges that he has spoken with a friend about shooting him if he were diagnosed with dementia—but the friend declined to do so. Mr. Armstrong notes that he feels emotionally close to his daughters and grandchildren, and he worries what effect it would have on his family if he died from suicide.

Mr. Armstrong describes no difficulties growing up. He has a bachelor's degree in civil engineering and worked for 40 years building roads and bridges; he retired 10 years ago. He has three adult daughters, all of whom live out of town. He and his wife divorced 5 years ago; she had said that if he did not stop drinking, she would leave him. He did not stop drinking and currently drinks 2–3 beers per day. He denies having had alcohol withdrawal and has never sought treatment or attended a 12-step program. He reports no use of cannabis or illicit substances. His family history is notable for Alzheimer's disease (sister), depression (mother), and excessive alcohol use (father). There is no family history of completed suicide. He himself has never attempted suicide or been hospitalized psychiatrically. He is fairly socially isolated, except for weekly phone calls with his daughters and an occasional dinner with former coworkers. He spends most days on social media or watching television. He reports no problems with his finances or housing.

Mr. Armstrong's medical history includes hyperlipidemia (for which he takes simvastatin), hypertension (which is treated with hydrochlorothiazide), obstructive sleep apnea (for which he has refused a continuous positive airway pressure device), glucose intolerance, obesity, benign prostatic hyperplasia (for which he takes finasteride), and chronic neuropathic pain (which is treated with gabapentin). He does not take any over-the-counter medications or nutraceuticals.

Mr. Armstrong's primary care provider had already completed a laboratory workup, including electrolytes; renal function; hepatic function; thyroid-stimulating hormone; and thiamine, B12, and folate levels. His St. Louis University Mental Status (SLUMS) examination score was 25. An MRI of the brain is pending.

The following suicide risk factors (as per Table 4–1) are identified:

- Age >65 years old
- Male
- White
- Socially isolated
- Chronic pain
- Divorced
- Anxiety
- Alcohol use
- Suicidal ideation

The following protective factors (as per Table 4–1) are identified:

- Engagement with medical care and mental health care
- Meaningful family relationships

Because of his multiple risk factors and few protective factors, Mr. Armstrong's risk of suicide is deemed to be moderate (see Table 4–2). He is diagnosed with generalized anxiety disorder, and the psychiatrist recommends treatment with a selective serotonin reuptake inhibitor and interpersonal psychotherapy, to begin immediately. Mr. Armstrong is counseled about reducing his intake of alcohol and is told that referral to a substance use disorder counselor is available. A safety plan is developed that includes calling his daughters more regularly, increasing his social activities with friends, and contacting the psychiatrist immediately if suicidal ideation intensifies. Follow-up is scheduled for 1 week, and the psychiatrist contacts the neurologist and primary care provider to coordinate care.

Given the concern that Mr. Armstrong has major neurocognitive disorder and heightened risk of suicide soon after a dementia diagnosis, he will need to be monitored especially closely for suicidal ideation in the ensuing months.

SUICIDE IN LONG-TERM CARE SETTINGS

For many patients living in long-term care facilities, transitioning to life in this type of setting is difficult. Loss of independence can lead to strong feelings of disappointment related not only to a change in lifestyle but also the acknowledgment that one's identity as a fully independent individual has changed. Many people's core values revolve around work and what society interprets as productivity; it is therefore not uncommon for patients to associate living in a long-term care setting with a sense of worthlessness or lost hope for a meaningful future.

Consistent with the difficulties of this transition, thoughts of dying or of suicide are considered common occurrences in long-term care facilities, as well as in the period before transitioning to the long-term care facility. However, suicide in long-term care is considered a rare event, with the prevalence rate estimated to be 1% (Mills et al. 2016). Although the reasons for this discrepancy are not entirely clear, the supervised and structured setting and the presence of regular social contact with staff, volunteers, and other residents may be protective. The implication of this is that although there is likely a protective element to being in a long-term care setting, many older adults still suffer from depression and suicidal ideation, and awareness of and treatment for these conditions is needed.

When a suicide does occur, the resulting distress in family and staff are high, and medicolegal issues can be problematic to navigate. All facilities are best served by having procedures in place with respect to screening and provision of treatment, as well as educating staff about suicide risk and having clear lines of communication among staff and providers. Retrospective reviews of suicides in skilled nursing facilities identified the following areas of improvement: staff education on suicide, communication of risk among staff, environmental problems, suicide assessment, and treatment of suicidal patients (Mills et al. 2016).

Legal and Ethical Considerations

INVOLUNTARY COMMITMENT

Although the criteria for involuntary hospitalization vary by jurisdiction, there are commonalities, at least in the United States. Civil commitment laws typically include these elements: 1) the person has a mental illness, 2) the person is a danger to self or others or has a grave disability,

3) treatment is required, 4) the person is experiencing deterioration, and 5) the person lacks competence around the decision to be hospitalized. Many jurisdictions also include a requirement to pursue less restrictive alternatives if possible and may provide procedures to facilitate commitment to a less restrictive alternative.

The approach I use to determine whether to proceed with involuntary treatment is related to the suicide risk assessment described earlier in the chapter. The first question to consider is whether the best form of treatment would be psychiatric hospitalization. If a patient is assessed at a high-risk level for suicide, then psychiatric hospitalization is indeed the more appropriate route, and voluntary hospitalization is recommended. At this level, a patient would also meet criteria for involuntary psychiatric hospitalization in most cases. Determining the best treatment is more problematic at the moderate-risk level for suicide. A voluntary psychiatric admission may be clinically appropriate, especially if outpatient resources are unavailable, but the patient may not meet imminent risk criteria for involuntary hospitalization either legally or ethically. In such cases, providing the best outpatient treatment available may be the only feasible option. From a medicolegal perspective, it is important to document carefully that hospitalization was recommended but declined by the patient and reasons why that patient did not meet criteria for involuntary treatment.

SUICIDE AT THE END OF LIFE

Addressing suicide risk at the end of life is a challenging issue and could take an entire chapter on its own. There are often complex ethical conflicts involved, such as the values of autonomy versus beneficence and a medical provider's directive to do no harm. That being said, these issues arise frequently in geriatric practice, so anyone caring for older adults will need to become familiar with this topic. Examples of such scenarios include advance directive discussion about goals of care; a patient stating that he would consider suicide an option if a certain pain or disability threshold is reached; a patient requesting discontinuation of life-prolonging treatment; and a patient asking for physician-assisted suicide, particularly in jurisdictions where this is legally allowed.

Although mental health providers can and often do evaluate ethical considerations and may be members of ethics committees in facilities, most often we are called on for a more pragmatic issue to address: Is depression influencing a patient's decisions? And if so, what course of action should be taken next? Questions arise around whether to proceed with a patient's decisions or whether to consider the patient unable to make these decisions because of depression (and therefore defer to a different decision-making process), or even to consider psychiatric hospitalization because of concern about risk for self-harm.

One factor to consider in determining suicide risk at end of life is to establish whether depression is present and to what severity, especially because depression is associated with cognitive distortions that can affect the will to live (Walaszek 2009). Psychological distress is normal and expected when a patient is faced with terminal illness, and it is important to distinguish between typical grief and distress apart from major depression, a distinct clinical disorder (Widera and Block 2012). If depression is present, treatment of depression is indicated at the very least to relieve suffering; treatment may also alter the patient's decision-making around suicide assuming this decision is being influenced by depression. The severity of depression is also important because if a patient has most or all symptoms of a major depressive episode, there is a greater likelihood that suicidal ideation is a symptom of the psychiatric disorder.

However, how individuals view their life and how they will die can be a distinct, values-driven perspective, separate from psychiatric illness. In many cases, someone's request to stop life-sustaining treatment or for physician-assisted suicide is driven by how he or she interprets issues of control, dignity, and autonomy. An inquiry into a person's longer-standing values and the overall context of his or her life history can provide some help in determining the person's perspective, and an interview that includes a discussion of these topics is essential. For example, someone who highly values independence and autonomy may express a desire to maintain control over the dying process and therefore may wish to consider physician-assisted suicide. In an opposite scenario, for a person whose life history is consistent with strongly held religious beliefs, including beliefs against suicide, a request for physician-assisted suicide could be contrary to his or her values and therefore is more likely to be due to depression. In addition, an advance directive completed when a patient's depression was less severe would provide confirmatory information about the patient's views on life-sustaining treatment and resuscitation. Information from family or friends can be helpful because these individuals can speak to the patient's past statements on the issue.

After determining a diagnosis of depression and separately to what degree depression is contributing to expressions about suicide, the next question to answer is how to proceed. If a patient is requesting physician-assisted suicide, areas where this is legal will have parameters that need to be followed, which usually include treatment of depression. In some situations, next steps are less clear, such as when patients are asking to discontinue life-sustaining treatment and are seeking a palliative approach.

The imperative to treat depression still exists in these situations. However, I have worked with cases of severe treatment-resistant depression in which depression treatment may worsen quality of life (e.g., medication side effects, burden of frequent psychotherapy visits in a frail patient, frequent hospital visits for ECT and associated cognitive-adverse effects). Psychiatric hospitalization could also be considered contrary to palliative care goals, particularly when involuntary psychiatric hospitalization is being considered. These types of cases are complicated, and different treatment team members often will have differing opinions: some may want to pursue an aggressive depression treatment course, whereas others may wish to proceed with the request to discontinue treatment. Communication about goals of care, with ongoing collaboration between the patient, family, spiritual advisors, and treatment team members, usually brings some degree of direction in these challenging situations.

Summary: Importance of Suicide Risk Assessment in Older Adults

Suicide is both a personal and a public health tragedy that disproportionately affects older adults. For health care providers who work with older adults, awareness of suicide screening, risk assessment, and intervention are core skills, and in this chapter we provide some approaches, tools, and resources to assist in our ongoing growth in this area. My hope is that with the work that we do in this field, whether we are working with a patient in the clinic, in an emergency room, or at a nursing home, we can identify patients at risk, reduce their suffering, and thereby save a life from suicide. Equally important are those of us in administrative positions and our partners in social services organizations where suicide risk is addressed at a system or public health level. Our efforts can and do change the lives of our patients and can reverse the trend of increasing numbers of suicides in the United States and elsewhere.

KEY POINTS

- The demographic that historically has had and continues to have the highest suicide rate in the United States is men ages 75 and older.

- Screening with a validated screening instrument is recommended. Commonly used screening tools include the Patient Health Questionnaire two-item version (PHQ-2) supplemented by item 9 from the nine-item version and the Columbia Suicide Severity Rating Scale (C-SSRS).

- A suicide risk assessment includes the following:
  - Identification of risk factors
  - Identification of protective factors
  - An inquiry about thoughts about suicide, including the nature of these thoughts, planning, and intent
  - Documentation of the assessment, rationale, and treatment or disposition plan

- Possible settings for intervention include psychiatric hospitalization (including involuntary hospitalization), intensive outpatient or partial hospitalization programs, and outpatient mental health treatment.

- Suicide risk reduction involves the following:
  - Risk factor reduction, including pharmacological, biological, and psychotherapeutic treatments for psychiatric illness
  - Means reduction
  - Enhancement of protective factors, particularly social connectedness
  - Safety planning

- Procedures at the clinic or hospital system level can help identify at-risk patients and help them access care. Resources to help implement these procedures include trainings on the collaborative care model from the American Psychiatric Association and toolkits from the Zero Suicide initiative.

- Area agencies on aging are a good resource for older adults to access free or low-cost services, including nutrition and health and wellness support, social opportunities, transportation services, and caregiver education and support.

- It is important to be comfortable with complex ethical situations such as suicide at end of life because they are not uncommon occurrences when working with older adults.

Resources for Patients, Families, and Caregivers

CRISIS NUMBERS AND CHATS

National Suicide Prevention Lifeline
https://suicidepreventionlifeline.org
Crisis Text Line
www.crisistextline.org
1-800-273-TALK (8255)
Text HOME to 741741

Friendship Line
www.ioaging.org/services/all-inclusive-health-care/friendship-line
1-800-971-0016

OTHER AGENCIES AND RESOURCES

National Association of Area Agencies on Aging
www.n4a.org
Suicide Prevention Resource Center
www.sprc.org
National Alliance on Mental Illness
www.nami.org

Resources for Clinicians

SUICIDE SCREENING INSTRUMENTS

Patient Health Questionnaire (PHQ)
www.phqscreeners.com
Columbia Suicide Severity Rating Scale (C-SSRS)
https://cssrs.columbia.edu

SUICIDE RISK ASSESSMENT AND SAFETY PLANNING TOOLS

SAFE-T Pocket Card: Suicide Assessment Five-Step Evaluation and Triage for Clinicians

https://store.samhsa.gov/product/SAFE-T-Pocket-Card-Suicide-Assessment-Five-Step-Evaluation-and-Triage-for-Clinicians/sma09-4432

Suicide Safety Plan

https:// suicidesafetyplan.com

COLLABORATIVE CARE

American Psychiatric Association Integrated Care

www.psychiatry.org/psychiatrists/practice/professional-interests/integrated-care

University of Washington Advancing Integrated Mental Health Solutions (AIMS) Center

http:// aims.uw.edu

OTHER AGENCIES AND RESOURCES

Zero Suicide

https://zerosuicide.edc.org

References

Alexopoulos GS, Reynolds CF 3rd, Bruce ML, et al: Reducing suicidal ideation and depression in older primary care patients: 24-month outcomes of the PROSPECT study. Am J Psychiatry 166(8):882–890, 2009 19528195

American Psychiatric Association: Practice Guideline for the Assessment and Treatment of Patients With Suicidal Behaviors. Washington, DC, American Psychiatric Association, 2010. Available at: https://psychiatryonline.org/pb/assets/raw/sitewide/practice_guidelines/guidelines/suicide.pdf. Accessed January 15, 2021.

Arias SA, Boudreaux ED, Segal DL, et al: Disparities in treatment of older adults with suicide risk in the emergency department. J Am Geriatr Soc 65(10):2272–2277, 2017 28752539

Betz ME, Arias SA, Segal DL, et al: Screening for suicidal thoughts and behaviors in older adults in the emergency department. J Am Geriatr Soc 64(10):e72–e77, 2016 27596110

Bozzay ML, Primack J, Barredo J, et al: Transcranial magnetic stimulation to reduce suicidality—a review and naturalistic outcomes. J Psychiatr Res 125:106–112, 2020 32251917

Chan SM, Chiu FK, Lam CW, et al: Elderly suicide and the 2003 SARS epidemic in Hong Kong. Int J Geriatr Psychiatry 21(2):113–118, 2006 16416469

Cooper C, Katona C, Lyketsos K, et al: A systematic review of treatments for refractory depression in older people. Am J Psychiatry 168(7):681–688, 2011 21454919

Department of Veterans Affairs: VA/DoD Clinical Practice Guideline for the Assessment and Management of Patients at Risk for Suicide. Washington, DC, Department of Veterans Affairs, May 2019. Available at: www.health quality.va.gov/guidelines/MH/srb/VADoDSuicideRiskFullCPGFinal 5088212019.pdf. Accessed January 15, 2021.

Günak MM, Barnes DE, Yaffe K, et al: Risk of suicide attempt in patients with recent diagnosis of mild cognitive impairment or dementia. JAMA Psychiatry March 24, 2021 Epub ahead of print 33760039

Gustavson KA, Alexopoulos GS, Niu GC, et al: Problem-solving therapy reduces suicidal ideation in depressed older adults with executive dysfunction. Am J Geriatr Psychiatry 24(1):11–17, 2016 26743100

Hedegaard H, Curtin SC, Warner M: Suicide mortality in the United States, 1999–2017. NCHS Data Brief (330):1–8, 2018a 30500324

Hedegaard H, Curtin SC, Warner M: Suicide rates in the United States continue to increase. NCHS Data Brief (309):1–8, 2018b 30312151

Heisel MJ: Suicide and its prevention among older adults. Can J Psychiatry 51(3):143–154, 2006 16618005

Heisel MJ, Talbot NL, King DA, et al: Adapting interpersonal psychotherapy for older adults at risk for suicide. Am J Geriatr Psychiatry 23(1):87–98, 2015 24840611

Jin HM, Khazem LR, Anestis MD: Recent advances in means safety as a suicide prevention strategy. Curr Psychiatry Rep 18(10):96, 2016 27629355

Kellner CH, Fink M, Knapp R, et al: Relief of expressed suicidal intent by ECT: a consortium for research in ECT study. Am J Psychiatry 162(5):977–982, 2005 15863801

Kiosses DN, Rosenberg PB, McGovern A, et al: Depression and suicidal ideation during two psychosocial treatments in older adults with major depression and dementia. J Alzheimers Dis 48(2):453–462, 2015 26402009

Leavey K, Hawkins R: Is cognitive behavioural therapy effective in reducing suicidal ideation and behaviour when delivered face-to-face or via e-health? A systematic review and meta-analysis. Cogn Behav Ther 46(5):353–374, 2017 28621202

LeFevre ML; U.S. Preventive Services Task Force: Screening for suicide risk in adolescents, adults, and older adults in primary care: U.S. Preventive Services Task Force recommendation statement. Ann Intern Med 160(10):719–726, 2014 24842417

Lepkifker E, Iancu I, Horesh N, et al: Lithium therapy for unipolar and bipolar depression among the middle-aged and older adult patient subpopulation. Depress Anxiety 24(8):571–576, 2007 17133442

Louzon SA, Bossarte R, McCarthy JF, et al: Does suicidal ideation as measured by the PHQ-9 predict suicide among VA patients? Psychiatr Serv 67(5):517–522, 2016 26766757

McDonald WM: Neuromodulation treatments for geriatric mood and cognitive disorders. Am J Geriatr Psychiatry 24(12):1130–1141, 2016 27889282

Meltzer HY, Alphs L, Green AI, et al: Clozapine treatment for suicidality in schizophrenia: International Suicide Prevention Trial (InterSePT). Arch Gen Psychiatry 60(1):82–91, 2003 12511175

Meyer JP, Swetter SK, Kellner CH: Electroconvulsive therapy in geriatric psychiatry: a selective review. Clin Geriatr Med 36(2):265–279, 2020 32222301

Mills PD, Gallimore BI, Watts BV, et al: Suicide attempts and completions in Veterans Affairs nursing home care units and long-term care facilities: a review of root-cause analysis reports. Int J Geriatr Psychiatry 31(5):518–525, 2016 26422195

Morgan ER, Gomez A, Rivara FP, et al: Household firearm ownership and storage, suicide risk factors, and memory loss among older adults: results from a statewide survey. Ann Intern Med 171(3):220–222, 2019 30986820

Nezu AM, Maguth Nezu C, D'Zurilla T: Problem-Solving Therapy: A Treatment Manual. New York, Springer, 2013

Ochs-Ross R, Daly EJ, Zhang Y, et al: Efficacy and safety of esketamine nasal spray plus an oral antidepressant in elderly patients with treatment-resistant depression—TRANSFORM-3. Am J Geriatr Psychiatry 28(2):121–141, 2020 31734084

Office of the Surgeon General (US); National Action Alliance for Suicide Prevention (US): 2012 National Strategy for Suicide Prevention: Goals and Objectives for Action: A Report of the U.S. Surgeon General and of the National Action Alliance for Suicide Prevention. Washington, DC, U.S. Department of Health and Human Services, 2012

Posner K, Brown GK, Stanley B, et al: The Columbia-Suicide Severity Rating Scale: initial validity and internal consistency findings from three multisite studies with adolescents and adults. Am J Psychiatry 168(12):1266–1277, 2011 22193671

Seyfried LS, Kales HC, Ignacio RV, et al: Predictors of suicide in patients with dementia. Alzheimers Dement 7(6):567–573, 2011 22055973

Simon GE, Rutter CM, Peterson D, et al: Does response on the PHQ-9 Depression Questionnaire predict subsequent suicide attempt or suicide death? Psychiatr Serv 64(12):1195–1202, 2013 24036589

Siu AL, Bibbins-Domingo K, Grossman DC, et al: Screening for depression in adults: US Preventive Services Task Force Recommendation statement. JAMA 315(4):380–387, 2016 26813211

Smith KA, Cipriani A: Lithium and suicide in mood disorders: updated meta-review of the scientific literature. Bipolar Disord 19(7):575–586, 2017 28895269

Stanley B, Brown GK: Safety planning intervention: a brief intervention to mitigate suicide risk. Cognit Behav Pract 19(2):256–264, 2012

Steele IH, Thrower N, Noroian P, et al: Understanding suicide across the lifespan: A United States perspective of suicide risk factors, assessment and management. J Forensic Sci 63(1):162–171, 2018 28639299

Stone M, Laughren T, Jones ML, et al: Risk of suicidality in clinical trials of antidepressants in adults: analysis of proprietary data submitted to US Food and Drug Administration. BMJ 339:b2880, 2009 19671933

Studdert DM, Zhang Y, Swanson SA, et al: Handgun ownership and suicide in California. N Engl J Med 382(23):2220–2229, 2020 32492303

Substance Abuse and Mental Health Services Administration: Suicide Assessment Five-Step Evaluation and Triage (SAFE-T) Pocket Card. HHS Publ No (SMA) 09-4432. Rockville MD, Substance Abuse and Mental Health Services Administration, 2009. Available at: https://store.samhsa.gov/sites/default/files/d7/priv/sma09-4432.pdf. Accessed May 18, 2021.

The Joint Commission: National Patient Safety Goal for Suicide Prevention. R3 Report. Oakbrook Terrace, IL, The Joint Commission, November 27, 2019. Available at: www.jointcommission.org/-/media/tjc/documents/standards/r3-reports/r3_18_suicide_prevention_hap_bhc_cah_11_4_19_final1.pdf. Accessed January 15, 2021.

Raue PJ, Ghesquiere AR, Bruce ML: Suicide risk in primary care: identification and management in older adults. Curr Psychiatry Rep 16(9):466, 2014 25030971

Unützer J, Tang L, Oishi S, et al; IMPACT Investigators: Reducing suicidal ideation in depressed older primary care patients. J Am Geriatr Soc 54(10):1550–1556, 2006 17038073

Vahia IV, Jeste DV, Reynolds CF 3rd: Older adults and the mental health effects of COVID-19. JAMA 324(22):2253–2254, 2020 33216114

Van Orden K, Deming C: Late-life suicide prevention strategies: current status and future directions. Curr Opin Psychol 22:79–83, 2018 28938218

Walaszek A: Clinical ethics issues in geriatric psychiatry. Psychiatr Clin North Am 32(2):343–359, 2009 19486818

Weissman MM, Markowitz JC, Klerman G: Comprehensive Guide to Interpersonal Psychotherapy. New York, Basic Books, 2000

Widera EW, Block SD: Managing grief and depression at the end of life. Am Fam Physician 86(3):259–264, 2012 22962989

Wilkinson ST, Ballard ED, Bloch MH, et al: The effect of a single dose of intravenous ketamine on suicidal ideation: a systematic review and individual participant data meta-analysis. Am J Psychiatry 175(2):150–158, 2018 28969441

World Health Organization: Suicide in the World: Global Health Estimates. Geneva, Switzerland, World Health Organization, 2019

Yeates C: Suicide later in life: challenges and priorities for prevention. Am J Prev Med 47(3 suppl 2):S244–S250, 2014 25145746

CHAPTER 5

Management of Late-Life Depression and Anxiety

Anna Borisovskaya, M.D.
Elizabeth Chmelik, M.D.
William Bryson, M.D., Ph.D.
Matthew Schreiber, M.D.
Marcella Pascualy, M.D.
Samantha May, M.D.
Courtney Roberts, M.D.

PRÉCIS

A variety of effective treatments exist for late-life depression and anxiety. Every treatment plan begins with psychoeducation of older adult patients and their families. There is strong evidence for psychotherapy, which patients often prefer and which is safer than pharmacotherapy; in some settings, psychotherapy (e.g., cognitive-behavioral therapy for insomnia, problem-solving therapy for patients with executive dysfunction) offers significant advantages over medications. Pharmacotherapy is generally effective and requires careful weighing of benefits and risks because older adults are more prone to side effects and drug-drug interactions than are younger adults. Exercise, bright light therapy, and alternative treatments such as art or music therapy serve as excellent augmentation strategies. For patients with severe depression, psychotic depression, or treatment-resistant depression, electroconvulsive therapy is the most effective treatment, and evidence is emerging for the efficacy of repetitive transcranial magnetic stimulation and ketamine. Collaborative care models are interventions that health care systems can implement to improve the care of older adults with mental illness. More research is urgently needed to understand how to effectively use and adapt these treatments for older adults.

Psychoeducation of Patients and Families

Treatment of late-life depression and anxiety begins with psychoeducation. Psychoeducation is a "learning experience designed to facilitate voluntary behavior changes that improve and maintain health" (Cho et al. 2016, p. 286). Key components of effective psychoeducation include early detection of symptoms, improved understanding of an illness and its treatment options, and promoting healthy lifestyle habits in a way that empowers individuals to become active participants in their own care; it is often most valuable during periods of euthymia when a person has optimal emotional and cognitive capacity to engage in thoughtful dialogue (Cho et al. 2016). Psychoeducation can include paper handouts, individual discussions, or groups. Cho et al. proposed a framework for psychoeducation that we believe is useful in the care of older adults (Table 5–1).

Psychoeducation about late-life depression and anxiety can also be useful as a preventive strategy for older adults who are at risk for negative beliefs about mental health care and stigma-related barriers to engagement and are vulnerable to social isolation, physical decline, reduced mobility, cognitive impairment, financial strain, and bereavement (Blais et al. 2015; O'Dwyer et al. 2012). Psychoeducation focused on positive experiences can improve the well-being of and reduce depression and insomnia in older adults (Friedman et al. 2017). Psychoeducation focused on modifiable risk factors for cognitive decline, including depression and anxiety, can help improve knowledge about healthy brain aging (Norrie et al. 2011).

Table 5–1. Framework for psychoeducational interventions

Component of psychoeducation	Example questions to guide discussion	Goal of intervention
Illness understanding	• What is your diagnosis, and do you agree with it? • How does this illness interfere with your life goals?	• Enhance insight • Reduce stigma
Pharmacological treatment	• What is getting in the way of you taking medications? • What have you or others noticed since you began to take medications?	• Identify treatment goals • Address barriers to adherence • Engage in motivational interviewing • Build alliance and rapport
Promoting a healthy lifestyle	• How are you managing stress? • What is your diet like? • What kinds of exercise do you enjoy? • Are you smoking or using other substances?	• Encourage healthy lifestyle habits to promote general physical and emotional wellness • Promote healthy coping skills
Involving family and caregivers	• What is your understanding of your family member's illness? • What have you noticed about your family member's response to medications? • What signs or symptoms do you notice when your family member is depressed or anxious, and what steps can you take to help him or her?	• Help family encourage and support appropriate treatment for the patient • Encourage family to partner with care teams to support the patient's recovery • Connect family with caregiver support groups if needed
Preventing relapse	• What are some of your warning signs for relapse? • What is your plan when you notice symptoms return?	• Reduce risk for relapse • Maintain symptom remission during the recovery phase of illness

Source.   Adapted from Cho et al. 2016.

Effective psychoeducation is tailored to an individual's specific situation, needs, preferences, and resources (Cho et al. 2016; O'Dwyer et al. 2012). The first step is to assess a person's unique explanatory model for his or her illness with attention to misconceptions, perceived need for care, and barriers to access (Cunningham et al. 2007; Srinivasan et al. 2003). For example, the Treatment Initiation Program (TIP), a psychoeducational model for older adults prescribed a new psychotropic medication, was designed to elicit barriers to treatment such as misconceptions about depression and its treatment, perceived stigma, cognitive distortions, and logistical barriers and then to address each barrier (Sirey et al. 2005). Individuals assigned to the TIP were more likely to accept and remain in treatment and showed greater decrease in depression severity compared with usual care, confirming the importance of psychoeducation in the treatment of older adults with depression and anxiety (Sirey et al. 2005).

There are several additional elements to consider in adapting psychoeducational interventions to older adults. It's important to adapt the way that audiovisual information is presented, given sensory changes that can occur with age, such as hearing loss or worsened eyesight. Larger fonts, increased spacing, and use of colors to emphasize key concepts may optimize visual learning, and a loud and clear voice is likely to enhance the auditory learning experience for older adults with hearing loss (O'Dwyer et al. 2012). For individuals who are self-conscious about sensory deficits or are unable to participate fully because of them, group settings may not be ideal. Finally, information that is presented succinctly and clearly is likely to promote best learning for those struggling with early cognitive impairment (Norrie et al. 2011).

Older adults may not have the skills, resources, or physical ability to benefit from technological advances such as internet-based apps and video appointments (telepsychiatry). In order to be effective, we must adapt technology to ensure it is learnable, efficient, and pleasant to use, with a low error rate (Helbostad et al. 2017).

Up to one-third of older adults present to their primary care appointments with a family member, providing an opportunity for family involvement in psychoeducation (Hinton et al. 2019). Partnering with family members can help the patient and clinician detect early signs of depression or anxiety and encourage persons to seek needed care. Family members can be helpful partners in reducing stigma, promoting access to prescribed treatments, and holding a patient accountable for enacting a recommended care plan (Hinton et al. 2019). Staying attuned to cultural factors (including expectations about family members' roles in the care of older adults) is essential for engaging and promoting productive family involvement. Collaboration with community partners to adapt and deliver psychoeducational interventions in settings likely to feel acceptable for a person and his or her community can overcome cultural barriers and improve access to effective treatments (Sadavoy et al. 2004). Alas, it is not universally true that family involvement is beneficial: for older adults with conflicted family relationships or complicated family dynamics, family involvement may interfere with care.

Psychotherapy

Psychotherapy for late-life depression and anxiety is a robust treatment with effect sizes matching those in younger adults. The efficacy of psychotherapy in late-life depression and anxiety has been substantiated in the context of such medical comorbidities as chronic obstructive pulmonary disease, heart failure, Parkinson's disease, and stroke, as well as in patients with cognitive impairment and suicide risk (Raue et al. 2017). Older adults generally express comparable or even higher interest in psychotherapy than in medications or combined treatment (Gum et al. 2006; Luck-Sikorski et al. 2017). In fact, older adults with depression who also have executive dysfunction or a high degree of neuroticism may benefit more from psychotherapy than medications (Steffens et al. 2018).

Patients with dementia or other types of cognitive impairment may benefit from psychotherapy that has been modified so as to increase structure and redundancy, to adapt the conversational flow to slower rates of cognitive processing, and to flexibly modify the length of sessions (Leyhe et al. 2017); we discuss these adaptations in greater detail later in the chapter. As in younger patients, the strength of the therapeutic relationship is key to treatment success. For example, in a randomized controlled trial of older patients with major depressive disorder (MDD) and executive dysfunction receiving problem-solving therapy (PST) or supportive therapy, the quality of the therapeutic relationship predicted reduction of depression in both interventions (Mace et al. 2017). Given the substantial medical burden of many elderly patients, collaborating with all of the patients' physicians is vital. Involving family members in therapy may promote efficacy; for example, a systematic review of interventions involving spouses and close family members demonstrated moderate effectiveness for treating late-life depression (Stahl et al. 2016).

Cognitive-behavioral therapy (CBT), interpersonal therapy (IPT), and PST are the most effective psychotherapeutic interventions for late-life depression and anxiety; thus, we cover them in detail in the following subsections. We strongly recommend psychotherapy for all older adults with depression of mild or moderate severity. See Table 5–2 for a summary of these and other psychotherapies and Table 5–3 for definitions of depression severity.

Table 5–2. Summary of psychotherapy in late-life depression and anxiety

Modality	Comments
CBT	CBT is generally effective for anxiety and depressive disorders. It may also be effective, with adaption, in older adults with cognitive impairment. It can be delivered via internet or telephone.
CBT-I	CBT-I should be considered as first-line treatment for insomnia in older adults. It can be helpful for reducing use of and discontinuing benzodiazepines and may help reduce depression.
Third-wave cognitive behavioral therapies	Overall, these therapies are not well studied in older adults. The strongest evidence base is for MBSR and MBCT for depression, anxiety, and insomnia. DBT may be helpful in chronic depression and depression comorbid with personality disorder. Not enough evidence is available regarding ACT.
IPT	Although results of controlled trials are somewhat mixed, there is evidence to support use of IPT (alone or combined with an antidepressant) for acute or maintenance treatment of depression, depression in primary care, and subsyndromal depression and for older adults at risk of suicide.
PST and PATH	Strong evidence exists for PST in older adults with depression, including those with medical illness or cognitive impairment. There is emerging evidence for PATH as effective for depressed elders with cognitive impairment.
Brief psychodynamic psychotherapy	This therapy may be effective, but it has a much smaller evidence base than other therapies.
Life review and reminiscence	Reminiscence therapy is effective at reducing depressive symptoms in older adults with and without dementia.

Note. See text for details.
Abbreviations. ACT=acceptance and commitment therapy; CBT=cognitive-behavioral therapy; CBT-I=cognitive-behavioral therapy for insomnia; DBT=dialectical behavior therapy; IPT=interpersonal psychotherapy; MBCT=mindfulness-based cognitive therapy; MBSR=mindfulness-based stress reduction; PATH=problem adaptation therapy; PST=problem-solving therapy.

Table 5–3. Describing the severity of depression

DSM-5 severity specifiers	PHQ-9 score range
Mild: Few, if any, symptoms in excess of those required to make the diagnosis are present, the intensity of the symptoms is distressing but manageable, and the symptoms result in minor impairment in social or occupational functioning.	5–9
Moderate: The number of symptoms, intensity of symptoms, and/or functional impairment are between those specified for "mild" and "severe."	10–14
Severe: The number of symptoms is substantially in excess of that required to make the diagnosis, the intensity of the symptoms is seriously distressing and unmanageable, and the symptoms markedly interfere with social and occupational functioning.	15–19 (moderately severe) or 20–27 (severe)

Abbreviation.   PHQ-9=Patient Health Questionnaire, nine-item version.
Source.   Adapted from American Psychiatric Association 2013; Kroenke et al. 2001.

There is a great need for developing and testing other psychotherapeutic interventions for older adults as well as promoting referrals and access, especially in ethnic minority older adults (Conner et al. 2010). We must ensure that physicians and psychotherapists are properly trained to care for the ever-increasing number of older adults, many of whom would benefit from psychotherapy for late-life depression and anxiety (Laidlaw 2013).

COGNITIVE-BEHAVIORAL THERAPY

The evidence supporting the use of CBT in older adults with anxiety disorders is strong. A systematic review and meta-analysis of studies comprising 297 patients showed that CBT is effective for late-life anxiety disorders (including generalized anxiety disorder [GAD], social phobia, and agoraphobia), with significant effects on anxiety symptoms, worrying, and depression (Hendriks et al. 2008). In GAD, CBT is more effective than no treatment, but benefits may not be sustained after 6 months (Hall et al. 2016). CBT may also augment response to antidepressants in GAD. For example, in a small open-label study, 10 patients received 12 weeks of escitalopram followed by 16 weeks of escitalopram augmented with modular CBT; adding CBT to escitalopram resulted in significant reduction of anxiety symptoms (Wetherell et al. 2011b). A modification of CBT, prolonged exposure therapy, may be helpful in the treatment of PTSD in older adults (Thorp et al. 2019).

There have been many studies of CBT in older adults with depression. The results have generally been positive, although several reviews (e.g., Jonsson et al. 2016) pointed out problems in the design of many of these studies. Despite these methodological limitations, it does appear that CBT is probably effective in late-life depression (Kiosses et al. 2011).

CBT has been adapted to the needs of patients with late-life depression in a variety of ways. For example, weekly group CBT sessions were shown to benefit older adults with depression who were also recovering from an acute medical illness (Hummel et al. 2017). Another example is Engage, a behavioral intervention meant to target brain circuit abnormalities primarily through "reward exposure," starting with simple social and physical activities and gradually stepping up their intensity and complexity (Alexopoulos et al. 2016a). A large clinical trial ($N=249$) of older adults with depression found that Engage had similar outcomes to PST (discussed in a later subsection) (Alexopoulos et al. 2020). Interestingly, even when Engage was employed successfully, there was evidence of impaired reward learning in some patients, which increased the risk of depression relapse (Victoria et al. 2018).

Behavioral activation, a component of CBT, may play a special role in the treatment of late-life depression. Intentional activity scheduling, particularly of social and family-related activities, has been associated with a decrease in depressive symptoms during the Improving Mood—Promoting Access to Collaborative Treatment (IMPACT) trial (Riebe et al. 2012). A systematic review of CBT for older adults living in residential facilities and experiencing depression and anxiety found evidence of efficacy in 8 out of 12 studies; the content of effective interventions included psychoeducation, behavioral activation, and problem-solving techniques; both residents and staff viewed CBT favorably (Chan et al. 2021).

With adaptations, CBT is effective in treating anxiety and depression in patients with dementia. A systematic review of 11 studies involving 116 older adults had promising results; the patients included in the studies had a Clinical Dementia Rating (CDR) score of 2 or less or Mini-Mental Status Examination (MMSE) score greater than 15 (Tay et al. 2019). Using a greater amount of repetition, simplifying homework, focusing on behavioral components, including caregivers in treatment, and using the spaced retrieval technique (Paukert et al. 2010) can improve learning in patients with cognitive impairment. *Spaced retrieval* pairs verbal learning with procedural memory (which remains intact later in the course of dementia). For example, the patient learns a self-soothing technique while at the same time picking up a note card on which that technique is written. The therapist has the patient retrieve learned information at increasing time intervals (e.g., from 1 minute to 2 minutes); if the patient has difficulty recalling the information, the therapist has the patient learn it again, and the next retrieval interval is shortened (e.g., from 2 minutes to 1 minute).

There is some controversy regarding whether executive dysfunction, a common feature of late-life depression, anxiety, and dementia, can improve or worsen the response to CBT. In one study, poor performance on the Wisconsin Card Sort Task performance, indicative of executive dysfunction, was associated with better response to CBT (Goodkind et al. 2016). In another study, poor cognitive flexibility, an aspect of executive functioning, was associated with poorer learning from *cognitive restructuring*, a CBT technique that helps patients identify and dispute maladaptive thoughts (Johnco et al. 2015). It has been suggested that psychotherapies that address the executive skill of switching, a trait that may be predicted by performance on the Trails B test, could augment treatment response in older patients with executive dysfunction (Beaudreau et al. 2015). From that perspective, PST, which addresses executive function, may offer advantages over CBT; we discuss PST in greater detail later in the chapter.

Access to CBT can be a challenge for older adults. CBT can be delivered at home, via the internet (ICBT), or over the phone. For example, a study of 134 rural-dwelling adults ages 65 years and older with anxious symptoms and decreased quality of life randomly assigned to CBT delivered at home or minimal support saw greater improvement in symptoms with CBT treatment (DiNapoli et al. 2017). ICBT has been shown to be effective for older adults with either late-life depression or GAD, with depressed older adults demonstrating better adherence than depressed younger adults (Hobbs et al. 2017, 2018). Telephone-delivered CBT has been demonstrated to be superior to supportive therapy in rural older adults with GAD, with gains maintained up to 1 year after completing treatment (Brenes et al. 2017). CBT can be delivered by non-expert lay providers working under expert supervision, with equivocal results (Freshour et al. 2016). CBT is also effective for treating late-life depression and anxiety when delivered as group therapy (Wuthrich and Rapee 2013; Wuthrich et al. 2016).

There are very few studies assessing the effectiveness of CBT in ethnic minority elders or evaluating whether making cultural adaptations in the delivery of therapy is beneficial (Fuentes and Aranda 2012). At the same time, physicians are less likely to refer ethnic minority elders than white elders to psychotherapy (Mansour et al. 2020). These are critical areas for psychotherapy research and public policy. In addition, it may be valuable to incorporate religion into CBT when treating older adults with depression and anxiety (Paukert et al. 2009).

CBT FOR INSOMNIA

Insomnia is a common complaint in the elderly, particularly those suffering from depression, anxiety, and poor overall health status. It is also a significant and underappreciated risk factor for onset of depression that is potentially treatable (Cole and Dendukuri 2003). Pharmacological treatment options such as benzodiazepines (BZDs) and hypnotics should be used cautiously in the elderly given the associated risks of sedation, confusion, falls, worsening depression, and suicide (Gooneratne and Vitiello 2014). Nonpharmacological approaches such as CBT-I have become first-line treatments for insomnia in older adults. CBT-I, which incorporates cognitive therapy, stimulus control, sleep restriction, sleep hygiene, and relaxation, has been demonstrated to improve several sleep-related measures (sleep onset latency, wake after sleep onset, total sleep time, and sleep efficiency) (Trauer et al. 2015). CBT-I is an effective treatment for adults with chronic insomnia, with effects sustained over time and therefore offering advantages over hypnotic medications (Trauer et al. 2015). Another advantage of CBT-I is that it can be delivered effectively over the internet. In a recent meta-analysis, it was found that CBT-I decreased the insomnia severity index and the severity of depression, effects maintained 4–48 weeks after the treatment (Seyffert et al. 2016).

CBT-I hasn't been studied as extensively in older adults, but the available evidence points to at least a moderate benefit. When compared with pharmacological treatments in older patients, CBT-I demonstrates equal efficacy, with more sustained improvement. In a randomized controlled trial (RCT) that compared CBT-I with temazepam or their combination versus placebo, CBT-I (alone or in combination) was rated as more effective than temazepam by the study subjects, their significant others, and clinicians (Morin et al. 1999). In another RCT that compared CBT-I with zopiclone or placebo in older adults with chronic primary insomnia who were followed for 6 months, CBT-I resulted in improved short-term and long-term outcomes as compared with zopiclone (Sivertsen et al. 2006).

CBT-I can lead not only to improved sleep quality but also to reduced hypnotic drug use, as demonstrated in an RCT of patients between ages 31 and 92 with chronic insomnia who were receiving repeat hypnotic drug prescriptions (Morgan et al. 2004). The patients were randomly assigned to "sleep-clinic" CBT versus a "no additional treatment" control group; those treated with CBT showed improved sleep measures and reduced frequency of drug use, with many CBT-treated patients reporting no hypnotic drug use at the end of treatment. In a study of 76 older outpatients with prolonged BZD use for chronic insomnia who were randomly assigned to a 10-week supervised BZD withdrawal program, CBT-I, or combination treatment, 85% of subjects in the combination treatment arm were BZD-free after the initial intervention; combination treatment was more effective than CBT-I alone, which was more effective than supervised BZD withdrawal (Morin et al. 2004). Similar results were seen in a larger RCT that compared CBT-I plus gradual tapering of BZDs prescribed for chronic insomnia versus gradual tapering of treatment only (Baillargeon et al. 2003).

An abbreviated form of CBT-I (4 weeks rather than 6–8 weeks) has also been found to be effective in older adults with insomnia (McCrae et al. 2018). CBT-I may also improve depressive symptoms in older adults (Tanaka et al. 2019). Finally, CBT-I can be delivered by nonclinician sleep coaches, making it an accessible and cost-effective treatment (Alessi et al. 2016).

THIRD-WAVE COGNITIVE-BEHAVIORAL THERAPIES

So-called third-wave CBTs incorporate mindfulness, emotions, acceptance, the therapeutic relationship, values, goals, and metacognition into CBT. Examples include *acceptance and commitment therapy* (ACT), *dialectical behavior therapy* (DBT), *mindfulness-based cognitive therapy* (MBCT), and *mindfulness-based stress reduction* (MBSR). A Cochrane review of these therapies for treatment of depression in adults of all ages found them to be more effective than treatment as usual, although the quality of evidence was thought to be low (Churchill et al. 2013). A meta-analysis of 10 third-wave CBT trials in older adults, typically delivered in group format, found a moderate effect on reducing depressive symptoms (0.55) and anxiety symptoms (0.58), although there was evidence of publication bias (i.e., negative studies may not have been published, inflating the effect size) (Kishita et al. 2017).

Among the third-wave therapies, MBSR and MBCT have been studied the most in older adults. MBSR was developed to relieve the stresses of living with chronic illness using meditation techniques in a structured group format; participants learn to incorporate mindfulness into their daily routine (Kabat-Zinn 1990). MBCT is an adaptation of MBSR to specific clinical conditions such as depression and anxiety (Hazlett-Stevens et al. 2019). A review of seven RCTs of MBSR or MBCT in older adults (including a community sample and clinical samples with insomnia, anxiety, depression, or chronic low back pain) found the interventions to be effective (Hazlett-Stevens et al. 2019). For example, a study of 60 adults ages 75 and older with chronic insomnia found that those who underwent MBSR experienced significant improvement in sleep quality and decrease in depressive symptoms relative to the control group (Zhang et al. 2015). However, except for the study by Zhang et al. (2015), all of the studies had predominantly white subjects, thus limiting generalizability.

Patients undergoing ACT learn to reduce attempts to control negative thoughts and emotions and instead focus on engaging more in meaningful life activities. A pilot study comparing ACT with CBT for treatment of GAD found that older adults benefited with both approaches; those in ACT were more likely to complete treatment than those in CBT (Wetherell et al. 2011a). An uncontrolled trial of telephone-based ACT in 15 dementia caregivers (mean age 69, 80% women, all non-Hispanic white) with significant anxiety found marked reduction in anxiety symptoms (Fowler et al. 2021).

DBT, which combines CBT; mindfulness; and training in distress tolerance, emotion regulation, and interpersonal skills, is effective for people with borderline personality disorder. Unfortunately, there have been just two RCTs of DBT in older adults, both reported by Lynch et al. (2007). In the first, older adults with chronic depression who were randomly assigned to DBT plus medication management were more likely to experience remission from depression (75%) than were those assigned to medication alone (31%). In the second study, older adults with depression and comorbid personality disorder who did not respond to 8 weeks of medication management were randomly assigned to DBT plus medication or to medication alone; there were no statistically significant differences between the groups, although the DBT plus medication group achieved remission faster (Lynch et al. 2007).

We clearly need more research on these newer approaches in older adults, especially in samples with more racial and ethnic diversity.

INTERPERSONAL PSYCHOTHERAPY

IPT is a time-limited therapy that focuses on the present circumstances rather than past life issues and on the role of interpersonal difficulties in the depressive episode. The treatment is manualized and offers a strong psychoeducational component whereby the therapist serves as an advocate and an educator. IPT seems well suited to older adults: two problem areas explored in IPT are grief and role transitions (e.g., retirement). Nevertheless, although clinical experience would seem to support the benefit of IPT, the results from controlled trials have been somewhat mixed.

IPT has been studied in combination with antidepressants for acute treatment of depression. Reynolds et al. (1999b) enrolled 80 patients ages 50 and older diagnosed with MDD in an RCT with four arms (nortriptyline with IPT, nortriptyline alone, placebo with IPT, and placebo alone). Nortriptyline combined with IPT led to the highest remission rate (69%). IPT with placebo led to remission in 29% of the patients, and the remission rate for nortriptyline alone was 45%; overall, there was mixed evidence for a synergistic effect between antidepressants and IPT (Reynolds et al. 1999b). Another RCT of partial responders to escitalopram did not demonstrate added benefit of IPT (Reynolds et al. 2010).

In the primary care setting, IPT has been studied in patients 55 and older who were diagnosed with MDD. Although there were no differences between IPT and the control group in response or remission rates, 51% of those who underwent IPT no longer met criteria for MDD at 6-month follow-up, compared with 34% in the control group (van Schaik et al. 2007).

IPT may have benefit as a maintenance treatment for late-life depression, that is, as a relapse prevention strategy. For example, a trial of 107 adults older than 59 years who had experienced remission from depression after treatment with IPT and nortriptyline were randomly assigned to maintenance IPT plus nortriptyline, IPT alone, nortriptyline alone, or neither. Over the course of 3 years, remission rates were lowest (20%) in the combined treatment group; treatment with IPT alone or nortriptyline was better than placebo (Reynolds et al. 1999a). In a trial following patients recovering from MDD, additional benefits were seen in social adjustment for patients treated with a combination of nortriptyline and IPT compared with those treated with either intervention alone (Lenze et al. 2002). The focus of IPT has an effect on outcome. In an RCT comparing IPT with monthly supportive clinical management (control group), subjects receiving IPT with a focus on role conflict were less likely than were control subjects to have a depressive recurrence; however, subjects receiving IPT with a focus on role transitions or abnormal grief had no better outcomes than did control subjects (Miller et al. 2003). However, in another RCT of older patients recovering from MDD, maintenance treatment with paroxetine was superior to placebo and to IPT (Reynolds et al. 2006).

As noted in Chapter 4, "Suicide Risk Reduction in Older Adults," IPT may be helpful in older adults at risk for suicide. Heisel and colleagues (2015) enrolled 17 adults ages 60 and older who reported current suicidal ideation or who had engaged in self-injurious behavior in the previous 2 years. After a 16-week course of IPT, which included extra support (access to a therapist through a cell phone, extension of the therapy session in cases of extreme distress and agitation, and ongoing monitoring of the risk for suicide), subjects experienced a substantial reduction in suicidal ideation and depressive symptoms and improvement in interpersonal functioning (Heisel et al. 2015).

An understudied area is the treatment of subsyndromal depression. Mossey and colleagues (1996) examined interpersonal counseling, derived from IPT, to address depression that did not fulfill criteria for MDD or dysthymia in medically hospitalized patients shortly after discharge, with significant improvement in the treatment group at 6 months.

In summary, clinical wisdom and a fair amount of research support the use of IPT (either alone or in combination with an antidepressant) in older adults, including for acute and maintenance treatment of MDD, for patients in primary care, for those at risk of suicide, and for those with subsyndromal depression.

PROBLEM-SOLVING THERAPY

PST is based on cognitive-behavioral principles and is focused particularly on helping patients identify problems in living and either find effective solutions for these problems or learn how to cope with them. A meta-analysis of 30 RCTs (including 3,530 subjects) found that PST was as effective in the treatment of depression as other psychotherapies and medications and more effective than control conditions (Cuijpers et al. 2018). In another meta-analysis, limited to studies of older adults with MDD (9 studies, 569 subjects), PST was found to be effective on measures of both depression and disability (Kirkham et al. 2016).

PST has been successfully used for patients with medical illness and functional impairment (macular degeneration, stroke), and it can be delivered via internet or phone (with or without video) (Kiosses and Alexopoulos 2014). A modification of PST in primary care was found to be effective for treatment of dysthymia and minor depression, although it was not as consistently effective as paroxetine (Williams et al. 2000). As mentioned in Chapter 4, PST can reduce suicidal ideation in adults with MDD and executive dysfunction (Gustavson et al. 2016).

PST may be particularly effective in older adults with depression and executive dysfunction, sometimes referred to as the depression-executive dysfunction syndrome of late life, which is associated with greater disability and is often resistant to treatment with pharmacotherapy (Areán et al. 2010). As noted in the subsection "Cognitive-Behavioral Therapy," PST has comparable efficacy to Engage, an adaptation of CBT for people with cognitive impairment (Alexopoulos et al. 2020). However, PST does not improve cognitive deficits in patients with depression-executive dysfunction syndrome (Mackin et al. 2014). Interestingly, a trial of clinical case management compared with PST combined with case management for low-income older adults with disability demonstrated no significant advantages, which indicates that for patients who may be too impaired to engage in PST, case management offers a viable alternative (Alexopoulos et al. 2016b).

Problem adaptation therapy (PATH) is a home-delivered psychotherapy that integrates PST with compensatory strategies, environmental adaptations, and caregiver participation. It aims to improve emotion regulation and thus is particularly useful for older patients with depression and cognitive impairment (Kiosses et al. 2015a). In a preliminary study of 35 adults older than 65 years with MDD and cognitive impairment who were randomly assigned to receive PATH or home-delivered supportive therapy, PATH participants had better depression, cognitive, and disability outcomes (Kanellopoulos et al. 2020). In another RCT, PATH led to greater remission of depression (38%) compared with supportive therapy (14%), even in patients who had treatment-resistant depression (Kiosses et al. 2015a). PATH may also reduce suicidal ideation, although not more so than supportive therapy (Kiosses et al. 2015b).

In summary, PST has a very strong evidence base for the treatment of depression in older adults, including those who are medically ill or who are being seen in primary care settings. PST and its cousin PATH may also be effective in individuals with comorbid depression and cognitive impairment or executive dysfunction.

PSYCHODYNAMIC PSYCHOTHERAPY

Psychodynamic psychotherapy, especially in its brief form, may offer benefit for late-life depression and anxiety. Brief psychodynamic psychotherapy focuses on the development of insight and relies on the value of transference and countertransference in the therapist-patient relationship. One study of brief psychodynamic psychotherapy in 91 older adults with MDD found benefits comparable to behavioral therapy and cognitive therapy; all subjects received 16–20 sessions of one of these therapies for twice a week for 4 weeks, then weekly thereafter (Thompson et al. 1987). At 1- and 2-year follow-up, there was no difference in relapse rates among the three interventions (Gallagher-Thompson et al. 1990). Another study of 66 caregivers (mean age 62) of frail elders found that brief psychodynamic psychotherapy and CBT were equally effective at treating depression (Gallagher-Thompson and Steffen 1994).

LIFE REVIEW AND REMINISCENCE

Life review, based on Erik Erikson's theory of life stages, was originally proposed as a way of helping older adults achieve ego integrity, an important developmental task (Butler 1963). Reminiscence and life review are often used interchangeably, but whereas reminiscence is a process of recalling the past that may lead to conflict resolution, life review is a structured treatment in which resolving conflicts or assessing coping responses is offered systematically, either individually or in groups (Fry 1983). A meta-analysis found an overall effect size of 0.84 for life review and reminiscence, indicating a significant benefit for depressive symptoms in older people (Bohlmeijer et al. 2003). Subsequently, several more studies demonstrated the effectiveness of life review and reminiscence on late-life depression (Lamers et al. 2015; Latorre et al. 2015; Serrano et al. 2004). However, reminiscence may not be as effective as PST in reducing depression (Areán et al. 1993). Group therapy using reminiscence and problem-solving can also help reduce depression (Djukanovic et al. 2016). Reminiscence has been studied extensively in persons with dementia and has been found to decrease depressive symptoms (Park et al. 2019).

Exercise

The role of exercise in treating late-life depression has long been of interest to geriatricians, given its benefits in the treatment of depression for adults (Rimer et al. 2012) and the suggested role of exercise in the prevention of cognitive decline (Alty et al. 2020). Several putative physiological mechanisms for how exercise can affect the aging brain and prevent or treat depression have been proposed, but the evidence substantiating these hypotheses is still limited. These mechanisms include increase of brain-derived neurotrophic factor and basic fibroblast growth factor levels in the hippocampus, exercise-induced enhancement of insulin growth factor 1 expression, increased production of tryptophan and dopamine, and modulation of proinflammatory factors (Farioli Vecchioli et al. 2018). A great deal of research on how exercise affects the function and integrity of the aging hippocampus comes from the animal literature, where robust evidence demonstrates the positive impact of physical activity on cell proliferation in the dentate gyrus of the hippocampus and increased vascularization of neural tissue, associated with volumetric and functional changes in the brain and improved mood and cognition (Erickson et al. 2013). However, similar studies in humans are still lacking. From the psychological perspective, exercise leads to increased self-efficacy and a sense of mastery, offers distraction, and leads to changes in self-concept (Ströhle 2009).

Exercise has been explored both as a stand-alone treatment for late-life depression and in combination with medications. A recent meta-analysis of exercise for late-life depression found a significant effect of moderate to vigorous physical activity on reducing depressive symptoms, although there was heterogeneity in the effect of physical exercise intervention (Klil-Drori et al. 2020). The authors cautioned that more work is needed to support the positive effects of exercise for adults ages 80 and older, as well as for those with MMSE score <23. An earlier umbrella review of exercise in older adults similarly found moderate effects of exercise on depression and no reported serious adverse events (Catalan-Matamoros et al. 2016). The authors concluded that exercise was safe and efficacious in reducing depressive symptoms in older people.

In a trial of primary care patients older than 65 years with MDD who were randomly assigned to 24 weeks of higher-intensity aerobic exercise with sertraline, lower-intensity aerobic exercise with sertraline, or sertraline alone, a significant proportion of patients in each group improved, with the best results in those who received higher-intensity exercise along with sertraline (Murri et al. 2015). Exercise appears to offer advantages for addressing the affective symptoms of depression rather than other dimensions of the illness, such as somatic symptoms, as demonstrated in a study comparing effectiveness of sertraline alone versus exercise combined with sertraline (Murri et al. 2018). In the same study, the patients in the sertraline combined with thrice-weekly progressive aerobic exercise group experienced improvement in cognition (Neviani et al. 2017).

Exercise is an inexpensive treatment with a more benign side-effect profile than that of antidepressants. Patients can engage in exercise with the help of physical therapists or at home; individually or in groups; and in activities tailor-made to their personal preferences, social circumstances, and preexisting conditions. Exercise may also improve cognition and reduce disability in older adults, and it should be recommended as part of a multidisciplinary treatment plan to patients experiencing late-life depression. Consideration should be given to recommending moderate to vigorous exercise as an augmentation of antidepressants in all older patients with mild or moderate depression.

Pharmacological Interventions

ANTIDEPRESSANTS

Antidepressants are a key component in the treatment of depression in older individuals (Kok and Reynolds 2017). Treatment of older adults, including with antidepressants, is often complicated by medical comorbidity, polypharmacy, and changes in physiology (Wallace and Paauw 2015). At the same time, uncertainty about antidepressant effectiveness and safety persists (Lenze and Ajam Oughli 2019). However, on balance, expert opinion has consistently recommended antidepressant use in older patients, especially for moderate to severe depression, along with nonpharmacological interventions (Mulsant et al. 2014; Taylor 2014).

Antidepressants are commonly prescribed to older adults, and their use has been increasing despite relatively stable incidence of depression (Arthur et al. 2020). However, older adults have not been included in antidepressant trials as frequently as younger or middle-age adults. Clinical trials often exclude subjects older than 65 years, and where elders are not explicitly excluded, they often may not qualify because of polypharmacy or comorbid medical conditions. Real-world clinical treatment is often complicated by these issues, and we need studies specifically focused on older adults (Krause et al. 2019). In addition, clinicians are less likely to prescribe antidepressants to ethnic minority elders, presenting a barrier to effective care for a substantial number of older adults (Mansour et al. 2020).

Efficacy of Antidepressants

Deciding whether or not to prescribe an antidepressant requires examination of benefits and risks. In general, antidepressants are modestly effective in the treatment of late-life depression, with about 51% of older adults responding to antidepressants (Gutsmiedl et al. 2020). The effects are not robust: the number needed to treat (NNT) is 6.7 for response and 14.4 for remission (Kok et al. 2012). The results are similar for studies of younger adults, which found an NNT for response of 6.1 (Kok and Reynolds 2017).

Older adults with comorbid medical conditions such as cerebrovascular disease, dementia, cardiovascular disease, executive dysfunction, or frailty may not benefit from antidepressants as much (Kok and Reynolds 2017). For example, a meta-analysis suggested that antidepressants are of questionable benefit and are of concern when used with frail older patients, finding response in 45.3% of patients versus 40.5% with placebo (Mallery et al. 2019). Antidepressants may not be effective in depressed older adults with dementia and thus should not be used as first-line treatment (Kok and Reynolds 2017).

Another factor affecting response rate is that clinicians may prescribe suboptimal doses of antidepressants to older adults (Kok and Reynolds 2017). Although we recommend following the guideline of "start low, go slow" (in other words, begin treatment at one-half or even one-quarter of the usual starting dose and titrate more slowly than one would in a younger adult), the effective dosages of most antidepressants are the same in older adults as in younger adults. This is especially true of selective serotonin reuptake inhibitors (SSRIs), serotonin-norepinephrine reuptake inhibitors (SNRIs), mirtazapine, bupropion, and vortioxetine. Although tricyclic antidepressants (TCAs) are prescribed less often because they are more likely to cause side effects, monitoring blood levels can help determine a therapeutic dosage. Trials of antidepressants should be of adequate duration, perhaps as long as 6–8 weeks on the maximally tolerated dosage.

No clear predictors of how an older adult might respond to an antidepressant have been found. For example, there is little evidence to support the use of pharmacogenomic testing to select an antidepressant in late-life depression. The most rigorous study to date is a post hoc analysis of 206 older adult subjects of the Genomics Used to Improve Depression Decisions (GUIDED) trial that used pharmacogenomic testing to inform medication selection in MDD treatment (Forester et al. 2020). The study found no statistically significant improvement in depression symptoms relative to treatment as usual but found higher response (29.6% versus 16.1%) and remission rates (20.1% versus 7.4%) at 8 weeks (Forester et al. 2020). We are not aware of any studies of pharmacogenomic testing in anxiety disorders in older adults. At this point we would not recommend widespread use of pharmacogenomic testing to guide the selection of antidepressants.

Note that most of the literature on using antidepressants in older adults pertains to the treatment of depression, with far fewer studies on anxiety disorders in older adults. A 2012 review that pooled results from five studies found evidence of modest efficacy for duloxetine, escitalopram, notriptyline, and venlafaxine (Gonçalves and Byrne 2012). The largest RCT to date of late-life GAD (291 subjects) demonstrated efficacy of duloxetine (Alaka et al. 2014). Finally, both escitalopram alone and escitalopram combined with CBT were found to be more effective than placebo at preventing relapse of an anxiety disorder (Wetherell et al. 2013). Because, as noted earlier, the evidence base for CBT in late-life anxiety disorders is strong, we would consider psychotherapy with or without antidepressant to be the first-line treatment.

Adverse Effects of Antidepressants

Cautious optimism about the benefits of antidepressants in older adults must be balanced with the concern for potential adverse effects. In general, older adults are less likely to be able to tolerate antidepressants and are more likely to experience drug-drug or drug-disease interactions. SSRIs appear to have a better safety profile than SNRIs (Sobieraj et al. 2019). Specifically, although SSRIs lead to higher discontinuation rates due to adverse events than placebo does, the rates of side effects do not differ; on the other hand, SNRIs are associated with more side effects than are placebo, with a number needed to harm (NNH) of 10 (Sobieraj et al. 2019). Side effects (especially anticholinergic effects, postural hypotension, and risk of cardiac arrhythmia) limit the use of TCAs; drug-drug interactions and dietary restrictions are challenges in the use of monoamine oxidase inhibitors (MAOIs; Kok and Reynolds 2017).

A recent network meta-analysis presented data comparing adverse events reported in clinical trials, showing how antidepressants differ relative to one another in side effects including anticholinergic effects, gastrointestinal effects, sedation, and dizziness—all of which are of heightened concern in an older population (Krause et al. 2019). In addition to these well-known potential side effects of antidepressants, more serious adverse events associated with antidepressants include hyponatremia, osteoporosis, and falls. For citalopram specifically, the FDA has issued a warning about limiting dosages in older patients because of the risk of prolongation of the QT interval leading to a potentially lethal arrhythmia. Hyponatremia has been associated with almost all antidepressants (bupropion seems to be least implicated); risk factors for experiencing hyponatremia with antidepressants include age, being female, using diuretics, low weight, and low baseline sodium (Jacob and Spinler 2006). For patients at higher risk of hyponatremia, we recommend checking a baseline plasma sodium level and then rechecking 2–3 weeks after each dose increase. Consideration should also be given to the increased risk of gastrointestinal bleeding with serotonergic antidepressants, especially in patients who are taking anticoagulation agents or are otherwise at higher risk (Wallace and Paauw 2015). Hyperhidrosis is more likely to occur with SNRIs than with other antidepressants (Krause et al. 2019). Nausea is among the most common of antidepressant side effects, although less frequently with mirtazapine (Krause et al. 2019). Sexual side effects are among the most common problems with antidepressants in younger adults, and we suspect this is the case with older adults, too; perhaps mirtazapine and bupropion are less likely to cause sexual side effects.

Antidepressants are included in the American Geriatrics Society Beers Criteria as potentially inappropriate medications in older patients because of safety considerations in two areas (American Geriatrics Society Beers Criteria Update Expert Panel 2019). First, sedating antidepressants (such as TCAs and paroxetine) are considered highly anticholinergic and should be avoided for all geriatric patients, with a strong recommendation based on high-quality evidence. Second, there is a strong recommendation to avoid antidepressants in patients with a history of falls and fractures, although allowance is made for patients for whom these medications might be considered essential (i.e., there are no safer alternatives). Because many older patients have a history of falls, this recommendation can greatly influence prescribing patterns for geriatric depression (Gebara et al. 2015). Rigorous, criteria-driven systematic review for both falls (Gebara et al. 2015) and overall bone health (Gebara et al. 2014) did not suggest a causal relationship between antidepressant (SSRI) treatment and these potentially serious adverse effects, and the authors concluded that prescribing likely should not be curtailed solely on these grounds. We would suggest that clinicians prescribe antidepressants with caution to patients who have fallen or are at risk of falling and monitor closely for any new problems with balance.

Because antidepressants can interact with other medications, we recommend that clinicians consult a reliable database of drug-drug interactions whenever prescribing a new antidepressant. Optimizing Outcomes of Treatment-Resistant Depression in Older Adults (OPTIMUM) is a large ongoing comparative effectiveness study that should add to our understanding of the risks associated with the use of antidepressants in older adults, with robust primary end points involving safety (Cristancho et al. 2019).

Augmentation Strategies

Because antidepressants may not resolve depression with initial treatment for many patients, augmentation of partial response to antidepressants is an important clinical consideration. As with late-life depression treatment itself, augmentation has been understudied. Currently, the most robust data are for aripiprazole, from the first RCT of augmentation in the geriatric population (Lenze et al. 2015). Follow-up to this study found that patients with preserved executive function responded better to aripiprazole augmentation following initial partial response to venlafaxine; patients performing worse on the Trail Making Test did not separate from placebo, and neither anxiety nor medical co-morbidity provided predictive information (Kaneriya et al. 2016). Inter-estingly, one study has demonstrated efficacy for quetiapine monotherapy in late-life depression (Katila et al. 2013) and another for late-life anxiety (Mezhebovsky et al. 2013), although we would have concerns about the tolerability of quetiapine in older adults.

Otherwise, there is very limited evidence on augmentation strate-gies. One review concluded that for patients ages 55 and older, the only treatment with replicated evidence is lithium (Cooper et al. 2011), but the challenges facing use of lithium with its narrow therapeutic level window and potential for thyroid and renal complications in an older population will likely always limit its use for this purpose. Addressing a related goal, accelerating the response to antidepressant treatment, a small trial showed that combining methylphenidate with citalopram led to both higher remission rates and shorter time to remission (Lavretsky et al. 2015). In this study there were no indications of a higher rate of adverse effects due to methylphenidate use, which is re-assuring because the subjects' mean age was near 70.

Antidepressant augmentation in late-life depression research has also been critiqued for not examining real-world practices such as combining antidepressants, a practice that likely occurs often in the community despite the lack of an evidence base for doing so (Maust et al. 2013). The Sequenced Treatment Alternatives to Relieve Depression (STAR*D) trial, which included subjects up to age 75 years, demon-strated some support for adding bupropion to an SSRI and for combin-ing venlafaxine and mirtazapine (Gaynes et al. 2008). A meta-analysis of studies of antidepressant combinations in subjects 18 years and older found evidence for combining mirtazapine with SSRIs (Henssler et al. 2016). Buspirone was included as an augmentation strategy in the STAR*D trial, with limited benefit. The only RCT of buspirone in older adults with GAD found comparable efficacy to sertraline (Mokhber et al. 2010).

OPTIMUM, the study described earlier, is under way to examine medication switch versus augmentation specifically in patients 60 and older (Cristancho et al. 2019). It will compare real-world practices of augmentation with lithium, bupropion, or aripiprazole and switching to bupropion or nortriptyline; it will also feature primary outcomes in both efficacy and, crucially, safety. Like STAR*D, this study will provide invaluable large-scale data in this very understudied area.

For information on the use of ketamine and esketamine in late-life depression, see the subsection "Ketamine and Esketamine."

Prescribing an Antidepressant

In summary, the evidence for using antidepressants in late life suggests that they are modestly effective and that they should, after careful weighing of the benefits and risks for individual patients, be used to treat moderate to severe MDD in older adults (see Table 5–3 for descriptions of depression severity). Antidepressants can also be used to treat anxiety disorders in late life. The role of antidepressants in bipolar depression is discussed in the subsection "Treating Bipolar Depression." Selecting a specific antidepressant depends on determining where the patient is in the treatment algorithm (i.e., is this the patient's first antidepressant, or have many antidepressants already been tried?), determining which side effects are most important to avoid (see the subsection "Adverse Effects of Antidepressants" for a guide), and perhaps matching antidepressants with specific clinical situations (Table 5–4). Admittedly, we make these recommendations primarily on the basis of clinical experience because the evidence base has not consistently demonstrated head-to-head differences in efficacy among antidepressants in late life. Furthermore, most of the literature pertains to late-life depression, with few studies in anxiety disorders.

Expert consensus recommends the use of SSRIs as first-line agents for late-life depression, given their overall balance of effectiveness and safety. We recommend citalopram, escitalopram, and sertraline over paroxetine (because of paroxetine's anticholinergic properties) and over fluoxetine (because of fluoxetine's long half-life). If first-line treatment is not effective, switching to another SSRI or switching to an SNRI, bupropion, mirtazapine, or vortioxetine are reasonable options. Anecdotally, mirtazapine is thought to be sedating, whereas bupropion and SNRIs are thought to be activating; thus, mirtazapine can be considered for depressed elders with prominent insomnia (and anorexia or weight loss), whereas bupropion and SNRIs can be considered for those with anergia and excess sleep. In general, we would recommend avoiding polypharmacy, although there are reasonable combination and augmentation strategies to try later in the treatment algorithm, as described in the previous subsection. When the patient has had a partial response to an antidepressant, combining with another antidepressant or augmenting with another agent can be considered. If the patient has not responded or has not tolerated an antidepressant, we advise switching to another antidepressant or to a nonpharmacological approach. Because of concerns about tolerability, TCAs and MAOIs come later in the treatment algorithm. Among the TCAs, nortriptyline is the best studied among older adults and may be better tolerated than amitriptyline.

Table 5–4.   Summary of medications for late-life depression

Clinical scenario	Treatment options	Initial dose	Target dosage
Typical depression	Citalopram	10 mg at breakfast	20–30 mg/day[a]
	Escitalopram	5 mg at breakfast	10–20 mg/day
	Sertraline	25 mg at breakfast	50–200 mg/day
Prominent fatigue, hypersomnia, and/or lack of motivation	Bupropion XL	150 mg at breakfast	300–450 mg/day
	Venlafaxine XR	37.5 mg at breakfast	75–225 mg/day
	Duloxetine	20 mg at breakfast	40–60 mg/day[b]
Prominent insomnia and/or weight loss	Mirtazapine	15 mg at bedtime	15–45 mg/day
	Notriptyline	25 mg at bedtime	Varies[c]
Treatment-resistant depression	Vortioxetine	5 mg at breakfast	5–20 mg/day
	Venlafaxine, duloxetine, nortripyline, MAOIs, combinations,[d] augmentation[e]		
Psychotic depression	Antidepressant plus antipsychotic[f]		
Bipolar depression[g]	Lithium	300 mg at bedtime	Varies[h]
	Lamotrigine	25 mg at breakfast	≥200 mg/day
	Quetiapine	25–50 mg at bedtime	300 mg/day

Table 5–4. Summary of medications for late-life depression *(continued)*

Clinical scenario	Treatment options	Initial dose	Target dosage
Bipolar depression[g] *(continued)*	Lurasidone	20 mg at bedtime	80 mg/day

[a]There is concern for QT prolongation at doses of citalopram >20 mg/day.

[b]Duloxetine can be titrated to 120 mg/day, but it has no evidence of further antidepressant efficacy beyond 60 mg/day.

[c]Target blood level of 80–120 mg/dL.

[d]Combinations include selective serotonin reuptake inhibitor (SSRI) plus bupropion, venlafaxine plus mirtazapine, SSRI plus mirtazapine.

[e]The strongest evidence is for aripiprazole (starting dose 2 mg qhs, target 5–15 mg/day), lithium, and methylphenidate as augmentation agents.

[f]Electroconvulsive therapy is the gold standard for psychotic depression; the best evidence for medication is the combination of sertraline 150–200 mg/day and olanzapine 15–20 mg/day.

[g]Note that there is controversy about effective treatments for bipolar depression; here we list the first-line recommendations of the CANMAT/ISBD guidelines. For detailed discussion, see subsection "Treating Bipolar Depression."

[h]Target blood level of 0.4–0.6 mEq/L.

Abbreviations. CANMAT=Canadian Network for Mood and Anxiety Treatments; ISBD=International Society for Bipolar Disorders=MAOIs=monoamine oxidase inhibitors.

Source. Adapted from Taylor 2014; Yatham et al. 2018.

Dosing should be done carefully because of changes in drug metabolism with age and the potential for drug interactions, but at the same time the aim should be to treat with full adult dosages of antidepressants if possible (Unützer and Park 2012). The recommendation to treat with antidepressants along with nonpharmacological interventions such as psychotherapy and other options discussed in this chapter has remained stable at least since as long ago as 2001 (Alexopoulos et al. 2001). Although there is evidence for maintenance treatment with an antidepressant to lessen the risk of relapse (in one study, for example, patients who continued placebo had a 2.4 higher risk of recurrence than did those continuing paroxetine) (Reynolds et al. 2006), overall it remains an open question in need of extensive additional studies. Although no definite recommendations can be made on when to discontinue antidepressants after resolution of depression (Wilkinson and Izmeth 2016), we recommend considering long-term treatment in patients who have chronic or recurrent MDD and who experience benefit from their medications. Patients who have experienced their first major depressive episode can be tapered off the antidepressant after 1 year of remission (Kok and Reynolds 2017). Finally, although conventional clinical trials focus on the statistical separation from placebo, in clinical practice benefit comes from additive drug and placebo effects, much to patients' advantage. As with most every consideration in geriatric patients, the risk of treatment should be carefully and thoughtfully balanced against the risk of not treating the patient.

SEDATIVE-HYPNOTICS FOR ANXIETY

In this subsection we focus on benzodiazepines (BZDs); use of other sedative-hypnotic medications to treat insomnia is covered in the following subsection. BZDs are commonly used to treat late-life anxiety despite significant risks and widespread recommendations to avoid their use. In fact, in 2020 the FDA strengthened its boxed warning on BZDs to highlight the risk of abuse, misuse, and physical dependence.

BZDs enhance the effect of γ-aminobutyric acid (GABA) through positive allosteric modulation of $GABA_A$ receptor complexes in the CNS (Saari et al. 2011). These properties give BZDs their benefits (anxiety and insomnia relief, muscle relaxation) and their adverse effects (addiction, cognitive impairment, ataxia). The GABA neurotransmitter system changes with age, rendering older adults more sensitive to these adverse effects (Hutchison and O'Brien 2007).

BZDs are listed in the Beers Criteria of potentially inappropriate medications for most older adults (American Geriatrics Society Beers Criteria Update Expert Panel 2019). Clinicians are strongly recommended to avoid BZDs because "older adults have increased sensitivity to BZDs and decreased metabolism of long-acting agents; in general, all BZDs increase the risk of cognitive impairment, delirium, falls, fractures, and motor vehicle crashes in older adults" (American Geriatrics Society Beers Criteria Update Expert Panel 2019, p. 7). While allowing that BZDs may be appropriate in certain contexts, such as severe GAD and alcohol withdrawal, the Beers Criteria also identify situations in which BZDs are particularly problematic and should be avoided: delirium, dementia or cognitive impairment, history of falls or fractures, and polypharmacy with two or more other CNS-active drugs. The criteria recommend against prescribing BZDs and opioids at the same time because of the risk of respiratory depression and death from overdose.

Risks associated with BZDs in older adults are significant. Short-term and long-term BZD use is associated with impairment across several cognitive domains, which can be long-lasting (Barker et al. 2004; Tannenbaum et al. 2012). Some studies have linked BZDs to the development of dementia (Zhong et al. 2015), but results are mixed (Gray et al. 2016). Several studies associate BZDs with falls and fractures, especially hip fractures, in older adults (Markota et al. 2016). The risk of fracture appears to be dose-dependent, beginning at the equivalent of 0.3 mg/day of lorazepam. Motor vehicle accidents happen more often among BZD users, likely because of cognitive impairment and sedation (Dassanayake et al. 2011). BZD use is linked to poor outcomes in older adults with chronic obstructive pulmonary disease (Vozoris et al. 2014). Finally, studies have associated BZD use with all-cause mortality, but it is unclear if the association is causal (Palmaro et al. 2015).

In contrast to the abundant evidence of risks associated with BZDs, there is little evidence to support their benefits for anxiety in older adults. One recent review article (Gerlach et al. 2018) identified a single RCT from 1982 that found that oxazepam reduced anxiety more than did placebo among 220 older adults with anxiety (Koepke et al. 1982). Otherwise, the benefits of BZDs to treat anxiety in older adults are extrapolated from evidence of their efficacy in younger age groups.

Despite significant risks and little evidence of benefit, BZDs are still commonly prescribed to older adults for anxiety and insomnia. Among U.S. older adults, 8.7% filled at least one prescription for a BZD in the preceding year, and approximately one-third of those with a prescription were taking BZDs on a chronic basis (Olfson et al. 2015).

Why might clinical practice diverge to such an extent from the available evidence and professional recommendations? Studies of patient and provider perspectives have found that both groups perceived BZDs to be effective, underestimated or were not aware of potential risks, and did not know what else to do (Cook et al. 2007a, 2007b).

Given the risks and questionable efficacy of this drug class, it may be prudent for providers to taper older adults off BZDs and use alternative treatments for anxiety. Several studies have demonstrated that older adults can be tapered off BZDs, and a combination of psychotherapy, education, and supervised tapering achieved the highest success rates (Gould et al. 2014). BZD doses can be tapered by 10%–20% every 1–2 weeks until discontinued. As noted earlier, safer alternatives to BZDs for late-life anxiety include antidepressants and psychotherapy.

If BZDs must be used to treat anxiety in older adults, the goal should be to minimize potential risks. Treatment duration should be limited to 2 weeks if possible. Age-related changes in oxidative metabolism slow the clearance of most BZDs, prolonging their effects and increasing the potential for drug-drug interactions. Three BZDs (lorazepam, oxazepam, and temazepam) are metabolized by glucuronidation, which is unaffected by age, resulting in no active metabolites and lower risk of interactions. Lorazepam, with its intermediate half-life, may be the best choice for most scenarios, but the total dosage should be limited to 0.5 mg/day to limit the risk of fractures.

SEDATIVE-HYPNOTICS AND OTHER MEDICATIONS FOR INSOMNIA

Insomnia is commonly comorbid with depression and anxiety, and it can contribute to cognitive impairment, dementia, cardiovascular disease, and mortality (Abad and Guilleminault 2018). Nonpharmacological approaches are the first-line treatments for insomnia, as described in the subsection "CBT for Insomnia," but medications are often used when preferred options are unavailable or fail to work. Suvorexant and low-dose doxepin are good choices for sleep maintenance, and ramelteon is a good choice for sleep initiation. Table 5–5 displays medications that are FDA approved and those that are used off-label for insomnia in older adults.

Suvorexant is the first FDA-approved dual orexin receptor antagonist. It inhibits the neuropeptide orexin, which promotes wakefulness. The recommended dosage range is 5–20 mg/day, and the usual starting dose is 10 mg at bedtime. Pooled data of the older adults in two 12-week RCTs found that suvorexant improved sleep maintenance and, to a lesser extent, reduced sleep onset latency (Herring et al. 2017). Risks are generally mild, but next-day somnolence appears to be dose-related, and suvorexant may affect driving at higher doses. Safety in older adults with sleep apnea is not well established, so caution should be used in this group.

Doxepin is a TCA that acts as a selective H_1 receptor antagonist at dosages in the 1–6 mg/day range. Three RCTs found that doxepin improves sleep maintenance with no effect on sleep onset latency (Krystal et al. 2010; Lankford et al. 2012; Scharf et al. 2008). Common side effects are somnolence, nausea, and dizziness. Cognitive impairment has not been observed at these doses. Doxepin is not recommended for insomnia in individuals with severe sleep apnea. Because of the high cost of the brand-name version of low-dose doxepin, clinicians in the United States can consider using generic doxepin at the slightly higher dose of 10 mg at bedtime.

Ramelteon is a highly selective melatonin MT_1 and MT_2 receptor agonist that does not cause CNS depression. Studies of ramelteon in older adults have had mixed results, but the consensus is that it may be modestly beneficial for sleep initiation (Kuriyama et al. 2014). It is generally considered safe in the context of comorbid chronic obstructive pulmonary disease (COPD) and sleep apnea. Standard dosing is 8 mg at bedtime.

Like the BZDs, the Z-drugs (zolpidem, eszopiclone, and zaleplon) bind to and stimulate $GABA_A$, except that they are more selective for α_1 subunits, which mediate sedative and hypnotic effects. Theoretically, this selectivity should reduce the risks associated with Z-drugs relative to BZDs. However, the Beers Criteria also strongly recommend avoiding

Table 5–5.   Medications for late-life insomnia

Medication	Benefits	Adverse effects	Recommendations and comments
FDA-approved medications for insomnia			
Suvorexant	Best evidence for sleep maintenance; modest benefit for sleep initiation	Somnolence; at higher doses, may affect driving	First-line option for sleep maintenance
Low-dose doxepin	Sleep maintenance	Somnolence, nausea, dizziness	First-line option for sleep maintenance
Ramelteon	Sleep initiation	Generally well tolerated	First-line option for sleep initiation
Z-drugs • Eszopiclone • Zolpidem • Zaleplon	Sleep initiation (eszopiclone, zolpidem IR, zaleplon) Sleep maintenance (eszopiclone, zolpidem ER)	Somnolence, delirium, falls and fractures, motor vehicle accidents	Strong recommendation to avoid
BZDs • Triazolam • Temazepam	Sleep initiation, sleep maintenance	Tolerance; sedation; cognitive impairment; possible increased risk of dementia, delirium, falls, and fractures; motor vehicle accidents; overdose mortality in combination with opioids; poor respiratory outcomes in COPD	Strong recommendation to avoid

Table 5–5.   Medications for late-life insomnia *(continued)*

Medication	Benefits	Adverse effects	Recommendations and comments
Medications commonly used off-label for insomnia			
Sedating antidepressants • Trazodone • Mirtazapine	Improvement in sleep with comorbid late-life depression and anxiety	Trazodone: somnolence, dizziness, orthostasis, falls Mirtazapine: somnolence, weight gain	May be good options for insomnia comorbid with depression and anxiety; insufficient evidence of benefit for primary insomnia
Antihistamines • Diphenhydramine • Hydroxyzine	Mixed results; benefits not well established	Anticholinergic tolerance develops to hypnotic effect	Risks outweigh benefits; strong recommendation to avoid
Melatonin	Sleep initiation	Generally well tolerated	May be helpful for sleep initiation with few side effects; product quality varies when purchased over the counter
Herbal supplements • Tryptophan • Valerian	Not well studied in older adults	Generally well tolerated	Benefits are not well established but is generally safe

Note.   See text for dosing.
Abbreviations.   COPD=chronic obstructive pulmonary disease; ER=extended release; IR=immediate release.
Source.   Adapted from Abad and Guilleminault 2018; Schroeck et al. 2016.

Z-drugs, citing that they "have adverse events similar to those of BZDs in older adults (e.g., delirium, falls, fractures); increased emergency room visits/hospitalizations; motor vehicle crashes; [and] minimal improvement in sleep latency and duration" (American Geriatrics Society Beers Criteria Update Expert Panel 2019, p. 7). The American College of Physicians agrees that evidence of benefit with Z-drugs for older adults is of low quality (Qaseem et al. 2016). If these medications must be used, doses should be limited to eszopiclone 2 mg for sleep initiation and maintenance, immediate-release zolpidem 5 mg for sleep initiation, extended-release zolpidem 6.25 mg for sleep maintenance, or zaleplon 5–10 mg for sleep initiation.

Two BZDs are FDA approved for the short-term treatment (7–10 days) of insomnia: triazolam and temazepam. Although available evidence from small studies suggests that these drugs may help with sleep initiation and maintenance in older adults, tolerance develops rapidly, and harms likely outweigh benefits (Abad and Guilleminault 2018). If these drugs must be used, doses should not exceed 0.125 mg of triazolam or 15 mg of temazepam.

For information about off-label use of medications for insomnia, see Table 5–5.

TREATING PSYCHOTIC DEPRESSION

Treating psychotic depression effectively is critical because of the high morbidity and mortality associated with this condition. Electroconvulsive therapy (ECT), described in detail later in the chapter, is the gold standard treatment for psychotic depression. An alternative is prescribing a combination of an antidepressant and an antipsychotic. Psychotherapy is unlikely to be effective.

In a study by Meyers et al. (2009), combining sertraline 150–200 mg/day and olanzapine 15–20 mg/day was found to be as effective for psychotic depression in older adults as in younger adults and more effective than olanzapine alone. Weight gain (mean increase of 7.3 pounds over 12 weeks among older adult subjects), hyperlipidemia, and hypertriglyceridemia were worrisome side effects (Meyers et al. 2009). A 36-week maintenance study of younger and older patients who had responded to this combination found that those randomly assigned to continue both olanzapine and sertraline had lower relapse rates than those continuing with sertraline alone (54.8% vs. 20.3%) but gained weight at a rate of about 1 pound per week (Flint et al. 2019). The combinations of olanzapine and fluoxetine and of quetiapine and venlafaxine have been found to be effective in studies of younger adults with psychotic depression and perhaps could be considered in older adults (Rothschild et al. 2004; Wijkstra et al. 2010). The dearth of studies of pharmacological treatment of late-life psychotic depression and the concerning side effects of antipsychotics reinforce the recommendation for ECT.

TREATING BIPOLAR DEPRESSION

The care of an older adult with bipolar depression poses significant challenges. Older adults with bipolar disorder often experience significant medical burden, including cardiovascular disease, diabetes, hypertension, hyperlipidemia, and obesity (Sajatovic and Chen 2011), which raises concerns about tolerability of many medications commonly used to treat bipolar disorder. Atypical antipsychotics, among the most commonly prescribed medications in bipolar disorder, pose particular risks with respect to metabolic syndrome and coronary heart disease (Correll et al. 2006). Older adults may be at higher risk of adverse events from lithium use due to decline in renal function and drug-drug interactions (Sajatovic et al. 2015). Valproate has been associated with motor side effects and metabolic effects and may also cause cerebral atrophy in older adults with dementia (Fleisher et al. 2011; Yatham et al. 2018).

Across all ages, treating bipolar depression remains challenging and even controversial. (Note that we do not cover treatment of mania or maintenance treatment of bipolar disorder here.) In the United States, the FDA has approved several agents specifically for bipolar depression, including olanzapine+fluoxetine combination, lurasidone, quetiapine, and cariprazine. But the evidence base and associated recommendations related to fundamental questions remain mixed and even contradictory:

Is lithium effective for bipolar depression? A recent systematic review and network meta-analysis of 50 RCTs comprising 11,448 participants of all ages concluded that lithium is no more effective than placebo in treatment of bipolar depression (Bahji et al. 2020). On the other hand, the Canadian Network for Mood and Anxiety Treatments (CANMAT) and International Society for Bipolar Disorders (ISBD) treatment guidelines list lithium as first-line treatment for bipolar depression (Yatham et al. 2018). A report from the ISBD Task Force on Older-Age Bipolar Disorders noted the "potential usefulness" of lithium in bipolar depression (Sajatovic et al. 2015). Lithium may also reduce the risk of suicide (Bobo 2017).

Are antidepressants effective for bipolar depression? The same network meta-analysis described above identified the antidepressants tranylcypromine, venlafaxine, fluoxetine, and imipramine as efficacious and well tolerated for the treatment of bipolar depression (Bahji et al. 2020). However, other systematic reviews have concluded that antidepressants are not effective (McGirr et al. 2016; Sidor and Macqueen 2011), and the CANMAT/ISBD guidelines relegate SSRIs and bupropion (combined with lithium, valproate, or an atypical antipsychotic) to second-line status (Yatham et al. 2018).

Do antidepressants increase the risk of switch from depression to mania? Bahji et al. (2020) concluded that no medication studied in bipolar disorder, including antidepressants, increases the risk of treatment-emergent mania relative to placebo (Bahji et al. 2020). McGirr et al. (2016)

raised the concern about a possible increase in risk of switch when antidepressants are used for an extended period of time, and the CANMAT/ISBD guidelines argue that there is a significant risk of treatment-emergent mania with SNRIs, TCAs, and MAOIs (Yatham et al. 2018).

So which medications are effective for bipolar depression? The CANMAT/ISBD guidelines recommend the following (FDA-approved agents for this indication appear in italics): *quetiapine*, lithium, lamotrigine, and *lurasidone* as first-line treatments and valproate, SSRI/bupropion (combined with lithium, valproate, or atypical antipsychotic), *cariprazine*, and *olanzapine/fluoxetine* as second-line treatments (Yatham et al. 2018).

Unfortunately, there is limited evidence on the agents described above for treating bipolar depression in older adults. For example, there are no RCTs on the use of quetiapine, cariprazine, or lurasidone in the treatment of late-life bipolar depression (Vasudev et al. 2018). The only RCT of lithium or valproate thus far in older-age bipolar disorder studied the treatment of mania, not depression (Young et al. 2017). Generally, recommendations for treatment in older adults are based on uncontrolled trials and on post hoc analyses of and extrapolations from studies of mixed-age populations with bipolar disorder. We recommend following the CANMAT/ISBD guidelines summarized in the previous paragraph.

Older adults prescribed lithium should have regular monitoring of lithium blood level (at least every 3 months, more frequently when titrating, with a target of 0.4–0.6 mEq/L), renal function (every 3 months), electrolytes (every 3 months), and thyroid function (every 6 months because the incidence of hypothyroidism in older adults taking lithium is 6% per year) (Sajatovic et al. 2015; Volkmann et al. 2020). Special attention should be paid to avoiding dehydration and to drug-drug interactions with angiotensin-converting enzyme inhibitors, angiotensin-receptor blockers, diuretics. and nonsteroidal anti-inflammatory drugs (Volkmann et al. 2020).

When using atypical antipsychotics in the treatment of bipolar depression, using the lowest effective dosage will reduce the risk of adverse effects–related discontinuation (Bartoli et al. 2017). This is particularly relevant for geriatric patients, who are more sensitive to the side effects of medications (including motor symptoms such as tremor and metabolic complications) and drug-disease interactions (Sajatovic et al. 2015).

ECT remains a valuable treatment option for bipolar depression when psychopharmacological options fail or when presence of suicidal ideation and psychosis as well as declining self-care necessitate fast treatment response (Bobo 2017). Response of bipolar depression to ECT is higher than that of MDD, based on the results of systematic review and meta-analysis of 19 studies examining patients whose average age was 51.2 years (Bahji et al. 2019). For a detailed discussion of the risks and benefits of ECT in older adults, see the subsection "Electroconvulsive Therapy."

Although the data can be called only preliminary at best, results of a systematic review of intravenous ketamine for bipolar depression suggest that it is a safe and effective treatment for this indication; however, the existing data concern younger adults rather than older adults (Alberich et al. 2017). Psychosocial interventions, particularly CBT, interpersonal social rhythm therapy (IPSRT), family-focused therapy, psychoeducation, and an integrated care model are recommended as ways to enhance and augment treatment of bipolar depression in the elderly population (Bobo 2017; Sajatovic and Chen 2011). Adding psychotherapy to medications in treatment of bipolar depression can reduce recurrence by 50% (Bobo 2017).

When breakthrough episodes of bipolar depression occur in patients established on a treatment regimen, it is important to evaluate contributing factors, such as inadequate doses or noncompliance with medications, drug-drug interactions contributing to medication inefficacy, use of concomitant medications that may destabilize mood such as antidepressants and psychostimulants, changes in thyroid functioning induced by lithium, substance use, and/or psychosocial stressors (Bobo 2017).

Finally, patients with bipolar disorder frequently experience anxiety or have comorbid anxiety disorders. There are no controlled trials of the treatment of anxiety in older-age bipolar disorder. In younger adults, quetiapine has the strongest evidence of efficacy, with some evidence for lamotrigine, olanzapine, olanzapine+fluoxetine, gabapentin, and topiramate (for obsessive-compulsive disorder) (Yatham et al. 2018). Limiting the use of antidepressants and especially of BZDs is a good idea.

AVOIDING AND ADDRESSING POLYPHARMACY

The physiological changes that accompany aging place individuals at risk for an increased burden of general medical conditions, increased number of prescribed medications, and increased risk of adverse side effects from these medications (Mangin et al. 2018; Poudel et al. 2016). Mental health comorbidities contribute to *polypharmacy* both directly (psychotropic prescriptions) and indirectly (depression is associated with higher rates of multimorbidity and higher odds of polypharmacy), such that the interplay has important impact on disease course (Holvast et al. 2017). Polypharmacy is often defined as the daily use of five or more medications and can increase risk of serious complications such as falls, functional and cognitive decline, hospitalization, and even mortality (Masnoon et al. 2017). For a summary of how polypharmacy comes into existence and its impacts on geriatric patients, refer to Figure 5–1.

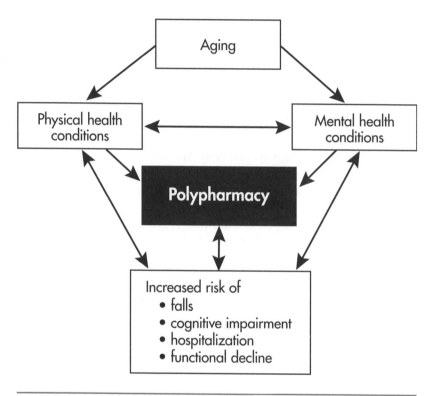

Figure 5–1. **Interplay among age, physical disorders, mental disorders, and polypharmacy.**

Explicit guidelines and lists such as the aforementioned Beers Criteria and the Screening Tool of Older Persons' Prescriptions and Screening Tool to Alert to Right Treatment (STOPP/START) exist to promote attention to medication burden in older adults. In these guidelines, psychotropic medications are described as "potentially inappropriate" or "high risk" because of their potential for anticholinergic and other CNS side effects. A number of psychotropic medications we have discussed have anticholinergic effects, including TCAs, paroxetine, and olanzapine—even citalopram and fluoxetine are slightly anticholinergic (Chew et al. 2008). This is not to say that antidepressant medications should be discontinued for all or even most older adults but rather to point out that these medications are not without risk. It's important to reevaluate the need for these medications over time because the risk-to-benefit ratio may change as a person ages and becomes more vulnerable to adverse effects.

Although algorithm-based guidelines are helpful resources, these tools rarely capture the complexity of multimorbidity, which often requires a higher level of clinical reasoning. It may be useful to follow a more general approach to medication review in older adults that applies to the review of prescribed psychotropics as well. Poudel et al. (2016) propose the following questions to consider when deciding whether to continue a potentially inappropriate medication in an older adult:

- Is there a valid and active indication for this medication?
- Is this medication offering relevant and meaningful benefit?
- Is this medication causing side effects?

Poudel et al. (2016) proposed that medications offering clinical benefit with minimal or no side effects should be continued in most cases. However, they also proposed that medications without a clear indication or meaningful benefit should be withdrawn or adjusted, with careful monitoring to reduce unnecessary polypharmacy and to reduce risk for adverse outcomes (Poudel et al. 2016). See Table 5–6 for a summary of addressing polypharmacy.

There are several options to consider when a person is taking a psychotropic such as an antidepressant that is not proving to be of sufficient benefit. A first step is to assess adherence because most psychotropics, including antidepressants, must be taken daily for best benefit. If a person is not taking medications regularly, interventions to bolster adherence are likely to be safer and more effective than adding another medication to the mix. Another factor to consider is dosage and duration of the trial. If a person is not finding benefit but the dosage is not optimized, the simplest and safest psychopharmacological step is to optimize benefit from one medication before adding second. When a medication produces benefit but also unacceptable side effects, options include 1) transitioning to a new dosage or changing the frequency of dose or formulation of the same drug or 2) transitioning to an alternative drug with less risk for problematic side effects, although one must be mindful to discontinue the ineffective medication in the process (Mangin et al. 2018). Finally, nonpharmacological options such as psychotherapy should also be employed when possible because these alternative evidence-based treatments are likely to reduce a person's need for psychotropic medication over time (Poudel et al. 2016).

Table 5–6. Reducing polypharmacy in older adults with depression or anxiety

For each potentially inappropriate medication, ask the following:

• Is there a valid and active indication? If not, taper or discontinue medication

• Is the patient getting meaningful benefit? If not,

  - Assess and address adherence.

  - Ensure adequate dosage and duration of medication trial.

  - Review the diagnosis and treatment plan.

  - If there is still no benefit, then taper or discontinue medication.

• Are there side effects? If so (but there is benefit):

  - Consider dose reduction before tapering or stopping.

  - Switch to another medication or nonpharmacological approach.

Be especially mindful of transitions of care, which increase the risk of medication errors and also present an opportunity to address polypharmacy.

Source.   Adapted from Poudel et al. 2016.

A final note includes the need for attention to care transitions that are a risky time for medication reconciliation errors. Older adults with more medically complex conditions are more likely to receive care in different settings such as a hospital or a nursing home in addition to outpatient care with multiple specialists (Zullo et al. 2018). Transitions between health care settings and health care providers open unfortunate opportunities for medication errors, especially when individuals are unable to accurately describe their current home medication regimen. Clinicians must vigilantly review and compare medication lists from the inpatient and outpatient settings and compare these lists to the person's actual home regimen. If an individual is unable to organize and adhere to his or her prescribed regimen, he or she is unlikely to benefit from it, such that assistance with medication organization and adherence becomes the top priority for effective psychopharmacological care.

Somatic Treatments

ELECTROCONVULSIVE THERAPY

ECT is the gold standard for treatment-resistant MDD. ECT is more effective than pharmacotherapy and more effective than sham ECT (Spaans et al. 2015; UK ECT Review Group 2003). There is a consensus on the primary use of ECT in severe MDD with psychotic features, mania with psychotic features, and catatonia. Patients should also be referred to ECT in cases of poor clinical response or intolerance of side effects with use of pharmacotherapy, emergence of suicidal ideation, or poor self-care (American Psychiatric Association Committee on Electroconvulsive Therapy 2001). As a group, elderly patients constitute a high proportion of those who receive ECT because they are more likely to have experienced intolerable side effects with medications and to have medical complications of depression that necessitate a more rapid response (American Psychiatric Association Committee on Electroconvulsive Therapy 2001).

Overall, older adults appear to derive greater benefit from ECT than do their younger counterparts (O'Connor et al. 2001). They also experience lower rates of psychiatric rehospitalization following a successful course of ECT (Rosen et al. 2016). A great deal is still unknown about who is most likely to benefit from ECT. Predictors of poor response to ECT include longer depressive episodes, greater number of pharmacotherapy failures, and medial temporal atrophy (American Psychiatric Association Committee on Electroconvulsive Therapy 2001; Oudega et al. 2011).

Increasing age and presence of a higher number of medical comorbidities may result in a greater likelihood of medical problems developing during ECT, which may require treatment or temporary halt of ECT. These problems include cardiovascular issues (exacerbation of congestive heart failure, hypertension, development of arrhythmias), CNS problems (greater degree of confusion and disorientation), and aspiration pneumonia (Alexopoulos et al. 1984). However, these problems are generally reversible (Alexopoulos et al. 1984). Interestingly, older patients and those with cardiac disease are less likely to experience asystole during ECT than are younger, healthier patients (Burd and Kettl 1998). Cardiovascular safety of ECT is further substantiated by a retrospective chart review of 35 patients, ages ranging from 54 to 92, all of whom were diagnosed with congestive heart failure and decreased left ventricular systolic ejection fraction. All of them tolerated ECT without death, decompensated heart failure, myocardial ischemia, or myocardial infarction during or within 24 hours of an ECT session (Rivera et al. 2011). Given the frequent comorbidity of COPD in older patients, particularly smokers, the management of COPD should be optimized prior to ECT, and the procedure should be avoided during acute COPD exacerbations (Schak et al. 2008).

Despite the prevailing concern among clinicians about the cognitive side effects of ECT, in geriatric patients, as in others, these effects are usually transient and should not be a barrier to receiving ECT (Geduldig and

Kellner 2016; Kumar et al. 2016). ECT does not place a person at greater risk of developing dementia (Osler et al. 2018). In fact, patients with dementia do not experience ECT-related decline in cognition, although they may experience more cognitive side effects in the acute phase of treatment (Hausner et al. 2011). ECT for late-life depression may improve cognitive functioning, at least in part because of improvement of depressive symptoms. For example, ECT improved cognitive domains such as information processing and perception in a study of 45 patients without dementia (mean age 57) followed up to 12 months after a course of ECT, with older patients showing more improvement than younger ones (Bosboom and Deijen 2006). One way to reduce the risk of cognitive side effects during the course of ECT is to use right unilateral instead of bilateral lead placement (Kumar et al. 2016). A review of five clinical trials of the use of acetylcholinesterase inhibitor through the course of treatment found modest benefit for memory (Henstra et al. 2017). Because these medications are indicated only for treatment of dementia, we recommend that they be prescribed only for this indication rather than to ameliorate the side effects of ECT—but they may offer cognitive benefits to patients with dementia during the ECT course. Note that cholinesterase inhibitors may prolong the action of succinylcholine, an agent used to induce paralysis during ECT.

Recommendations for use of ECT in older adults are summarized in Table 5–7. As far as the technical aspects of ECT administration, older patients have a higher seizure threshold, which may cause problems with eliciting a seizure. Although the consideration of preventing cognitive side effects favors right unilateral over bilateral lead placement, an increase in stimulus or a switch to a bilateral method of administration of ECT may be necessary to achieve good quality seizures and ensure response to treatment (Kumar et al. 2016; Meyer et al. 2018). It may be wise to begin treatment bilaterally, foregoing a trial of the right unilateral method altogether, if the patient is so ill as to exhibit refusal to eat, catatonic features, acute suicidal ideation with a plan, severe psychosis, or other distressing symptoms related to his or her affective disorder. As noted earlier, ECT is also an effective treatment for bipolar depression.

Relapse rates following a successful course of ECT are high. For example, in an RCT that evaluated continuation pharmacotherapy following ECT, all participants in the study relapsed within 6 months of stopping ECT, although the combination of lithium and nortriptyline had some efficacy in preventing relapse (Sackeim et al. 2001). Unfortunately, evidence for continuation and maintenance ECT in depressed elderly patients is lacking. A systematic review found that maintenance

---

Table 5–7.   Recommendations for electroconvulsive use in late-life
                    depression

---

1. ECT is not a last-resort treatment and should be offered to severely
   depressed patients for whom pharmacotherapy was unsuccessful,
   particularly those with psychosis, suicidal ideation, and poor self-care.

2. A thorough history and physical should be done for any elderly patient
   about to have ECT, with all comorbidities addressed and stabilized if time
   permits.

3. The consent process should include family and caregivers if available. A
   discussion of the cognitive side effects should emphasize likely short-term
   problems but also potential long-term benefits and lack of long-term impact
   on cognition.

4. Medical problems during the index course of ECT in elderly patients are
   common. In addition to appropriate treatment, patients may benefit from
   reducing procedure frequency and stimulus intensity (although the latter
   may have a cost to efficacy).

5. Reduce or eliminate any medications that may have an impact on cognition
   (sedatives, anticholinergics, benzodiazepines) and seizure threshold
   (anticonvulsants).

6. Start with right unilateral stimulus but switch to bilateral stimulus if needed
   to achieve efficacy.

7. Consider maintenance ECT for patients with refractory depression who
   have not responded to other treatment modalities. Consider continuation
   pharmacotherapy with lithium and nortriptyline combination to increase
   chances for successful recovery. Consider maintenance ECT for patients who
   did not have success with continuation pharmacotherapy.

8. Clinicians should advocate for improved access to ECT, especially for ethnic
   minority older adults.

Note.   ECT=electroconvulsive therapy.

ECT is as effective as continuation medication and is generally well tolerated, leading the study's authors to recommend it if continuation pharmacotherapy is ineffective (van Schaik et al. 2012). Other experts (e.g., Geduldig and Kellner 2016) recommend continuation and maintenance ECT more wholeheartedly. In clinical practice, it is common to offer maintenance ECT to patients with chronic and severe late-life depression that does not respond to treatments other than ECT.

Novel procedures using electrical current, such as transcranial direct current stimulation and low-charge electrotherapy, are being investigated as potential alternative treatments to ECT, the latter showing promising results when administered bitemporally (Kong et al. 2019). However, so far none of them can boast of efficacy comparable with that of ECT. For now, ECT remains the undisputed champion and the prime treatment to offer to severely depressed elderly patients with treatment-resistant illness. Unfortunately, it is underused, as evidenced by the falling use of ECT in the United States (Case et al. 2013), with ethnic minority elders being less likely to receive ECT during inpatient hospitalization (Jones et al. 2019). It is up to all clinicians, particularly those with specialization in geriatrics, to advocate for all patients who may benefit from ECT to be referred to this often life-saving treatment.

REPETITIVE TRANSCRANIAL MAGNETIC STIMULATION

Repetitive transcranial magnetic stimulation (rTMS) is an FDA-approved treatment for adults with treatment-resistant MDD. Currently, in the United States it can be recommended for use in adults if they have a failed trial of one antidepressant. rTMS works by using an electric current to generate rapidly alternating magnetic fields, which pass through the skull when the device is placed on the scalp (Perera et al. 2016). Electric currents are then induced in localized areas of the cerebral cortex. The most commonly targeted cortical region is the dorsolateral prefrontal cortex (DLPFC), which is known to be involved in emotion regulation. Although more research is necessary, there is a great deal of interest in the potential of rTMS for enhancing cognition and executive functioning in late-life depression (Ilieva et al. 2018).

rTMS should be considered as a treatment option in older adults with depression who are intolerant of pharmacotherapy or who have relative contraindications for ECT and/or general anesthesia. Older adults appear to respond to rTMS as well as do younger adults. For example, a naturalistic study of 231 adults (75 of them ages 60 years and older and 156 of them younger than 60 years) did not demonstrate a difference in outcomes on the basis of age (Conelea et al. 2017). Although some early RCTs did not find efficacy of rTMS in older adults, more recent studies using higher stimulation intensity showed efficacy. Parameters now commonly used are 10 Hz frequency, 120% motor threshold stimulation over the left DLPFC, 3,000 pulses per session, and five sessions per week for at least 4 weeks (Iriarte and George 2018). There is some evidence supporting the use of bilateral rTMS and deep rTMS with a coil that allows stimulation of deeper and larger brain volumes (Kaster et al. 2018; Trevizol et al. 2019). rTMS may be effective in patients with vascular depression (late-life depression with evidence of cerebrovascular disease). Older age and smaller frontal gray matter volume, but not white matter hyperintensities, are associated with poorer response to rTMS (Jorge et al. 2008).

Significant advantages of rTMS over ECT are that it does not cause cognitive side effects and does not require anesthesia, and patients do not need an escort to return home after procedures. Still, there are safety considerations with rTMS. There is a small risk of generalized tonic-clonic seizures (incidence of less than 1 in 10,000), usually occurring in neurologically compromised patients or with parameters outside recommended standards (Iriarte and George 2018). This highlights the importance of a full neurological exam and screening for seizure risk factors prior to starting a course of treatment. Emergence of mania and hypomania is rare; more common side effects include vasovagal syncope; headache; a temporary increase in auditory threshold; and localized scalp discomfort, to which patients typically develop a tolerance after 2 weeks (Iriarte and George 2018; Perera et al. 2016).

BRIGHT LIGHT THERAPY

Bright light therapy (BLT) can be used alone or as an adjunct for patients with seasonal affective disorder (i.e., major depressive disorder with seasonal variation). There is also growing evidence that BLT may be effective for patients who have depression without seasonal variation. The mechanism of action of BLT is unclear, but it is thought to involve the suprachiasmatic nucleus of the hypothalamus, which helps regulate circadian rhythm. Dysfunction of the suprachiasmatic nucleus and associated circadian rhythm disruption may underlie sleep disturbance and diurnal variation in mood in people with depression (Lieverse et al. 2011).

A review and meta-analysis of BLT found efficacy similar to that of other augmentation strategies when used with standard antidepressant pharmacotherapy in treatment of MDD and bipolar depression (Penders et al. 2016). The American Psychiatric Association practice guideline for MDD recommends BLT as a monotherapy for acute MDD (American Psychiatric Association 2010). A meta-analysis that included six trials with 359 subjects 2–4 weeks in duration found that BLT was effective for nonseasonal depression in older adults (Zhao et al. 2018). BLT may be effective for bipolar depression, perhaps at a lower dosage and/or with midday timing to reduce the risk of a switch to mania (note that these studies were conducted in younger adults) (Hirakawa et al. 2020). A small RCT of light therapy among institutionalized patients with depression found substantial improvement in depressive symptoms (Sumaya et al. 2001).

We recommend a dose of 10,000 lux for 30 minutes each morning (lower and during the midday for bipolar depression). Please advise your patients to carefully review the specifications of a light box before buying one. The intensity of light drops off exponentially with distance, so the device should state at what distance the user should sit to receive 10,000 lux. The editor of this book has found light boxes for sale online that deliver 10,000 lux at a distance of 4 inches, which is not practical; he recommends light boxes from The Sunbox Company (www.sunbox.com) or Northern Light Technologies (https:// northernlighttechnologies.com). Unfortunately, Medicare does not cover the cost of a light box. The most common side effect is headache.

KETAMINE AND ESKETAMINE

Evidence from several clinical trials demonstrated that ketamine can produce a rapid although short-lived antidepressant effect, leading to widespread adoption of this agent for treatment-resistant depression (Newport et al. 2015). Today, it is not unusual to find ketamine clinics in many metropolitan centers, advertising directly to consumers and accepting cash payments. However, it's worth remembering that the evidence for using intravenous ketamine infusions is limited, especially in older adults, and that we lack long-term studies to assess the safety and efficacy of ketamine over time (Bratsos and Saleh 2019). We lack evidence that this treatment works when used as maintenance. We should also be concerned about long-term treatment on the basis of what we know of the impact of repeated ketamine use in recreational drug users, who experience profound urinary, hepatic, and cognitive side effects (Loo 2018). Ketamine's potential for abuse raises another concern, and it has been argued that ketamine's clinical benefits are due to its effects on the opioid system (Williams et al. 2018). Nevertheless, the great need for effective and versatile treatments in this arena is such that if ECT is unavailable or contraindicated, ketamine should be considered as a viable option.

The FDA has approved intranasal esketamine (in combination with an antidepressant) for MDD in patients with at least two failed antidepressant trials; intravenous and subcutaneous ketamine has not been FDA approved for any psychiatric indication. The American Psychiatric Association Council on Research Task Force on Novel Biomarkers and Treatments subgroup has made recommendations regarding the use of intravenous ketamine in the treatment of mood disorders, which range from training of clinicians administering the treatment to dosing of the medication to considering continuation and maintenance treatment (Sanacora et al. 2017); we highly recommend reviewing this article before recommending or administering such treatment to any patient, adult or geriatric. CANMAT has also published recommendations that cover both ketamine and esketamine in MDD (Swainson et al. 2021). Ketamine may also be effective in comorbid MDD and PTSD (Albott et al. 2018), in combination with ECT to accelerate the antidepressant effect (Ren et al. 2018), and perhaps as a single dose of (es)ketamine to rapidly reduce suicidal ideation (Canuso et al. 2018; Swainson et al. 2021).

Dosing for esketamine is as follows: The starting dose is 56 mg for adults younger than 65 years and 28 mg for adults ages 65 and older. Subsequent doses (56 mg or 84 mg for adults younger than 65 and 28 mg, 56 mg, or 84 mg for those ages 65 and older) are given twice a week for 4 weeks, followed by once a week for 4 weeks, and then once a week or once every 2 weeks from week 9, with treatment recommended for at least 6 months after symptoms improve (Drug Therapy Bulletin 2020). We recommend also reviewing the information at the manufacturer's website, www.spravatohcp.com/trd/dosing-and-administration.

Most protocols for intravenous ketamine infusions use a dose of 0.5 mg/kg, which produces moderate sedation, administered over 40 minutes, twice a week, for total of 6 treatments. On the basis of the lack of data regarding the long-term outcomes of ketamine infusions, this treatment should be considered a short-term "jump start," hopefully leading the patient to eventually engage in other forms of treatment for depression described in this chapter that offer long-term benefits.

Although there are studies of other ketamine administration routes demonstrating efficacy in treatment-resistant depression, such as subcutaneous and oral routes, no guidelines have been created for their use (Andrade 2017). Therefore, we do not discuss these types of treatments in detail here.

There is little literature regarding the use of (es)ketamine in older adults. One small RCT (16 subjects) of subcutaneous ketamine using midazolam as an active control, followed by open-label ketamine for those who did not remit and for those who relapsed, found that ketamine was effective at reducing depression (George et al. 2017). An RCT of intranasal esketamine plus antidepressant that used a similar design to a study that had demonstrated efficacy (Popova et al. 2019) and instead recruited older adults (N=138) did not find benefit, especially in subjects 75 years and older (Ochs-Ross et al. 2020). It is possible that the study was underpowered and that esketamine may have been underdosed. A case series of geriatric patients hospitalized with a relapse of MDD reported failure of intravenous ketamine infusions in three out of four patients, with the one relative success experiencing incomplete but notable improvement in depressive symptoms. Significantly, the patients described in this series had substantial treatment resistance (having had protracted courses of MDD through their lives and having not had positive outcomes with ECT) and comorbidities such as GAD and Parkinson's disease; therefore, this experience may not be applicable in patients with less treatment-resistant illness. In this series, one patient discontinued treatment because of psychotomimetic side effects and lack of efficacy, and another patient was frightened of his experiences (Szymkowicz et al. 2014).

Ketamine administration has a set of common side effects, including psychotomimetic and dissociative effects as well as impacts on blood pressure and heart rate. Although psychiatric side effects may be brief, the patients may experience them as highly unpleasant and, in our clinical experience, refuse further treatments because of them. In longer-term use, patients should be monitored for urinary symptoms (cystitis), cognitive impairment, and substance misuse (Swainson et al. 2021).

Complementary and Alternative Medicine

As people age, they tend to increase their use of complementary and alternative medicine (Nyer et al. 2013). Additionally, there is a movement in favor of natural remedies in the United States and Europe. Stigma surrounding mental health treatment may result in patients opting for mind-body strategies over psychotropic medications and psychotherapy (Meeks et al. 2007; Nyer et al. 2013). Although there have not been a great deal of well-designed RCTs exploring complementary and alternative treatments, some evidence in their favor exists. Supplements that have been studied in older adults include St. John's wort; fish oil; *S*-adenosyl methionine; folic acid; and a Chinese herbal medicine, shuganjieyu (Meeks et al. 2007; Nyer et al. 2013; Xie et al. 2015). For a summary of complementary and alternative treatments and recommendations for using them, see Table 5–8.

Creative expression, such as engaging in art or musical performance, can provide an outlet for emotions and a distraction from everyday stressors. In a systematic review of 12 studies, art therapy was found to be an acceptable treatment for most patients with nonpsychotic mental health disorders (Scope et al. 2017). Available evidence also suggests that this treatment is cost-effective and has clinical efficacy, although the data are of low quality (Uttley et al. 2015). In an RCT of older women with MDD who were stable with pharmacotherapy, those allocated to receive art therapy as adjuvant treatment had significant improvement on a depression scale after 20 weekly sessions as compared with control subjects (Ciasca et al. 2018).

Table 5–8.   Complementary and alternative treatments and
recommendations for their use

Therapy	Outcomes	Recommendations
Yoga	Plausible improvement in anger, self-control, depression, and anxiety Increased perception of self-control	Low-impact stretches and yoga exercises as tolerated at least weekly
Tai chi	Improved balance and physical function Reduced symptoms of depression, stress, and anxiety	Tai chi daily to weekly in addition to medication or in combination with art therapy, music reminiscence, and mindfulness awareness practice
St. John's wort	Cytochrome P450 inducer Possible antidementia effects Possible improvement in depressive symptoms	900–1800 mg/day Use caution with other medications Do not combine with SSRIs
Fish oil	Limited interactions with other drugs Improvement in depressive symptoms	Monotherapy or therapy augmented with standard antidepressants 3:2 ratio of EPA:DHA, 1000 mg/day
S-adenosyl methionine (SAMe)	Improvement in depressive symptoms Side effects of GI upset Possible improvement in cognition Improved joint health	SAMe monotherapy or with a TCA 800–1600 mg/day
Folic acid or L-methylfolate	Plausible improvement in depressive symptoms Possible antidementia affects	15 mg/day plus antidepressant
Massage	Possible mild benefits in depressive symptoms Side effect of soreness	Variable Low- to medium-pressure massage as tolerated
Music therapy	Plausible decrease in depressive symptoms Provides a comfortable alternative for emotional expression	Independent, home-based therapy sessions in addition to antidepressant

Table 5–8. Complementary and alternative treatments and recommendations for their use *(continued)*

Therapy	Outcomes	Recommendations
Chinese herbal medicine (shuganjieyu)	Safety and efficacy found in an RCT when shuganjieyu was administered with rTMS vs. sham rTMS; rTMS did not have additional benefit	Four capsules of shuganjieyu daily for 6 weeks
Art therapy	Decrease in depressive symptoms Positive results include understanding the self, finding perspective, distraction from everyday stressors, personal achievement, expression, relaxation, and empowerment	Recommended as adjuvant treatment in combination with other treatment modalities

Note. See text for discussion and references.
Abbreviations. DCA=docosahexaenoic acid; EPA=eicosapentaenoic acid; RCT = randomized controlled trial; SAMe=S-adenosyl methionine; rTMS=repetitive transcranial magnetic stimulation; SSRIs=selective serotonin reuptake inhibitors; TCA=tricyclic antidepressant.

Music therapy is an area of emerging research that has produced encouraging results. In an RCT of 134 community-dwelling adults older than 65 years who were at risk for falls, those who engaged in weekly supervised group classes of multitask exercises set to piano music experienced reductions in anxiety and improvement in cognition as compared with control subjects (Hars et al. 2014). Listening to music has been found effective for reducing anxiety for older adults admitted to an emergency department (Belland et al. 2017). A systematic review of music therapy among elders found a statistically significant reduction in depressive symptoms, although not when compared with standard treatments. Importantly, there was no support for the use of music therapy as treatment for depression in dementia (Zhao et al. 2016).

In a study conducted in Singapore, older adults with subsyndromal depression and anxiety participated in tai chi, art therapy, mindfulness awareness practice, and music reminiscence therapy (combination of music therapy and reminiscence therapy), at first as single interventions and then in combination, leading to significant reduction of anxious and depressive symptoms in both phases of treatment (Rawtaer et al. 2015). A community program using the same intervention for elderly individuals older than 60 years led to improved sleep quality, independent of changes in depressive and anxiety symptoms (Rawtaer et al. 2018). Tai chi, when added to escitalopram, led to additional benefits in treatment of depression as compared with medication alone (Lavretsky et al. 2011).

Yoga has been evaluated in several trials. In a small RCT, Sudarshan Kriya yoga, a breathing-based meditative technique, had demonstrated efficacy for patients with MDD who did not respond adequately to antidepressants (Sharma et al. 2017). Sahaj Samadhi, another meditation technique, has been found to improve depressive symptoms in patients ages 60–85 years with mild to moderate depression who were randomly assigned to receive this novel intervention or treatment as usual (Ionson et al. 2019).

Overall, the available evidence for use of complementary and alternative medicine in late-life depression and anxiety is encouraging. Music therapy, art therapy, tai chi, yoga, and other treatment modalities can be recommended as augmentation strategies for patients who are interested in them and who can access them.

Public Health Interventions

Even though late-life depression and anxiety are common and consequential, they remain underrecognized and undertreated in the general population (Ciechanowski et al. 2004; Tapia-Munoz et al. 2015; Unützer et al. 2002). Barriers to effective detection, diagnosis, and treatment exist at multiple levels, including the patient, the clinician, and the health care organization as a whole (Table 5–9) (Bruce and Pearson 1999; McEvoy and Barnes 2007).

Despite barriers to effective care, a strong and growing body of evidence has consistently shown that public health interventions with emphasis on the redesign of health care systems are both effective and resource-efficient for late-life depression and anxiety (Bruce and Pearson 1999; Hegel et al. 2005; Hunkeler et al. 2006; Unützer and Park 2012; Unützer et al. 2002). Much research on this topic stems from the *chronic care model* that was developed in the 1990s with the aim of effectively managing long-term chronic physical health conditions (McEvoy and Barnes 2007). The chronic care model calls for a systems delivery redesign to more proactively screen for and monitor chronic physical health conditions, uses clinical care managers to coordinate care for patients with complex needs, and includes decision support to guide evidence-

Table 5–9. Barriers to effective identification and treatment of older adults with depression and anxiety

	Patient-level barriers	Clinician-level barriers	Organizational barriers
Barriers to diagnosis and detection	• Assumption that symptoms are a normal part of aging • Assumption that symptoms are caused by comorbid physical health conditions • Fear of being stigmatized • Being embarrassed to talk about mental health symptoms	• Assumption that symptoms are a normal part of aging • Assumption that symptoms are caused by comorbid physical health conditions • Fear of stigmatizing the patient • Do not want to embarrass patient by talking about mental health symptoms	
Barriers to effective treatment	• Mistrust of the mental health system and treatments • Unaware of or misinformed about the risks and benefits of various treatment options	• Insufficient time to address mental health comorbidities • Mental health comorbidities given low priority during visit • Insufficient knowledge of or comfort with prescribing treatment for mental health conditions • Inadequate dosage or duration of antidepressant	• Most older adults prefer to access mental health care within primary care, but systems are often not set up to deliver effective care in this way • Health care systems were historically designed to be reactive rather proactive, which is not ideal for chronic health conditions such as depression and anxiety

Table 5–9. Barriers to effective identification and treatment of older adults with depression and anxiety *(continued)*

	Patient-level barriers	Clinician-level barriers	Organizational barriers
Barriers to effective treatment *(continued)*			• Older adults are at risk for logistical barriers to usual care, including limited finances, mobility problems, limited access to transportation, cognitive decline, sensory changes (eyesight, hearing) that are not routinely discussed but can interfere with access to care, and other structural barriers affecting minority elders

Note. See text for discussion and references.

based treatment protocols when problems are detected (McEvoy and Barnes 2007). The chronic care model emphasizes a need for leadership support at the organization level, inclusion of community partners to support and maintain health and wellness, and regular communication among care managers, patients, primary care providers, and consulting specialists to collaborate on care plans (McEvoy and Barnes 2007).

COLLABORATIVE CARE

More recently, a large body of evidence has grown to support *collaborative care* as an adaptation of the chronic care model to specifically address mental health conditions in the primary care setting. This is relevant because most older adults prefer to receive care within primary care rather than more specialized clinics, because more than half of depression care occurs within the primary care setting, and because studies have consistently shown depression care to be somewhat inadequate in this setting (Bruce and Pearson 1999; Hall and Reynolds 2014). The collaborative care model adds to the primary care team a behavioral health case manager who works directly with patients to proactively monitor mental health symptoms, provide support, and deliver evidence-based psychotherapy treatments. The case manager meets regularly with a psychiatric consultant to review the caseload and optimize treatment planning for patients, which might include recommendations for a psychotropic prescription or referral to a higher level of care when indicated. The primary care provider remains an active participant in the collaborative care model and commonly prescribes psychotropics when they are recommended by the behavioral health team (see the Advancing Integrated Mental Health Solutions (AIMS) Center website, http://aims.uw.edu). The key components to a successful collaborative care program include the following:

1. *A patient-centered care team*: primary care and behavioral health providers collaborate to address both physical and mental health care within the primary care setting
2. *Population-based care*: patients are tracked in a registry and proactively monitored
3. *Measurement-based treatment to target*: the program incorporates objective measures to monitor progress, and treatments are adjusted accordingly
4. *Evidence-based care*: the program uses scientifically proven psychotherapy and psychopharmacology interventions to treat mental health disorders
5. *Accountable care*: providers are accountable and are reimbursed for quality of care and outcomes (AIMS Center 2011)

The collaborative care model specifically requires systematic screening, follow-up, treatment adjustment, and relapse prevention as indicated (also known as *stepped care*) and regular communication and care coordination between the patient and all members of the health care team (AIMS Center 2011).

There are several key studies that have supported use of the chronic care model and specifically collaborative care as superior to usual care in the treatment of depressive and anxiety disorders in older adults. See Table 5–10 for a summary; we present the details next.

The most robust evidence stems from the Improving Mood—Promoting Access to Collaborative Care Treatment (IMPACT) study in which patients ages 60 and older with MDD, dysthymic disorder, or both were randomly assigned to receive usual care or a year-long intentional collaborative care intervention (Unützer et al. 2002). Patients receiving a collaborative care intervention were given access to a case manager who

Table 5–10. Summary of evidence for collaborative care in treatment of older adults with depression

Study	Primary target(s)	Primary intervention options with stepped-care application	Relevant outcomes for intervention group
IMPACT (Unützer et al. 2002)	Major depressive disorder Dysthymic disorder	• Problem-solving therapy • Antidepressant medication	• Increased access to appropriate treatment • Greater reduction in depressive symptoms • Less functional impairment • Better quality of life
PROSPECT (Bruce and Pearson 1999; Bruce et al. 2004)	Major depressive disorder Minor depression	• Interpersonal therapy • Antidepressant medications	• Increased access to appropriate treatment • More rapid and robust reduction in depressive symptoms • Reduced suicidal ideation
PEARLS (Ciechanowski et al. 2004)	Minor depression Dysthymia	• Problem-solving therapy • Behavioral activation (social and physical activation) • Antidepressant medications	• Increased response and remission rates for depressive symptoms • Improved functional and emotional well-being

Table 5–10. Summary of evidence for collaborative care in treatment of older adults with depression *(continued)*

Study	Primary target(s)	Primary intervention options with stepped-care application	Relevant outcomes for intervention group
I-TEAM (Gellis et al. 2014)	Depression (positive screen) in combination with significant medical comorbidity and high health care utilization	•Problem-solving therapy	•Greater reduction in depressive symptoms •Better problem-solving skills •Fewer ED visits
Healthy IDEAS (Casado et al. 2008; Quijano et al. 2007)	Low-income medically ill older adults with positive depression screen	•Psychoeducation •Behavioral activation	•Greater reduction in depressive symptoms •Improved pain •Increased activity
SUSTAIN (Mavandadi et al. 2015)	Depression or anxiety treated with newly prescribed antidepressant or anxiolytic for depression or anxiety symptoms	•Psychoeducation •Problem-solving therapy •Motivational interviewing •Antidepressant or anxiolytic medication	•Greater reduction in depressive symptoms •Greater reduction in anxiety symptoms •Improved overall mental health functioning

Abbreviations. ED=emergency department; IMPACT=Improved Mood—Promoting Access to Collaborative Care Treatment; Healthy IDEAS=Identifying Depression, Empowering Activities for Seniors; I-TEAM=Integrated Telehealth Education and Activation of Mood; PEARLS=Program to Encourage Active, Rewarding Lives for Seniors; PROSPECT=Prevention of Suicide in Primary Care Elderly: Collaborative Trial; SUSTAIN=Supporting Seniors Receiving Treatment and Intervention.

helped them develop a personalized treatment plan and provided proactive monitoring for progress. The case manager had access to a psychiatric consultant and a protocol for evidence-based stepped care. Treatment options included PST and/or SSRI antidepressants, and treatment plans were adjusted according to patient preference and clinical status. Significantly more intervention patients were prescribed an appropriate evidence-based treatment (psychotherapy and/or an antidepressant) compared with usual care, and intervention patients also had significantly lower depression scores, higher rates of treatment response and remission, and increased satisfaction with treatment (Unützer et al. 2002). The benefits also extended beyond the depressive disorders alone, and the intervention group showed better overall functioning and better quality of life (Unützer et al. 2002). There is also evidence that significant health benefits are sustained for a year or more after the treatment episode ends (Hunkeler et al. 2006).

A similar collaborative care study, Prevention of Suicide in Primary Care Elderly: Collaborative Trial (PROSPECT) aimed to use the collaborative care model to minimize barriers to depression treatment and improve access to effective depression care with the goal of reducing suicide risk in older adults (Bruce and Pearson 1999). The PROSPECT intervention uses guideline management, a strategy to increase the use by primary care providers of an evidence-based treatment algorithm for depression. The model requires a health specialist (often a nurse, social worker, or clinical psychologist) to be embedded in the primary care setting and to proactively recognize at-risk patients in need of screening. The health specialist is responsible for helping primary care providers identify depression, providing at-risk patients with psychoeducation, and assisting in linking the patient with appropriate treatment interventions. The PROSPECT treatment algorithm includes psychoeducation, interpersonal psychotherapy, and/or antidepressant medications based on patient preference and clinical needs (Bruce and Pearson 1999). Similar to IMPACT, PROSPECT incorporates stepped care, decision support algorithms, case management, and regular communication and collaboration between behavioral health specialists and primary care (Bruce and Pearson 1999). The study found that individuals in the intervention group experienced more rapid and robust improvement to depressive symptoms and also more rapid reduction and resolution of suicidal thoughts compared with usual care, with a trend toward greater benefit for those with more significant depressive symptoms at baseline (Bruce et al. 2004).

Although there is strong evidence to support collaborative care programs to diagnose and treat late-life depression and anxiety, there is likely even more value in collaborative care programs aimed at prevention (Kenning et al. 2019). Efforts to identify older adults at risk for developing a depressive or anxiety disorder in combination with a preventive stepped-care intervention can reduce the incidence of major depressive episodes by as much as half (Hall and Reynolds 2014). Psychoeducation, health coaching, and PST for subsyndromal depressive symptoms have all shown value for this purpose (Hall and Reynolds 2014). There is also evidence that interventions aimed at improving the psychological well-being of older adults (*well-being therapy*, which incorporates elements of psychoeducation and CBT to promote life purpose and improve social relations) in the general community can reduce depressive symptoms and improve life satisfaction in a way that is likely protective against development of more serious disorders (Friedman et al. 2017). Thus, prevention may improve quality of life for older adults with subthreshold symptoms and may result in cost saving by preventing downstream consequences (Friedman et al. 2017; Kenning et al. 2019).

Collaborative care also benefits older adults with anxiety. Follow-up from the IMPACT study showed that older adults with depression and comorbid anxiety disorders benefited from the intervention, albeit less quickly and robustly (Hegel et al. 2005). This suggests that individuals with comorbid anxiety may need longer and more aggressive collaborative care interventions to achieve the best benefit.

COMMUNITY-BASED INTERVENTIONS

Collaborative care interventions as described in the previous subsection have been applied outside the research setting and have been shown to be feasible, effective, and well-liked by patients and health care providers (Penkunas and Hahn-Smith 2015). For example, the IMPACT intervention was implemented as part of a publicly funded initiative for low-income individuals in California and was proven effective regardless of age, education, or marital status (Penkunas and Hahn-Smith 2015). Most older adults in the study (85%) experienced some improvement in depressive symptoms, and almost half achieved a 50% or greater reduction in depressive symptoms (Penkunas and Hahn-Smith 2015). Factors shown to increase the likelihood of response included male sex, adherence to follow-up, and absence of comorbid substance use (Penkunas and Hahn-Smith 2015).

A similar collaborative care program was instituted in the state of Pennsylvania via the Supporting Seniors Receiving Treatment and Intervention (SUSTAIN) program and also demonstrated that measurement-based care paired with active care management (defined as a structured reaction to measurement-based care results, often in the form of brief psychotherapy, in this case by telephone) improved treatment outcomes (Mavandadi et al. 2015). The study found that intervention patients reported greater improvement in overall mental health functioning and greater reduction in both depressive and anxiety symptoms over the course of the program compared with monitoring alone without support of an active case manager (Mavandadi et al. 2015).

The Program to Encourage Active, Rewarding Lives for Seniors (PEARLS) intervention focused on medically ill, low-income, home-dwelling older adults with minor depression or dysthymia (Ciechanowski et al. 2004). This intervention included a course of PST adapted to emphasize behavioral activation, including promotion of physical activity and social engagement, as well as a psychiatry consultant to guide antidepressant prescriptions when indicated. PEARLS proved to be cost-effective and beneficial, with the intervention group showing a reduced depression severity, higher remission rates, and improved functional and emotional well-being compared with usual care (Ciechanowski et al. 2004).

Other studies have examined various adaptations of the collaborative care model in different settings with similarly positive results. For example, the Integrated Telehealth Education and Activation of Mood (I-TEAM) study used telephone outreach for home-dwelling older adults with chronic medical illness and comorbid depression. The goal was to promote functioning and independence for this community population with early detection of mood problems and rapid connection with a treatment intervention (Gellis et al. 2014). The I-TEAM intervention included regular telephone monitoring, a care manager for both medical illness and depression, and a course of PST. The study found that intervention patients had fewer emergency department visits and a 50% reduction in depression scores at multiple follow-up points (Gellis et al. 2014). Healthy IDEAS (Identifying Depression, Empowering Activities for Seniors) combined elements of IMPACT and PEARLS to identify and treat depressive symptoms in older adults with chronic health conditions and functional limitations (Casado et al. 2008; Quijano et al. 2007). This program, which included psychoeducation, behavioral activation, and telephone outreach for monitoring, demonstrated efficacy for reduced depression severity and pain and also an increase in activity level in the intervention group (Casado et al. 2008; Quijano et al. 2007).

Community-based interventions for older adults may be especially helpful for addressing barriers to effective care. For example, as described previously in the subsection "Problem-Solving Therapy," using PST along with social services such as care management can have a synergistic impact on depression and self-efficacy.

In summary, there is robust evidence that creative and systematic public health interventions are effective for older adults with depression and anxiety. These programs significantly improve access to evidence-based care for late-life depression and anxiety and offer significant benefits for both mental and physical health and well-being for those who participate. In the next subsection, we explore the potential role of telepsychiatry in further addressing barriers to care.

TELEPSYCHIATRY

The coronavirus SARS-CoV-2 disease (COVID-19) pandemic accelerated the adoption of telepsychiatry and led to changes in the regulation and funding of telepsychiatry around the world (Kinoshita et al. 2020). Telepsychiatry may help older adults overcome barriers to care associated with geography (e.g., living in rural and other underserved areas), transportation, financial challenges, and physical disability (Gentry et al. 2019). At the same time, older adults may face challenges with telepsychiatry, especially those who are not technologically literate; those who cannot afford the necessary technology; and those with cognitive, sensory, or motor barriers (Gentry et al. 2019).

The literature studying the use of telepsychiatry in depressed or anxious elders is limited but promising. CBT delivered by phone or internet has been found to be effective in older adults with depression and GAD (for more details, see the subsection "Cognitive-Behavioral Therapy") (Brenes et al. 2017; Hobbs et al. 2017, 2018). An RCT of telephone-based PST found comparable acute efficacy with in-person PST in low-income homebound older adults, with telephone-based therapy actually having more sustained benefit on depression and disability (Choi et al. 2014). As noted in the previous subsection, telephone outreach was built into three collaborative care models: I-TEAM, Healthy IDEAS, and SUSTAIN (Casado et al. 2008; Gellis et al. 2014; Mavandadi et al. 2015; Quijano et al. 2007). Another collaborative care model, Telemedicine Enhanced Antidepressant Management (TEAM), was not specifically designed for older adults, but a study of its efficacy enrolled primarily elderly white male U.S. veterans (Fortney et al. 2007). Subjects receiving TEAM were more likely to experience depression response and remission than those receiving usual care (Fortney et al. 2007). Telepsychiatry delivered to nursing homes and inpatient medical settings appears to be feasible and acceptable to older adult patients (Gentry et al. 2019).

Further research is needed on the use of telepsychiatry in outpatient geriatric mental health. Nevertheless, the genie is out of the bottle, and the rapid widespread adoption of telepsychiatry will likely persist. We of course recommend that our readers pay careful attention to regulatory and reimbursement issues in the jurisdictions where they practice and where their patients live. Psychiatrists in the United States may benefit from the American Psychiatric Association's online telepsychiatry resources (see "Resources for Clinicians" at the end of the chapter).

Monitoring and Addressing the Risk of Suicide

We devote Chapter 4 to an in-depth discussion of the epidemiology of suicide, screening for suicidality, conducting a suicide risk assessment, strategies to reduce risk, systems-level interventions, suicide in people with dementia and in nursing home residents, and legal and ethical issues. We return now to the topic to emphasize the importance of addressing suicidality as part of the care of all older adults with depression and anxiety.

Depression is intricately related to suicide, especially in older adults. In psychological autopsy studies of elders who died from suicide, MDD and other mood disorders are the most common comorbidities (Conwell et al. 2002). This highlights the critical importance of adequately treating depression, as we have discussed throughout this chapter. In addition, substance use disorders, social isolation, bereavement, family discord, physical illness, pain, anxiety, and insomnia are suicide risk factors, suggesting further avenues for intervention (Conwell et al. 2002; Kay et al. 2016; Li and Conwell 2010). For a comprehensive list of risk and protective factors, see Table 4–1 in Chapter 4.

Assessment of suicide requires a multipronged approach to screening and risk assessment to develop a need-based evaluation, accurate triage, and an individually tailored and comprehensive intervention plan. Here we summarize the steps involved in addressing the risk of suicide in older adults with depression or anxiety.

SCREEN FOR SUICIDALITY

Suicide screening tools can be used as an aid to the overall clinical assessment. Screening in the primary care setting can be particularly useful because more than 75% of older adults who died from suicide had contact with a primary care provider the year before their death (Andersen et al. 2000; Luoma et al. 2002). No suicide screening tool meets gold standards of perfect sensitivity, reliability, and validity. However, the C-SSRS and the PHQ-2+9 can be used for assessment of older adults. For discussion of these tools, see Chapter 4, subsection "Screening Tools."

INTERVIEW THE PATIENT

All patients being assessed for depression or anxiety should be queried about suicidal ideation. It is particularly important to screen in person for warning signs, suicidal ideation, and any steps considered or taken toward planning. Tact, patience, and a listening stance are most likely to help develop a therapeutic alliance and yield an accurate assessment of the patient's perceived circumstances and intentions. When evaluating a patient, it is important to do so in an environment that allows for privacy. Older adults may be less likely to report suicidal ideation, and the evaluation should be conducted both sensitively and comprehensively (Duberstein et al. 1999). If the patient has completed a depression or suicide questionnaire, these responses should be carefully reviewed during the interview. For a suggested approach to inquiring about suicidal ideation, see Chapter 4, subsection "The Suicide Inquiry."

ESTIMATE THE RISK OF SUICIDE

Most suicide risk stratification tools (e.g., structured clinical interviews, self-reported measures, predictive analytical models) on their own are unable to provide a reliable association between clinical prediction and subsequent suicidal behavior. It is best to use several methods to gather information along with a comprehensive clinical interview and chart review to identify risk and protective factors and to determine the patient's risk. Past history of a suicide attempt is the most powerful predictor of suicide, but it is important to be aware that most elders who die from suicide did *not* have a prior history of attempt. Additional risk and protective factors can be found in Chapter 4, Table 4–1. It is essential to document your clinical reasoning in detail to justify your clinical assessment and recommendations. For a model for estimating the level of suicide risk, see Table 4–2.

DETERMINE THE APPROPRIATE LEVEL OF CARE

Appropriate triage to ensure safety and allow time for intervention is essential. Hospitalization of the individual to ensure his or her safety and to provide time for diagnostic clarification and stabilization is preferred when suicide risk is high and perhaps when risk is moderate (see Table 4–2). Involuntary commitment may be necessary, although the voluntary route is always the preferred option when possible. See Chapter 4, subsection "Involuntary Commitment," for detailed discussion of psychiatric hospitalization, including involuntary commitment for patients with increased risk of suicide. In general, our threshold for admitting geriatric patients is lower than that for younger patients because of older adults' risk of rapid physical decompensation with inadequately treated depression. Referral to an intensive outpatient or partial hospitalization program may be appropriate, in particular for patients with moderate risk. For those patients who return home following evaluation, a next-day (or as soon as possible) outpatient appointment is advisable.

REDUCE ACCESS TO MEANS OF SUICIDE

The home environment needs to be made as safe as possible by addressing lethal means safely. Firearms are the most common means of suicide in older men in the United States (74% of those 65–74 years old, 81% of those 75 and older) (Hedegaard et al. 2018). Poisoning is most common in older women (41% of those 65–74 years old, 37% of those 75 and older), and firearms are the second most common means (38% and 33%) (Hedegaard et al. 2018). Firearms should be removed from the home, at least on a temporary basis. Other options that can be considered include disabling the weapon and storing the firearm in a locked cabinet and having another person safeguard the key. In tandem, it is important to remove poisons and medications that can be used in overdose even if the individual has stated that the firearms would be his or her preferred mode for attempting suicide. Consideration of removing alcohol and other drugs is important because doing so can reduce the possibility of disinhibition and impulsivity.

DEVELOP A SUICIDE SAFETY PLAN

A suicide safety plan or crisis intervention plan should be developed collaboratively with patients. Patients may benefit from recognizing warning signs, being reminded to access self-management skills, and reaching out to preidentified individuals and systems in their social support network. Include the number for the National Suicide Prevention Lifeline, 1-800-273-TALK (8255), in the safety plan. We urge our readers to carefully review Table 4–4 for the elements of a suicide safety plan.

IMPLEMENT INTERVENTIONS TO REDUCE THE RISK OF SUICIDE

Psychotherapy and medications not only may help reduce depression and anxiety but also may reduce the risk of suicide. As discussed previously in the subsection "Problem-Solving Therapy" and in Chapter 4, subsection "Screening Tools," IPT, PST, and PATH appear to reduce suicidal ideation in depressed older adults (Gustavson et al. 2016; Heisel et al. 2015; Kiosses et al. 2015b). The collaborative care models IMPACT and PROSPECT have been shown to reduce suicidal ideation in depressed elders (Alexopoulos et al. 2009; Unützer et al. 2006).

In terms of pharmacology, antidepressants have been found to reduce the risk of suicidality in older adults, with an odds ratio of 0.37 among those at least 65 years old and 0.22 among those at least 75 years old (Stone et al. 2009). Lithium, discussed previously in the context of antidepressant augmentation, may decrease the risk of suicide and mortality in both bipolar and unipolar depressed patients, regardless of sex and age. This effect might be independent of its mood stabilization effect (Cipriani et al. 2005). Clozapine decreases suicidal behaviors in patients with schizophrenia and schizoaffective disorder, although some researchers have raised the question of whether this effect might be mediated in part by the close surveillance required to monitor the medication (Alphs et al. 2004). Clozapine is the only antipsychotic that is FDA approved for suicide prevention. ECT should be considered for patients with severe depression and associated suicidality. Ketamine infusions also appear to decrease suicidal ideation, with a meta-analysis finding that 55% of patients were free of suicidal ideation within 24 hours of one ketamine infusion and that 81% were free of suicidal ideation at the end of the course of ketamine (mean 7.5 infusions) (Wilkinson et al. 2018). Alas, two subsequent studies of esketamine designed specifically to address effect on suicidality did not find evidence of efficacy (although depression improved) (Fu et al. 2020; Ionescu et al. 2021).

CONTINUE TO MONITOR SUICIDE RISK

Suicidality can wax and wane as stressors and symptoms fluctuate. Thus, it is essential to monitor the response to treatment, regularly reassess suicide risk, and adjust the treatment plan accordingly.

Summary: Implementing a Treatment Algorithm for Late-Life Depression and Anxiety

Late-life depression and anxiety are eminently treatable conditions. By recommending evidence-based treatments to our older adult patients with depression and anxiety, we can reduce symptoms, improve quality of life, and even save lives. Comorbid medical conditions and substance use disorders should be identified and addressed. Given the

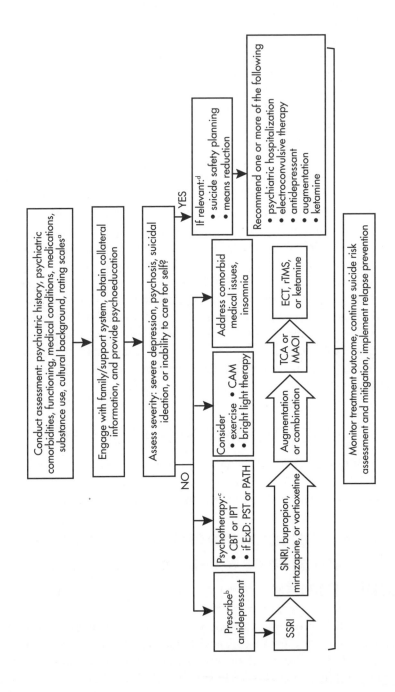

Figure 5–2.   Algorithm for treatment of late-life depression. *(opposite page)*

ECT should be earlier in the algorithm for severe depression, psychotic depression, and catatonia. Medication options are different for bipolar disorder. See text for more details.
ªFor outline of assessment, see Figure 3–2 in Chapter 3, "Assessment of Late-Life Depression and Anxiety."
ᵇFor moderate to severe depression.
ᶜFor mild to moderate depression.
ᵈFor detailed discussion of suicide safety planning and means reduction, see Chapter 4, subsection "Suicide and Safety Planning," Table 4–3, and Table 4–4.
Abbreviations.   CAM=complementary and alternative medicine; CBT=cognitive-behavioral therapy; ECT=electroconvulsive therapy; ExD=executive dysfunction (or cognitive impairment); IPT=interpersonal psychotherapy; MAOI=monoamine oxidase inhibitor; PATH=problem adaptation therapy; PST=problem-solving therapy; rTMS=repetitive transcranial magnetic stimulation; SNRI=serotonergic-noradrenergic reuptake inhibitor; SSRI=selective serotonin reuptake inhibitor; TCA=tricyclic antidepressant.

high risk of suicide among older adults, a thorough suicide risk assessment must shape the treatment plan, including consideration of psychiatric hospitalization, means reductions, and suicide safety planning.

The evidence base for treatment of late-life depression is strongest for psychoeducation (all patients), psychotherapy (mild to moderate depression), antidepressant medications (moderate to severe depression), and ECT (severe depression, including with psychosis or catatonia) (Figure 5–2). Among the psychotherapies, CBT, CBT-I (for insomnia), IPT, and PST appear to be the most effective for late-life depression, with PST and PATH helpful for older adults who also have cognitive impairment. Medications should be prescribed with caution because older adults are at greater risk of drug-drug interactions and side effects, including falls, hyponatremia, and gastrointestinal bleeding. Polypharmacy should be avoided, especially medications with anticho linergic and sedating properties. Other treatments that may be effective in late-life depression include rTMS, ketamine, exercise, and complementary and alternative medicine approaches.

The approach to the patient with bipolar depression is somewhat different, including probably avoiding antidepressants and instead using lithium, lamotrigine, an atypical antipsychotic, or ECT; with respect to psychotherapy, CBT and IPSRT appear to be most effective.

The evidence base for treatment of late-life anxiety is strongest for psychotherapy, especially CBT, which we recommend as the gold standard for both anxiety and insomnia (Figure 5–3). If medications are considered, we recommend SSRIs and SNRIs; we try to avoid BZDs because of safety concerns in older adults. Buspirone, TCAs, or quetiapine can be considered, although there are significant risks associated with the latter two. Treatment plans will vary somewhat on the basis of the specific diagnosis (e.g., GAD, PTSD, obsessive-compulsive disorder).

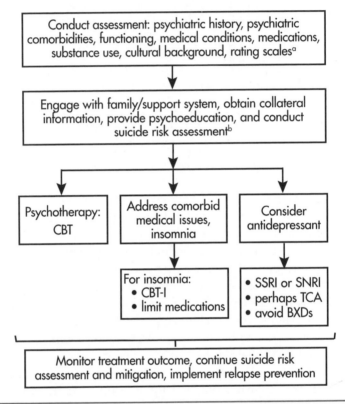

Figure 5–3. Algorithm for treatment of late-life anxiety.

See text for details, which vary somewhat depending on the anxiety diagnosis.
[a]See Chapter 3, Figure 3.2, for outline of assessment.
[b]For detailed discussion of suicide safety planning and means reduction, see Chapter 4, subsection "Suicide Safety Planning," Table 4–3, and Table 4–4.
Abbreviations. BZDs=benzodiazepines; CBT=cognitive-behavioral therapy; CBT-I = cognitive-behavioral therapy for insomnia; SNRI=serotonergic-noradrenergic reuptake inhibitor; SSRI=selective serotonin reuptake inhibitor; TCA=tricyclic antidepressant.

Systems-level interventions have been studied extensively in late-life depression, especially collaborative care models such as IMPACT. For clinicians who wish to effect change at a population level, we recommend working with your health care system to implement one of these models.

Finally, the literature on the treatment of depression and anxiety in ethnic, racial, and sexual minority elders is woefully inadequate. We do know that minority older adults face significant barriers to care, including stigma, racism, homophobia, and transphobia. It's our responsibility as mental health professionals to provide culturally sensitive care and to ensure that all our patients can get evidence-based care.

KEY POINTS

- Psychoeducation about late-life depression and anxiety should be included in every treatment plan. Family members may need education and support, too.

- Psychotherapy is an effective treatment for late-life depression of mild to moderate severity and is the gold standard for late-life anxiety.
  - Cognitive-behavioral therapy (CBT) has the strongest evidence for both late-life depression and anxiety.
  - CBT for insomnia (CBT-I) is a first-line treatment for insomnia in older adults and offers the opportunity to taper off benzodiazepines.
  - Problem-solving therapy (PST) and problem adaptation therapy (PATH) offer advantages in the treatment of depression and executive dysfunction.
  - PST and interpersonal therapy (IPT) offer benefits in reduction of suicidal ideation.

- Antidepressants are an effective treatment for moderate to severe late-life depression and can be considered for late-life anxiety. Selective serotonin reuptake inhibitors and serotonergic-noradrenergic reuptake inhibitors likely have the best risk-to-benefit profile in older adults.

- Avoidance of polypharmacy is paramount in older adults, who often have a greater burden of medical comorbidities and are more sensitive to medication side effects and drug interactions. Special attention should be paid to avoiding anticholinergic and sedating medications.

- Benzodiazepines should be used sparingly and only in the short term to prevent side effects and dependence. Good pharmacological alternatives to benzodiazepines for insomnia include ramelteon, suvorexant, and doxepin.

- Electroconvulsive therapy (ECT) is an effective and generally safe treatment for older adults with severe depression, including those with psychosis, catatonia, suicidality, and decreased inability to care for themselves. It remains a gold standard treatment for treatment-resistant major depressive disorder.

- Repetitive transcranial magnetic stimulation, bright light therapy, intravenous ketamine, and esketamine are promising treatment modalities for late-life depression, although research about how to adjust these treatments for geriatric patients is still needed.

- Effective treatments for late-life bipolar depression include lithium, lamotrigine, lurasidone, quetiapine, lithium, and ECT. Controversy remains about the efficacy of antidepressants and about the risk of switch to mania.

- Moderate to vigorous exercise can be used as an augmentation treatment strategy.

- Suicide is a global health problem to which older adults are especially vulnerable.

    - A comprehensive assessment is necessary to evaluate the individual's suicide risk and to develop an appropriate treatment plan, including means reduction and suicide safety planning.

    - Treating depression and anxiety should help reduce the risk of suicide. Interventions that may be particularly helpful include IPT, PST, PATH, antidepressants, lithium, clozapine, ECT, and perhaps ketamine.

    - Clinicians should monitor suicidality continually and modify the risk assessment and treatment plan accordingly.

- Strong evidence of efficacy exists for collaborative care models, and we recommend that health care systems implement a collaborative care model to improve the care of older adults with depression.

- Telepsychiatry offers significant benefits, as well as some challenges, for the care of older adults.

- We as clinicians must advocate for more research in the treatment of late-life depression and anxiety and improved access to care for all older adults.

Resources for Patients, Families, and Caregivers

LATE-LIFE DEPRESSION AND ANXIETY: A STARTING POINT FOR PATIENTS

HelpGuide

"Depression in Older Adults: Signs, Symptoms, Treatment"

www.helpguide.org/articles/depression/depression-in-older-adults.htm

Mental Health America
   "Anxiety in Older Adults"
   www.mhanational.org/anxiety-older-adults
   "Depression in Older Adults"
   www.mhanational.org/depression-older-adults
Psycom
   "Depression in the Elderly"
   www.psycom.net/depression.central.elderly.html
National Institute of Mental Health
   "Older Adults and Depression"
   www.nimh.nih.gov/health/publications/older-adults-and-depression/index.shtml

BIPOLAR DEPRESSION: A STARTING POINT FOR PATIENTS

National Institute of Mental Health
   www.nimh.nih.gov/health/publications/bipolar-disorder/index.shtml
National Alliance on Mental Illness
   www.nami.org/About-Mental-Illness/Mental-Health-Conditions/Bipolar-Disorder

BOOKS ON LATE-LIFE DEPRESSION

Miller MD, Reynolds CF III: Depression and Anxiety in Later Life: What Everyone Needs to Know, Baltimore, ND, (Johns Hopkins University Press, 2012

Serani D: Depression in Later Life: An Essential Guide. Lanham, MD, Rowman and Littlefield, 2016

TREATMENT EDUCATION

Medication Safety in Older Adults

American Geriatrics Society
   "Choosing Wisely"
   www.choosingwisely.org/societies/american-geriatrics-society

Health in Aging
"Medications & Older Adults"
www.healthinaging.org/medications-older-adults

ECT, rTMS, and Ketamine

International Society for ECT and Neurostimulation
"The Five B's for Dealing With Loved Ones Who Are Depressed"
https://isen-ect.org/educational-content

Mayo Clinic
"Transcranial Magnetic Stimulation"
www.mayoclinic.org/tests-procedures/transcranial-magnetic-stimulation/about/pac-20384625

Harvard Medical School
"Ketamine for Major Depression: New Tool, New Questions"
www.health.harvard.edu/blog/ketamine-for-major-depression-new-tool-new-questions-2019052216673

Light Therapy

Mayo Clinic
www.mayoclinic.org/tests-procedures/light-therapy/about/pac-20384604

Exercise for Depression and Anxiety

Mayo Clinic
www.mayoclinic.org/diseases-conditions/depression/in-depth/depression-and-exercise/art-20046495

SUICIDE PREVENTION

Suicide Prevention Resources Center
www.sprc.org/populations/older-adults

AgingInPlace
https://aginginplace.org/elderly-suicide-risks-detection-how-to-help

National Suicide Prevention Lifeline
https://suicidepreventionlifeline.org
1-800-273-8255

GeriatricsCareOnline

https://geriatricscareonline.org/ProductAbstract/ags-patient-handouts/H001

- Patient handouts, including handouts on alternatives to potentially problematic medications, concern about sleeping pills, and tips for healthy aging (subscription required)

Resources for Clinicians

PSYCHOPHARMACOLOGY

American Geriatrics Society, Beers Criteria (paid content)

https://geriatricscareonline.org/toc/american-geriatrics-society-updated-beers-criteria/CL001Psychotherapy

PSYCHOTHERAPY

Books

Hinrichsen GA, Clougherty KF: Interpersonal Psychotherapy for Depressed Older Adults. Washington, DC, American Psychological Association, 2006

Nezu AM, Nezu CM, D'Zurilla T: Problem-Solving Therapy: A Treatment Manual. New York, Springer, 2012

Mynors-Wallis L: Problem-Solving Treatment for Anxiety and Depression: A Practical Guide. New York, Oxford University Press, 2005

Collaborative Care

Healthy IDEAS

http://healthyideasprograms.org

PEARLS

"Help Older Adults With Depression Create Happier, Healthier Lives"

https://depts.washington.edu/hprc/evidence-based-programs/pearls-program

IMPACT

"IMPACT: Improving Mood—Promoting Access to Collaborative Treatment"

http://aims.uw.edu/impact-improving-mood-promoting-access-collaborative-treatment

Addressing Racial Disparities in the Provision of Mental Health Care

National Alliance on Mental Illness

"NAMI Sharing Hope: Mental Wellness in the Black Community"

https://nami.org/Support-Education/Mental-Health-Education/NAMI-Sharing-Hope-Mental-Wellness-in-the-Black-Community

"NAMI Compartiendo Esperanza: Speaking With Latinos About Mental Health"

https://nami.org/Support-Education/Mental-Health-Education/NAMI-Compartiendo-Esperanza-Speaking-with-Latinos-about-Mental-Health

Telepsychiatry Resources for Psychiatrists in the United States

American Psychiatric Association

www.psychiatry.org/psychiatrists/practice/telepsychiatry

• Membership may be required to access some materials.

References

Abad VC, Guilleminault C: Insomnia in elderly patients: recommendations for pharmacological management. Drugs Aging 35(9):791–817, 2018 30058034

AIMS Center: Advancing Integrated Mental Health Solutions Principles of Collaborative Care. Seattle, Psychiatry and Behavioral Sciences, University of Washington, 2011. Available at: https://aims.uw.edu/collaborative-care/principles-collaborative-care. Accessed May 19, 2021.

Alaka KJ, Noble W, Montejo A, et al: Efficacy and safety of duloxetine in the treatment of older adult patients with generalized anxiety disorder: a randomized, double-blind, placebo-controlled trial. Int J Geriatr Psychiatry 29(9):978–986, 2014 24644106

Alberich S, Martínez-Cengotitabengoa M, López P, et al: Efficacy and safety of ketamine in bipolar depression: a systematic review. Rev Psiquiatr Salud Ment 10(2):104–112, 2017 27387226

Albott CS, Lim KO, Forbes MK, et al: Efficacy, safety, and durability of repeated ketamine infusions for comorbid posttraumatic stress disorder and treatment-resistant depression. J Clin Psychiatry 79(3):17m11634, 2018 29727073

Alessi C, Martin JL, Fiorentino L, et al: Cognitive behavioral therapy for insomnia in older veterans using nonclinician sleep coaches: randomized controlled trial. J Am Geriatr Soc 64(9):1830–1838, 2016 27550552

Alexopoulos GS, Shamoian CJ, Lucas J, et al: Medical problems of geriatric psychiatric patients and younger controls during electroconvulsive therapy. J Am Geriatr Soc 32(9):651–654, 1984 6470382

Alexopoulos GS, Katz IR, Reynolds CF 3rd, et al: Pharmacotherapy of depression in older patients: a summary of the expert consensus guidelines. J Psychiatr Pract 7(6):361–376, 2001 15990550

Alexopoulos GS, Reynolds CF 3rd, Bruce ML, et al: Reducing suicidal ideation and depression in older primary care patients: 24-month outcomes of the PROSPECT study. Am J Psychiatry 166(8):882–890, 2009 19528195

Alexopoulos GS, Raue PJ, Gunning F, et al: "Engage" therapy: behavioral activation and improvement of late-life major depression. Am J Geriatr Psychiatry 24(4):320–326, 2016a 26905044

Alexopoulos GS, Raue PJ, McCulloch C, et al: Clinical case management versus case management with problem-solving therapy in low-income, disabled elders with major depression: a randomized clinical trial. Am J Geriatr Psychiatry 24(1):50–59, 2016b 25794636

Alexopoulos GS, Raue PJ, Banerjee S, et al: Comparing the streamlined psychotherapy "Engage" with problem-solving therapy in late-life major depression. A randomized clinical trial. Mol Psychiatry July 1, 2020 [Epub ahead of print] 32612251

Alphs L, Anand R, Islam MZ, et al: The International Suicide Prevention Trial (interSePT): rationale and design of a trial comparing the relative ability of clozapine and olanzapine to reduce suicidal behavior in schizophrenia and schizoaffective patients. Schizophr Bull 30(3):577–586, 2004 15631247

Alty J, Farrow M, Lawler K: Exercise and dementia prevention. Pract Neurol 20(3):234–240, 2020 31964800

American Geriatrics Society Beers Criteria Update Expert Panel: American Geriatrics Society 2019 updated AGS Beers Criteria for potentially inappropriate medication use in older adults. J Am Geriatr Soc 67(4):674–694, 2019 30693946

American Psychiatric Association: Practice Guideline for the Treatment of Patients with Major Depressive Disorder, 3rd edition. Washington, DC, American Psychiatric Association, 2010. Available at: https://psychiatryonline.org/pb/assets/raw/sitewide/practice_guidelines/guidelines/mdd.pdf. Accessed May 19, 2021.

American Psychiatric Association: Diagnostic and Statistical Manual of Mental Disorders, 5th Edition. Arlington, VA, American Psychiatric Association, 2013

American Psychiatric Association Committee on Electroconvulsive Therapy: The Practice of Electroconvulsive Therapy: Recommendations for Treatment, Training, and Privileging: A Task Force Report of the American Psychiatric Association. Washington, DC, American Psychiatric Association, 2001

Andersen UA, Andersen M, Rosholm JU, et al: Contacts to the health care system prior to suicide: a comprehensive analysis using registers for general and psychiatric hospital admissions, contacts to general practitioners and practising specialists and drug prescriptions. Acta Psychiatr Scand 102(2):126–134, 2000 10937785

Andrade C: Ketamine for depression, 4: in what dose, at what rate, by what route, for how long, and at what frequency? J Clin Psychiatry 78(7):e852–e857, 2017 28749092

Areán PA, Perri MG, Nezu AM, et al: Comparative effectiveness of social problem-solving therapy and reminiscence therapy as treatments for depression in older adults. J Consult Clin Psychol 61(6):1003–1010, 1993 8113478

Areán PA, Raue P, Mackin RS, et al: Problem-solving therapy and supportive therapy in older adults with major depression and executive dysfunction. Am J Psychiatry 167(11):1391–1398, 2010 20516155

Arthur A, Savva GM, Barnes LE, et al: Changing prevalence and treatment of depression among older people over two decades. Br J Psychiatry 216(1):49–54, 2020 31587673

Bahji A, Hawken ER, Sepehry AA, et al: ECT beyond unipolar major depression: systematic review and meta-analysis of electroconvulsive therapy in bipolar depression. Acta Psychiatr Scand 139(3):214–226, 2019 30506992

Bahji A, Ermacora D, Stephenson C, et al: Comparative efficacy and tolerability of pharmacological treatments for the treatment of acute bipolar depression: a systematic review and network meta-analysis. J Affect Disord 269:154–184, 2020 32339131

Baillargeon L, Landreville P, Verreault R, et al: Discontinuation of benzodiazepines among older insomniac adults treated with cognitive-behavioural therapy combined with gradual tapering: a randomized trial. CMAJ 169(10):1015–1020, 2003 14609970

Barker MJ, Greenwood KM, Jackson M, et al: Persistence of cognitive effects after withdrawal from long-term benzodiazepine use: a meta-analysis. Arch Clin Neuropsychol 19(3):437–454, 2004 15033227

Bartoli F, Dell'Osso B, Crocamo C, et al: Benefits and harms of low and high second-generation antipsychotics doses for bipolar depression: a meta-analysis. J Psychiatr Res 88:38–46, 2017 28086127

Beaudreau SA, Rideaux T, O'Hara R, et al: Does cognition predict treatment response and remission in psychotherapy for late-life depression? Am J Geriatr Psychiatry 23(2):215–219, 2015 25441055

Belland L, Rivera-Reyes L, Hwang U: Using music to reduce anxiety among older adults in the emergency department: a randomized pilot study. J Integr Med 15(6):450–455, 2017 29103414

Blais RK, Tsai J, Southwick SM, et al: Barriers and facilitators related to mental health care use among older veterans in the United States. Psychiatr Serv 66(5):500–506, 2015 25639990

Bobo WV: The diagnosis and management of bipolar I and II disorders: clinical practice update. Mayo Clin Proc 92(10):1532–1551, 2017 28888714

Bohlmeijer E, Smit F, Cuijpers P: Effects of reminiscence and life review on late-life depression: a meta-analysis. Int J Geriat Psychiatry 18(12):1088–1094, 2003 14677140

Bosboom PR, Deijen JB: Age-related cognitive effects of ECT and ECT-induced mood improvement in depressive patients. Depress Anxiety 23(2):93–101, 2006 16400627

Bratsos S, Saleh SN: Clinical efficacy of ketamine for treatment-resistant depression. Cureus 11(7):e5189, 2019 31565597

Brenes GA, Danhauer SC, Lyles MF, et al: Long-term effects of telephone-delivered psychotherapy for late-life GAD. Am J Geriatr Psychiatry 25(11):1249–1257, 2017 28673741

Bruce ML, Pearson JL: Designing an intervention to prevent suicide: PROSPECT (Prevention of Suicide in Primary Care Elderly: Collaborative Trial). Dialogues Clin Neurosci 1(2):100–112, 1999 22033641

Bruce ML, Ten Have TR, Reynolds CF 3rd, et al: Reducing suicidal ideation and depressive symptoms in depressed older primary care patients: a randomized controlled trial. JAMA 291(9):1081–1091, 2004 14996777

Burd J, Kettl P: Incidence of asystole in electroconvulsive therapy in elderly patients. Am J Geriatr Psychiatry 6(3):203–211, 1998 9659953

Butler RN: The life review: an interpretation of reminiscence in the aged. Psychiatry 26:65–76, 1963 14017386

Canuso CM, Singh JB, Fedgchin M, et al: Efficacy and safety of intranasal esketamine for the rapid reduction of symptoms of depression and suicidality in patients at imminent risk for suicide: results of a double-blind, randomized, placebo-controlled study. Am J Psychiatry 175(7):620–630, 2018 29656663

Casado BL, Quijano LM, Stanley MA, et al: Healthy IDEAS: implementation of a depression program through community-based case management. Gerontologist 48(6):828–838, 2008 19139256

Case BG, Bertollo DN, Laska EM, et al: Declining use of electroconvulsive therapy in United States general hospitals. Biol Psychiatry 73(2):119–126, 2013 23059049

Catalan-Matamoros D, Gomez-Conesa A, Stubbs B, et al: Exercise improves depressive symptoms in older adults: an umbrella review of systematic reviews and meta-analyses. Psychiatry Res 244:202–209, 2016 27494042

Chan P, Bhar S, Davison TE, et al: Characteristics and effectiveness of cognitive behavioral therapy for older adults living in residential care: a systematic review. Aging Ment Health 25(2):187–205, 2021 31707790

Chew ML, Mulsant BH, Pollock BG, et al: Anticholinergic activity of 107 medications commonly used by older adults. J Am Geriatr Soc 56(7):1333–1341, 2008 18510583

Cho SH, Torres-Llenza V, Budnik K, et al: The integral role of psychoeducation in clinical care. Psychiatr Ann 46(5):286–292, 2016

Choi NG, Marti CN, Bruce ML, et al: Six-month postintervention depression and disability outcomes of in-home telehealth problem-solving therapy for depressed, low-income homebound older adults. Depress Anxiety 31(8):653–661, 2014 24501015

Churchill R, Moore THM, Furukawa TA, et al: "Third wave" cognitive and behavioural therapies versus treatment as usual for depression. Cochrane Database Syst Rev (10):CD008705, 2013 24142810

Ciasca EC, Ferreira RC, Santana CLA, et al: Art therapy as an adjuvant treatment for depression in elderly women: a randomized controlled trial. Br J Psychiatry 40(3):256–263, 2018 29412335

Ciechanowski P, Wagner E, Schmaling K, et al: Community-integrated home-based depression treatment in older adults: a randomized controlled trial. JAMA 291(13):1569–1577, 2004 15069044

Cipriani A, Pretty H, Hawton K, Geddes JR: Lithium in the prevention of suicidal behavior and all-cause mortality in patients with mood disorders: a systematic review of randomized trials. Am J Psychiatry 162(10):1805–1819, 2005 16199826

Cole MG, Dendukuri N: Risk factors for depression among elderly community subjects: a systematic review and meta-analysis. Am J Psychiatry 160(6):1147–1156, 2003 12777274

Conelea CA, Philip NS, Yip AG, et al: Transcranial magnetic stimulation for treatment-resistant depression: naturalistic treatment outcomes for younger versus older patients. J Affect Disord 217:42–47, 2017 28388464

Conner KO, Copeland VC, Grote NK, et al: Mental health treatment seeking among older adults with depression: the impact of stigma and race. Am J Geriatr Psychiatry 18(6):531–543, 2010 20220602

Conwell Y, Duberstein PR, Caine ED: Risk factors for suicide in later life. Biol Psychiatry 52(3):193–204, 2002 12182926

Cook JM, Biyanova T, Masci C, et al: Older patient perspectives on long-term anxiolytic benzodiazepine use and discontinuation: a qualitative study. J Gen Intern Med 22(8):1094–1100, 2007a 17492325

Cook JM, Marshall R, Masci C, et al: Physicians' perspectives on prescribing benzodiazepines for older adults: a qualitative study. J Gen Intern Med 22(3):303–307, 2007b 17356959

Cooper C, Katona C, Lyketsos K, et al: A systematic review of treatments for refractory depression in older people. Am J Psychiatry 168(7):681–688, 2011 21454919

Correll CU, Frederickson AM, Kane JM, et al: Metabolic syndrome and the risk of coronary heart disease in 367 patients treated with second-generation antipsychotic drugs. J Clin Psychiatry 67(4):575–583, 2006 16669722

Cristancho P, Lenard E, Lenze EJ, et al: Optimizing outcomes of treatment-resistant depression in older adults (OPTIMUM): study design and treatment characteristics of the first 396 participants randomized. Am J Geriatr Psychiatry 27(10):1138–1152, 2019 31147244

Cuijpers P, de Wit L, Kleiboer A, et al: Problem-solving therapy for adult depression: an updated meta-analysis. Eur Psychiatry 48:27–37, 2018 29331596

Cunningham J, Sirey JA, Bruce ML: Matching services to patients' beliefs about depression in Dublin, Ireland. Psychiatr Serv 58(5):696–699, 2007 17463352

Dassanayake T, Michie P, Carter G, Jones A: Effects of benzodiazepines, antidepressants and opioids on driving: a systematic review and meta-analysis of epidemiological and experimental evidence. Drug Saf 34(2):125–156, 2011 21247221

DiNapoli EA, Pierpaoli CM, Shah A, et al: Effects of home-delivered cognitive behavioral therapy (CBT) for depression on anxiety symptoms among rural, ethnically diverse older adults. Clin Gerontol 40(3):181–190, 2017 28452665

Djukanovic I, Carlsson J, Peterson U: Group discussions with structured reminiscence and a problem-based method as an intervention to prevent depressive symptoms in older people. J Clin Nurs 25(7–8):992–1000, 2016 26813881

Drug and Therapeutics Bulletin: DTB drug review: esketamine for treatment-resistant depression. Drug and Therapeutics Bulletin 58(12):183–188, 2020

Duberstein PR, Conwell Y, Seidlitz L, et al: Age and suicidal ideation in older depressed inpatients. Am J Geriatr Psychiatry 7(4):289–296, 1999 10521160

Erickson KI, Gildengers AG, Butters MA: Physical activity and brain plasticity in late adulthood. Dialogues Clin Neurosci 15(1):99–108, 2013 23576893

Farioli Vecchioli S, Sacchetti S, Nicolis di Robilant V, et al: The role of physical exercise and omega-3 fatty acids in depressive illness in the elderly. Curr Neuropharmacol 16(3):308–326, 2018 28901279

Fleisher AS, Truran D, Mai JT, et al: Chronic divalproex sodium use and brain atrophy in Alzheimer disease. Neurology 77(13):1263–1271, 2011 21917762

Flint AJ, Meyers BS, Rothschild AJ, et al: Effect of continuing olanzapine vs placebo on relapse among patients with psychotic depression in remission: the STOP-PD II randomized clinical trial. JAMA 322(7):622–631, 2019 31429896

Forester BP, Parikh SV, Weisenbach S, et al: Combinatorial pharmacogenomic testing improves outcomes for older adults with depression. Am J Geriatr Psychiatry 28(9):933–945, 2020 32513518

Fortney JC, Pyne JM, Edlund MJ, et al: A randomized trial of telemedicine-based collaborative care for depression. J Gen Intern Med 22(8):1086–1093, 2007 17492326

Fowler NR, Judge KS, Lucas K, et al: Feasibility and acceptability of an acceptance and commitment therapy intervention for caregivers of adults with Alzheimer's disease and related dementias. BMC Geriatr 21(1):127, 2021 33593296

Freshour JS, Amspoker AB, Yi M, et al: Cognitive behavior therapy for late-life generalized anxiety disorder delivered by lay and expert providers has lasting benefits. Int J Geriatr Psychiatry 31(11):1225–1232, 2016 26923925

Friedman EM, Ruini C, Foy R, et al: Lighten UP! A community-based group intervention to promote psychological well-being in older adults. Aging Ment Health 21(2):199–205, 2017 26460594

Fry PS: Structured and unstructured reminiscence training and depression among the elderly. Clinical Gerontologist 1(3):15–37, 1983

Fu DJ, Ionescu DF, Li X, et al: Esketamine nasal spray for rapid reduction of major depressive disorder symptoms in patients who have active suicidal ideation with intent: double-blind, randomized study (ASPIRE I). J Clin Psychiatry 81(3):19m13191, 2020 32412700

Fuentes D, Aranda MP: Depression interventions among racial and ethnic minority older adults: a systematic review across 20 years. Am J Geriatr Psychiatry 20(11):915–931, 2012 22828202

Gallagher-Thompson D, Steffen AM: Comparative effects of cognitive-behavioral and brief psychodynamic psychotherapies for depressed family caregivers. J Consult Clin Psychol 62(3):543–549, 1994 8063980

Gallagher-Thompson D, Hanley-Peterson P, Thompson LW: Maintenance of gains versus relapse following brief psychotherapy for depression. J Consult Clin Psychol 58(3):371–374, 1990 2365900

Gaynes BN, Rush AJ, Trivedi MH, et al: The STAR*D study: treating depression in the real world. Cleve Clin J Med 75(1):57–66, 2008 18236731

Gebara MA, Shea ML, Lipsey KL, et al: Depression, antidepressants, and bone health in older adults: a systematic review. J Am Geriatr Soc 62(8):1434–1441, 2014 25039259

Gebara MA, Lipsey KL, Karp JF, et al: Cause or effect? Selective serotonin reuptake inhibitors and falls in older adults: a systematic review. Am J Geriatr Psychiatry 23(10):1016–1028, 2015 25586602

Geduldig ET, Kellner CH: Electroconvulsive therapy in the elderly: new findings in geriatric depression. Curr Psychiatry Rep 18(4):40, 2016 26909702

Gellis ZD, Kenaley BL, Ten Have T: Integrated telehealth care for chronic illness and depression in geriatric home care patients: the Integrated Telehealth Education and Activation of Mood (I-TEAM) study. J Am Geriatr Soc 62(5):889–895, 2014 24655228

Gentry MT, Lapid MI, Rummans TA: Geriatric telepsychiatry: systematic review and policy considerations. Am J Geriatr Psychiatry 27(2):109–127, 2019 30416025

George D, Gálvez V, Martin D, et al: Pilot randomized controlled trial of titrated subcutaneous ketamine in older patients with treatment-resistant depression. Am J Geriatr Psychiatry 25(11):1199–1209, 2017 28739263

Gerlach LB, Wiechers IR, Maust DT: Prescription benzodiazepine use among older adults: a critical review. Harv Rev Psychiatry 26(5):264–273, 2018 30188338

Gonçalves DC, Byrne GJ: Interventions for generalized anxiety disorder in older adults: systematic review and meta-analysis. J Anxiety Disord 26(1):1–11, 2012 21907538

Goodkind MS, Gallagher-Thompson D, Thompson LW, et al: The impact of executive function on response to cognitive behavioral therapy in late-life depression. Int J Geriatr Psychiatry 31(4):334–339, 2016 26230057

Gooneratne NS, Vitiello MV: Sleep in older adults: normative changes, sleep disorders, and treatment options. Clin Geriatr Med 30(3):591–627, 2014 25037297

Gould RL, Coulson MC, Patel N, et al: Interventions for reducing benzodiazepine use in older people: meta-analysis of randomised controlled trials. Br J Psychiatry 204(2):98–107, 2014 24493654

Gray SL, Dublin S, Yu O, et al: Benzodiazepine use and risk of incident dementia or cognitive decline: prospective population based study. BMJ 352:i90, 2016 26837813

Gum AM, Areán PA, Hunkeler E, et al: Depression treatment preferences in older primary care patients. Gerontologist 46(1):14–22, 2006 16452280

Gustavson KA, Alexopoulos GS, Niu GC, et al: Problem-solving therapy reduces suicidal ideation in depressed older adults with executive dysfunction. Am J Geriatr Psychiatry 24(1):11–17, 2016 26743100

Gutsmiedl K, Krause M, Bighelli I, et al: How well do elderly patients with major depressive disorder respond to antidepressants: a systematic review and single-group meta-analysis. BMC Psychiatry 20(1):102, 2020 32131786

Hall CA, Reynolds CF III: Late-life depression in the primary care setting: challenges, collaborative care, and prevention. Maturitas 79(2):147–152, 2014 24996484

Hall J, Kellett S, Berrios R, et al: Efficacy of cognitive behavioral therapy for generalized anxiety disorder in older adults: systematic review, meta-analysis, and meta-regression. Am J Geriatr Psychiatry 24(11):1063–1073, 2016 27687212

Hars M, Herrmann FR, Gold G, et al: Effect of music-based multitask training on cognition and mood in older adults. Age Ageing 43(2):196–200, 2014 24212920

Hausner L, Damian M, Sartorius A, et al: Efficacy and cognitive side effects of electroconvulsive therapy (ECT) in depressed elderly inpatients with coexisting mild cognitive impairment or dementia. J Clin Psychiatry 72(1):91–97, 2011 21208587

Hazlett-Stevens H, Singer J, Chong A: Mindfulness-based stress reduction and mindfulness-based cognitive therapy with older adults: a qualitative review of randomized controlled outcome research. Clin Gerontol 42(4):347–358, 2019 30204557

Hedegaard H, Curtin SC, Warner M: Suicide rates in the United States continue to increase. NCHS Data Brief (309):1–8, 2018 30312151

Hegel MT, Unützer J, Tang L, et al: Impact of comorbid panic and posttraumatic stress disorder on outcomes of collaborative care for late-life depression in primary care. Am J Geriatr Psychiatry 13(1):48–58, 2005 15653940

Heisel MJ, Talbot NL, King DA, et al: Adapting interpersonal psychotherapy for older adults at risk for suicide. Am J Geriatr Psychiatry 23(1):87–98, 2015 24840611

Helbostad JL, Vereijken B, Becker C, et al: Mobile health applications to promote active and healthy ageing. Sensors (Basel) 17(3):1–13, 2017 28335475

Hendriks GJ, Oude Voshaar RC, Keijsers GPJ, et al: Cognitive-behavioural therapy for late-life anxiety disorders: a systematic review and meta-analysis. Acta Psychiatr Scand 117(6):403–411, 2008 18479316

Henssler J, Bschor T, Baethge C: Combining antidepressants in acute treatment of depression: a meta-analysis of 38 studies including 4511 patients. Can J Psychiatry 61(1):29–43, 2016 27582451

Henstra MJ, Jansma EP, van der Velde N, et al: Acetylcholinesterase inhibitors for electroconvulsive therapy-induced cognitive side effects: a systematic review. Int J Geriatr Psychiatry 32(5):522–531, 2017 28295591

Herring WJ, Connor KM, Snyder E, et al: Suvorexant in elderly patients with insomnia: pooled analyses of data from phase III randomized controlled clinical trials. Am J Geriatr Psychiatry 25(7):791–802, 2017 28427826

Hinton L, La Frano E, Harvey D, et al: Feasibility of a family centered intervention for depressed older men in primary care. Int J Geriatr Psychiatry 34(12):1808–1814, 2019 31414506

Hirakawa H, Terao T, Muronaga M, et al: Adjunctive bright light therapy for treating bipolar depression: A systematic review and meta-analysis of randomized controlled trials. Brain Behav 10(12):e01876, 2020 33034127

Hobbs MJ, Mahoney AEJ, Andrews G: Integrating iCBT for generalized anxiety disorder into routine clinical care: Treatment effects across the adult lifespan. J Anxiety Disord 51:47–54, 2017 28926805

Hobbs MJ, Joubert AE, Mahoney AEJ, et al: Treating late-life depression: Comparing the effects of internet-delivered cognitive behavior therapy across the adult lifespan. J Affect Disord 226:58–65, 2018 28963865

Holvast F, van Hattem BA, Sinnige J, et al: Late-life depression and the association with multimorbidity and polypharmacy: a cross-sectional study. Fam Pract 34(5):539–545, 2017 28369380

Hummel J, Weisbrod C, Boesch L, et al: AIDE—Acute Illness and Depression in Elderly Patients. Cognitive behavioral group psychotherapy in geriatric patients with comorbid depression: a randomized, controlled trial. J Am Med Dir Assoc 18(4):341–349, 2017 27956074

Hunkeler EM, Katon W, Tang L, et al: Long term outcomes from the IMPACT randomised trial for depressed elderly patients in primary care. BMJ 332(7536):259–263, 2006 16428253

Hutchison LC, O'Brien CE: Changes in pharmacokinetics and pharmacodynamics in the elderly patient. J Pharm Pract 20:4–12, 2007

Ionescu DF, Fu DJ, Qiu X, et al: Esketamine nasal spray for rapid reduction of depressive symptoms in patients with major depressive disorder who have active suicide ideation with intent: results of a phase 3, double-blind, randomized study (ASPIRE II). Int J Neuropsychopharmacol 24(1):22–31, 2021 32861217

Ilieva IP, Alexopoulos GS, Dubin MJ, et al: Age-related repetitive transcranial magnetic stimulation effects on executive function in depression: a systematic review. Am J Geriatr Psychiatry 26(3):334–346, 2018 29111132

Ionson E, Limbachia J, Rej S, et al: Effects of Sahaj Samadhi meditation on heart rate variability and depressive symptoms in patients with late-life depression. Br J Psychiatry 214(4):218–224, 2019 30482255

Iriarte IG, George MS: Transcranial magnetic stimulation (TMS) in the elderly. Curr Psychiatry Rep 20(1):6, 2018 29427050

Jacob S, Spinler SA: Hyponatremia associated with selective serotonin-reuptake inhibitors in older adults. Ann Pharmacother 40(9):1618–1622, 2006 16896026

Johnco C, Wuthrich VM, Rapee RM: The impact of late-life anxiety and depression on cognitive flexibility and cognitive restructuring skill acquisition. Depress Anxiety 32(10):754–762, 2015 26014612

Jones KC, Salemi JL, Dongarwar D, et al: Racial/ethnic disparities in receipt of electroconvulsive therapy for elderly patients with a principal diagnosis of depression in inpatient settings. Am J Geriatr Psychiatry 27(3):266–278, 2019 30587412

Jonsson U, Bertilsson G, Allard P, et al: Psychological treatment of depression in people aged 65 years and over: a systematic review of efficacy, safety, and cost-effectiveness. PLoS One 11(8):e0160859, 2016 27537217

Jorge RE, Moser DJ, Acion L, et al: Treatment of vascular depression using repetitive transcranial magnetic stimulation. Arch Gen Psychiatry 65(3):268–276, 2008 18316673

Kabat-Zinn J: Full Catastrophe Living: Using the Wisdom of Your Mind and Body to Face Stress, Pain, and Illness. New York, Delacorte, 1990

Kanellopoulos D, Rosenberg P, Ravdin LD, et al: Depression, cognitive, and functional outcomes of problem adaptation therapy (PATH) in older adults with major depression and mild cognitive deficits. Int Psychogeriatr 32(4):485–493, 2020 31910916

Kaneriya SH, Robbins-Welty GA, Smagula SF, et al: Predictors and moderators of remission with aripiprazole augmentation in treatment-resistant late-life depression: an analysis of the IRL-GRey randomized clinical trial. JAMA Psychiatry 73(4):329–336, 2016 26963689

Kaster TS, Daskalakis ZJ, Noda Y, et al: Efficacy, tolerability, and cognitive effects of deep transcranial magnetic stimulation for late-life depression: a prospective randomized controlled trial. Neuropsychopharmacology 43(11):2231–2238, 2018 29946106

Katila H, Mezhebovsky I, Mulroy A, et al: Randomized, double-blind study of the efficacy and tolerability of extended release quetiapine fumarate (quetiapine XR) monotherapy in elderly patients with major depressive disorder. Am J Geriatr Psychiatry 21(8):769–784, 2013 23567397

Kay DB, Dombrovski AY, Buysse DJ, et al: Insomnia is associated with suicide attempt in middle-aged and older adults with depression. Int Psychogeriatr 28(4):613–619, 2016 26552935

Kenning C, Blakemore A, Bower P, et al: Preventing depression in the community by voluntary sector providers (PERSUADE): intervention development and protocol for a parallel randomised controlled feasibility trial. BMJ Open 9(10):e023791, 2019 31585966

Kinoshita S, Cortright K, Crawford A, et al: Changes in telepsychiatry regulations during the COVID-19 pandemic: 17 countries and regions' approaches to an evolving healthcare landscape. Psychol Med November 27, 2020 Epub ahead of print 33243311

Kiosses DN, Leon AC, Areán PA: Psychosocial interventions for late-life major depression: evidence-based treatments, predictors of treatment outcomes, and moderators of treatment effects. Psychiatr Clin North Am 34(2):377–401, viii, 2011 21536164

Kiosses DN, Alexopoulos GS: Problem-solving therapy in the elderly. Curr Treat Options Psychiatry 1(1):15–26, 2014 24729951

Kiosses DN, Ravdin LD, Gross JJ, et al: Problem adaptation therapy for older adults with major depression and cognitive impairment: a randomized clinical trial. JAMA Psychiatry 72(1):22–30, 2015a 25372657

Kiosses DN, Rosenberg PB, McGovern A, et al: Depression and suicidal ideation during two psychosocial treatments in older adults with major depression and dementia. J Alzheimers Dis 48(2):453–462, 2015b 26402009

Kirkham JG, Choi N, Seitz DP: Meta-analysis of problem solving therapy for the treatment of major depressive disorder in older adults. Int J Geriatr Psychiatry 31(5):526–535, 2016 26437368

Kishita N, Takei Y, Stewart I: A meta-analysis of third wave mindfulness-based cognitive behavioral therapies for older people. Int J Geriatr Psychiatry 32(12):1352–1361, 2017 27862293

Klil-Drori S, Klil-Drori AJ, Pira S, et al: Exercise intervention for late-life depression: a meta-analysis. J Clin Psychiatry 81(1):19r12877, 2020 31967748

Koepke HH, Gold RL, Linden ME, et al: Multicenter controlled study of oxazepam in anxious elderly outpatients. Psychosomatics 23(6):641–645, 1982 6750675

Kok RM, Reynolds CF 3rd: Management of depression in older adults: a review. JAMA 317(20):2114–2122, 2017 28535241

Kok RM, Nolen WA, Heeren TJ: Efficacy of treatment in older depressed patients: a systematic review and meta-analysis of double-blind randomized controlled trials with antidepressants. J Affect Disord 141(2–3):103–115, 2012 22480823

Kong XM, Xie XH, Xu SX, et al: Low-charge electrotherapy in geriatric major depressive disorder patients: a case series. Psychiatry Investig 16(6):464–468, 2019 31247706

Krause M, Gutsmiedl K, Bighelli I, et al: Efficacy and tolerability of pharmacological and non-pharmacological interventions in older patients with major depressive disorder: A systematic review, pairwise and network meta-analysis. Eur Neuropsychopharmacol 29(9):1003–1022, 2019 31327506

Kroenke K, Spitzer RL, Williams JB: The PHQ-9: validity of a brief depression severity measure. J Gen Intern Med 16(9):606–613, 2001 11556941

Krystal AD, Durrence HH, Scharf M, et al: Efficacy and safety of doxepin 1 mg and 3 mg in a 12-week sleep laboratory and outpatient trial of elderly subjects with chronic primary insomnia. Sleep 33(11):1553–1561, 2010 21102997

Kumar S, Mulsant BH, Liu AY, et al: Systematic review of cognitive effects of electroconvulsive therapy in late-life depression. Am J Geriatr Psychiatry 24(7):547–565, 2016 27067067

Kuriyama A, Honda M, Hayashino Y: Ramelteon for the treatment of insomnia in adults: a systematic review and meta-analysis. Sleep Med 15(4):385–392, 2014 24656909

Laidlaw K: A deficit in psychotherapeutic care for older people with depression and anxiety. Gerontology 59(6):549–556, 2013 23838157

Lamers SMA, Bohlmeijer ET, Korte J, et al: The efficacy of life-review as online-guided self-help for adults: a randomized trial. J Gerontol B Psychol Sci Soc Sci 70(1):24–34, 2015 24691155

Lankford A, Rogowski R, Essink B, et al: Efficacy and safety of doxepin 6 mg in a four-week outpatient trial of elderly adults with chronic primary insomnia. Sleep Med 13(2):133–138, 2012 22197474

Latorre JM, Serrano JP, Ricarte J, et al: Life review based on remembering specific positive events in active aging. J Aging Health 27(1):140–157, 2015 25005172

Lavretsky H, Alstein LL, Olmstead RE, et al: Complementary use of tai chi chih augments escitalopram treatment of geriatric depression: a randomized controlled trial. Am J Geriatr Psychiatry 19(10):839–850, 2011 21358389

Lavretsky H, Reinlieb M, St Cyr N, et al: Citalopram, methylphenidate, or their combination in geriatric depression: a randomized, double-blind, placebo-controlled trial. Am J Psychiatry 172(6):561–569, 2015 25677354

Lenze EJ, Ajam Oughli H: Antidepressant treatment for late-life depression: considering risks and benefits. J Am Geriatr Soc 67(8):1555–1556, 2019 31140584

Lenze EJ, Dew MA, Mazumdar S, et al: Combined pharmacotherapy and psychotherapy as maintenance treatment for late-life depression: effects on social adjustment. Am J Psychiatry 159(3):466–468, 2002 11870013

Lenze EJ, Mulsant BH, Blumberger DM, et al: Efficacy, safety, and tolerability of augmentation pharmacotherapy with aripiprazole for treatment-resistant depression in late life: a randomised, double-blind, placebo-controlled trial. Lancet 386(10011):2404–2412, 2015 26423182

Leyhe T, Reynolds CF 3rd, Melcher T, et al: A common challenge in older adults: classification, overlap, and therapy of depression and dementia. Alzheimers Dement 13(1):59–71, 2017 27693188

Li LW, Conwell Y: Pain and self-injury ideation in elderly men and women receiving home care. J Am Geriatr Soc 58(11):2160–2165, 2010 21054298

Lieverse R, Van Someren EJ, Nielen MM, et al: Bright light treatment in elderly patients with nonseasonal major depressive disorder: a randomized placebo-controlled trial. Arch Gen Psychiatry 68(1):61–70, 2011 21199966

Loo C: Can we confidently use ketamine as a clinical treatment for depression? Lancet Psychiatry 5(1):11–12, 2018 29277196

Luck-Sikorski C, Stein J, Heilmann K, et al: Treatment preferences for depression in the elderly. Int Psychogeriatr 29(3):389–398, 2017 27890036

Luoma JB, Martin CE, Pearson JL: Contact with mental health and primary care providers before suicide: a review of the evidence. Am J Psychiatry 159(6):909–916, 2002 12042175

Lynch TR, Cheavens JS, Cukrowicz KC, et al: Treatment of older adults with co-morbid personality disorder and depression: a dialectical behavior therapy approach. Int J Geriatr Psychiatry 22(2):131–143, 2007 17096462

Mace RA, Gansler DA, Suvak MK, et al: Therapeutic relationship in the treatment of geriatric depression with executive dysfunction. J Affect Disord 214:130–137, 2017 28288407

Mackin RS, Nelson JC, Delucchi K, et al: Cognitive outcomes after psychotherapeutic interventions for major depression in older adults with executive dysfunction. Am J Geriatr Psychiatry 22(12):1496–1503, 2014 24378255

Mallery L, MacLeod T, Allen M, et al: Systematic review and meta-analysis of second-generation antidepressants for the treatment of older adults with depression: questionable benefit and considerations for frailty. BMC Geriatr 19(1):306, 2019 31718566

Mangin D, Bahat G, Golomb BA, et al: International Group for Reducing Inappropriate Medication Use and Polypharmacy (IGRIMUP): position statement and 10 recommendations for action. Drugs Aging 35(7):575–587, 2018 30006810

Mansour R, Tsamakis K, Rizos E, et al: Late-life depression in people from ethnic minority backgrounds: differences in presentation and management. J Affect Disord 264:340–347, 2020 32056770

Masnoon N, Shakib S, Kalisch-Ellett L, et al: What is polypharmacy? A systematic review of definitions. BMC Geriatr 17(1):230, 2017 29017448

Markota M, Rummans TA, Bostwick JM, et al: Benzodiazepine use in older adults: dangers, management, and alternative therapies. Mayo Clin Proc 91(11):1632–1639, 2016 27814838

Maust DT, Oslin DW, Thase ME: Going beyond antidepressant monotherapy for incomplete response in nonpsychotic late-life depression: a critical review. Am J Geriatr Psychiatry 21(10):973–986, 2013 23567381

Mavandadi S, Benson A, DiFilippo S, et al: A telephone-based program to provide symptom monitoring alone vs symptom monitoring plus care management for late-life depression and anxiety: a randomized clinical trial. JAMA Psychiatry 72(12):1211–1218, 2015 26558530

McCrae CS, Curtis AF, Williams JM, et al: Efficacy of brief behavioral treatment for insomnia in older adults: examination of sleep, mood, and cognitive outcomes. Sleep Med 51:153–166, 2018 30195661

McEvoy P, Barnes P: Using the chronic care model to tackle depression among older adults who long-term physical conditions. J Psychiatr Ment Health Nurs 14(3):233–238, 2007 17430445

McGirr A, Vöhringer PA, Ghaemi SN, et al: Safety and efficacy of adjunctive second-generation antidepressant therapy with a mood stabiliser or an atypical antipsychotic in acute bipolar depression: a systematic review and meta-analysis of randomised placebo-controlled trials. Lancet Psychiatry 3(12):1138–1146, 2016 28100425

Meeks TW, Wetherell JL, Irwin MR, et al: Complementary and alternative treatments for late-life depression, anxiety, and sleep disturbance: a review of randomized controlled trials. J Clin Psychiatry 68(10):1461–1471, 2007 17960959

Meyer JP, Swetter SK, Kellner CH: Electroconvulsive therapy in geriatric psychiatry: a selective review. Psychiatr Clin North Am 41(1):79–93, 2018 29412850

Meyers BS, Flint AJ, Rothschild AJ, et al: A double-blind randomized controlled trial of olanzapine plus sertraline vs olanzapine plus placebo for psychotic depression: the study of pharmacotherapy of psychotic depression (STOP-PD). Arch Gen Psychiatry 66(8):838–847, 2009 19652123

Mezhebovsky I, Mägi K, She F, et al: Double-blind, randomized study of extended release quetiapine fumarate (quetiapine XR) monotherapy in older patients with generalized anxiety disorder. Int J Geriatr Psychiatry 28(6):615–625, 2013 23070803

Miller MD, Frank E, Cornes C, et al: The value of maintenance interpersonal psychotherapy (IPT) in older adults with different IPT foci. Am J Geriatr Psychiatry 11(1):97–102, 2003 12527545

Mokhber N, Azarpazhooh MR, Khajehdaluee M, et al: Randomized, single-blind, trial of sertraline and buspirone for treatment of elderly patients with generalized anxiety disorder. Psychiatry Clin Neurosci 64(2):128–133, 2010 20132529

Morgan K, Dixon S, Mathers N, et al: Psychological treatment for insomnia in the regulation of long-term hypnotic drug use. Health Technol Assess 8(8):iii–iv, 1–68, 2004 14960254

Morin CM, Colecchi C, Stone J, et al: Behavioral and pharmacological therapies for late-life insomnia: a randomized controlled trial. JAMA 281(11):991–999, 1999 10086433

Morin CM, Bastien C, Guay B, et al: Randomized clinical trial of supervised tapering and cognitive behavior therapy to facilitate benzodiazepine discontinuation in older adults with chronic insomnia. Am J Psychiatry 161(2):332–342, 2004 14754783

Mossey JM, Knott KA, Higgins M, et al: Effectiveness of a psychosocial intervention, interpersonal counseling, for subdysthymic depression in medically ill elderly. J Gerontol A Biol Sci Med Sci 51(4):M172–M178, 1996 8681000

Mulsant BH, Blumberger DM, Ismail Z, et al: A systematic approach to pharmacotherapy for geriatric major depression. Clin Geriatr Med 30(3):517–534, 2014 25037293

Murri MB, Amore M, Menchetti M, et al: Physical exercise for late-life major depression. Br J Psychiatry 207(3):235–242, 2015 26206864

Murri MB, Ekkekakis P, Menchetti M, et al: Physical exercise for late-life depression: effects on symptom dimensions and time course. J Affect Disord 230:65–70, 2018 29407540

Neviani F, Belvederi Murri M, Mussi C, et al: Physical exercise for late life depression: effects on cognition and disability. Int Psychogeriatr 29(7):1105–1112, 2017 28412979

Newport DJ, Carpenter LL, McDonald WM, et al: Ketamine and other NMDA antagonists: early clinical trials and possible mechanisms in depression. Am J Psychiatry 172(10):950–966, 2015 26423481

Norrie LM, Diamond K, Hickie IB, et al: Can older "at risk" adults benefit from psychoeducation targeting healthy brain aging? Int Psychogeriatr 23(3):413–424, 2011 20670460

Nyer M, Doorley J, Durham K, et al: What is the role of alternative treatments in late-life depression? Psychiatr Clin North Am 36(4):577–596, 2013 24229658

O'Connor MK, Knapp R, Husain M, et al: The influence of age on the response of major depression to electroconvulsive therapy: a C.O.R.E. report. Am J Geriatr Psychiatry 9(4):382–390, 2001 11739064

O'Dwyer S, Burke D, Malusa L: Potentiating patient participation: the "Homeward Bound" psychoeducation programme for depression in old age. Psychiatry of Old Age 20(5):397–400, 2012

Ochs-Ross R, Daly EJ, Zhang Y, et al: Efficacy and safety of esketamine nasal spray plus an oral antidepressant in elderly patients with treatment-resistant depression–TRANSFORM-3. Am J Geriatr Psychiatry 28(2):121–141, 2020 31734084

Olfson M, King M, Schoenbaum M: Benzodiazepine use in the United States. JAMA Psychiatry 72(2):136–142, 2015 25517224

Osler M, Rozing MP, Christensen GT, et al: Electroconvulsive therapy and risk of dementia in patients with affective disorders: a cohort study. Lancet Psychiatry 5(4):348–356, 2018 29523431

Oudega ML, van Exel E, Wattjes MP, et al: White matter hyperintensities, medial temporal lobe atrophy, cortical atrophy, and response to electroconvulsive therapy in severely depressed elderly patients. J Clin Psychiatry 72(1):104–112, 2011 20816035

Palmaro A, Dupouy J, Lapeyre-Mestre M: Benzodiazepines and risk of death: results from two large cohort studies in France and UK. Eur Neuropsychopharmacol 25(10):1566–1577, 2015 26256008

Park K, Lee S, Yang J, et al: A systematic review and meta-analysis on the effect of reminiscence therapy for people with dementia. Int Psychogeriatr 31(11):1581–1597, 2019 30712519

Paukert AL, Calleo J, Kraus-Schuman C, et al: Peaceful Mind: an open trial of cognitive-behavioral therapy for anxiety in persons with dementia. Int Psychogeriatr 22(6):1012–1021, 2010 20550745

Paukert AL, Phillips L, Cully JA, et al: Integration of religion into cognitive-behavioral therapy for geriatric anxiety and depression. J Psychiatr Pract 15(2):103–112, 2009 19339844

Penders TM, Stanciu CN, Schoemann AM, et al: Bright light therapy as augmentation of pharmacotherapy for treatment of depression: a systematic review and meta-analysis. Prim Care Companion CNS Disord 18(5), 2016 27835725

Penkunas MJ, Hahn-Smith S: An evaluation of IMPACT for the treatment of late-life depression in a public mental health system. J Behav Health Serv Res 42(3):334–345, 2015 24177923

Perera T, George MS, Grammer G, et al: The Clinical TMS Society consensus review and treatment recommendations for TMS therapy for major depressive disorder. Brain Stimul 9(3):336–346, 2016 27090022

Popova V, Daly EJ, Trivedi M, et al: Efficacy and safety of flexibly dosed esketamine nasal spray combined with a newly initiated oral antidepressant in treatment-resistant depression: a randomized double-blind active-controlled study. Am J Psychiatry 176(6):428–438, 2019 31109201

Poudel A, Ballokova A, Hubbard RE, et al: Algorithm of medication review in frail older people: Focus on minimizing the use of high-risk medications. Geriatr Gerontol Int 16(9):1002–1013, 2016 26338275

Qaseem A, Kansagara D, Forciea MA, et al: Management of chronic insomnia disorder in adults: a clinical practice guideline from the American College of Physicians. Ann Intern Med 165(2):125–133, 2016 27136449

Quijano LM, Stanley MA, Peterson NJ, et al: Healthy IDEAS: a depression intervention delivered by community-based case managers serving older adults. J Appl Gerontol 26(2):139–156, 2007

Raue PJ, McGovern AR, Kiosses DN, et al: Advances in psychotherapy for depressed older adults. Curr Psychiatry Rep 19(9):57, 2017 28726061

Rawtaer I, Mahendran R, Yu J, et al: Psychosocial interventions with art, music, Tai Chi and mindfulness for subsyndromal depression and anxiety in older adults: a naturalistic study in Singapore. Asia-Pac Psychiatry 7(3):240–250, 2015 26178378

Rawtaer I, Mahendran R, Chan HY: A nonpharmacological approach to improve sleep quality in older adults. Asia Pac Psychiatry 10e:12301, 2018 28994200

Ren L, Deng J, Min S, et al: Ketamine in electroconvulsive therapy for depressive disorder: a systematic review and meta-analysis. J Psychiatr Res 104:144–156, 2018 30077114

Reynolds CF3rd, Frank E, Perel JM, et al: Nortriptyline and interpersonal psychotherapy as maintenance therapies for recurrent major depression: a randomized controlled trial in patients older than 59 years. JAMA 281(1):39–45, 1999a 9892449

Reynolds CF3rd, Miller MD, Pasternak RE, et al: Treatment of bereavement-related major depressive episodes in later life: a controlled study of acute and continuation treatment with nortriptyline and interpersonal psychotherapy. Am J Psychiatry 156(2):202–208, 1999b 9989555

Reynolds CF3rd, Dew MA, Pollock BG, et al: Maintenance treatment of major depression in old age. N Engl J Med 354(11):1130–1138, 2006 16540613

Reynolds CF3rd, Dew MA, Martire LM, et al: Treating depression to remission in older adults: a controlled evaluation of combined escitalopram with interpersonal psychotherapy versus escitalopram with depression care management. Int J Geriatr Psychiatry 25(11):1134–1141, 2010 20957693

Riebe G, Fan MY, Unützer J, et al: Activity scheduling as a core component of effective care management for late-life depression. Int J Geriatr Psychiatry 27(12):1298–1304, 2012 22367982

Rimer J, Dwan K, Lawlor DA, et al: Exercise for depression. Cochrane Database Syst Rev 7(7):CD004366, 2012 22786489

Rivera FA, Lapid MI, Sampson S, et al: Safety of electroconvulsive therapy in patients with a history of heart failure and decreased left ventricular systolic heart function. J ECT 27(3):207–213, 2011 21865957

Rosen BH, Kung S, Lapid MI: Effect of age on psychiatric rehospitalization rates after electroconvulsive therapy for patients with depression. J ECT 32(2):93–98, 2016 26308147

Rothschild AJ, Williamson DJ, Tohen MF, et al: A double-blind, randomized study of olanzapine and olanzapine/fluoxetine combination for major depression with psychotic features. J Clin Psychopharmacol 24(4):365–373, 2004 15232326

Saari TI, Uusi-Oukari M, Ahonen J, et al: Enhancement of GABAergic activity: neuropharmacological effects of benzodiazepines and therapeutic use in anesthesiology. Pharmacol Rev 63(1):243–267, 2011 21245208

Sackeim HA, Haskett RF, Mulsant BH, et al: Continuation pharmacotherapy in the prevention of relapse following electroconvulsive therapy: a randomized controlled trial. JAMA 285(10):1299–1307, 2001 11255384

Sadavoy J, Meier R, Ong AYM: Barriers to access to mental health services for ethnic seniors: the Toronto study. Can J Psychiatry 49(3):192–199, 2004 15101502

Sajatovic M, Chen P: Geriatric bipolar disorder. Psychiatr Clin North Am 34(2):319–333, vii, 2011 21536161

Sajatovic M, Strejilevich SA, Gildengers AG, et al: A report on older-age bipolar disorder from the International Society for Bipolar Disorders Task Force. Bipolar Disord 17(7):689–704, 2015 26384588

Sanacora G, Frye MA, McDonald W, et al: A consensus statement on the use of ketamine in the treatment of mood disorders. JAMA Psychiatry 74(4):399–405, 2017 28249076

Schak KM, Mueller PS, Barnes RD, et al: The safety of ECT in patients with chronic obstructive pulmonary disease. Psychosomatics 49(3):208–211, 2008 18448774

Scharf M, Rogowski R, Hull S, et al: Efficacy and safety of doxepin 1 mg, 3 mg, and 6 mg in elderly patients with primary insomnia: a randomized, double-blind, placebo-controlled crossover study. J Clin Psychiatry 69(10):1557–1564, 2008 19192438

Schroeck JL, Ford J, Conway EL, et al: Review of safety and efficacy of sleep medicines in older adults. Clin Ther 38(11):2340–2372, 2016 27751669

Scope A, Uttley L, Sutton A: A qualitative systematic review of service user and service provider perspectives on the acceptability, relative benefits, and potential harms of art therapy for people with non-psychotic mental health disorders. Psychol Psychother 90(1):25–43, 2017 27257043

Serrano JP, Latorre JM, Gatz M, et al: Life review therapy using autobiographical retrieval practice for older adults with depressive symptomatology. Psychol Aging 19(2):270–277, 2004 15222820

Seyffert M, Lagisetty P, Landgraf J, et al: Internet-delivered cognitive behavioral therapy to treat insomnia: a systematic review and meta-analysis. PLoS One 11(2):e0149139, 2016 26867139

Sharma A, Barrett MS, Cucchiara AJ, et al: A breathing-based meditation intervention for patients with major depressive disorder following inadequate response to antidepressants: a randomized pilot study. J Clin Psychiatry 78(1):e59–e63, 2017 27898207

Sidor MM, Macqueen GM: Antidepressants for the acute treatment of bipolar depression: a systematic review and meta-analysis. J Clin Psychiatry 72(2):156–167, 2011 21034686

Sirey JA, Bruce ML, Alexopoulos GS: The Treatment Initiation Program: an intervention to improve depression outcomes in older adults. Am J Psychiatry 162(1):184–186, 2005 15625220

Sivertsen B, Omvik S, Pallesen S, et al: Cognitive behavioral therapy vs zopiclone for treatment of chronic primary insomnia in older adults: a randomized controlled trial. JAMA 295(24):2851–2858, 2006 16804151

Sobieraj DM, Martinez BK, Hernandez AV, et al: Adverse effects of pharmacologic treatments of major depression in older adults. J Am Geriatr Soc 67(8):1571–1581, 2019 31140587

Spaans HP, Sienaert P, Bouckaert F, et al: Speed of remission in elderly patients with depression: electroconvulsive therapy v. medication. Br J Psychiatry 206(1):67–71, 2015 25323140

Srinivasan J, Cohen NL, Parikh SV: Patient attitudes regarding causes of depression: implications for psychoeducation. Can J Psychiatry 48(7):493–495, 2003 12971021

Stahl ST, Rodakowski J, Saghafi EM, et al: Systematic review of dyadic and family oriented interventions for late-life depression. Int J Geriatr Psychiatry 31(9):963–973, 2016 26799782

Steffens DC, Wu R, Grady JJ, et al: Presence of neuroticism and antidepressant remission rates in late-life depression: results from the Neurobiology of Late-Life Depression (NBOLD) study. Int Psychogeriatr 30(7):1069–1074, 2018 29198213

Stone M, Laughren T, Jones ML, et al: Risk of suicidality in clinical trials of antidepressants in adults: analysis of proprietary data submitted to US Food and Drug Administration. BMJ 339:b2880, 2009 19671933

Ströhle A: Physical activity, exercise, depression and anxiety disorders. J Neural Transm (Vienna) 116(6):777–784, 2009 18726137

Sumaya IC, Rienzi BM, Deegan JF 2nd, et al: Bright light treatment decreases depression in institutionalized older adults: a placebo-controlled crossover study. J Gerontol A Biol Sci Med Sci 56(6):M356–M360, 2001 11382795

Swainson J, McGirr A, Blier P, et al: The Canadian Network for Mood and Anxiety Treatments (CANMAT) task force recommendations for the use of racemic ketamine in adults with major depressive disorder: recommandations du Groupe de Travail du Réseau Canadien Pour les Traitements de l'Humeur et de l'Anxiété (CANMAT) concernant l'utilisation de la kétamine racémique chez les adultes souffrant de trouble dépressif majeur. Can J Psychiatry 66(2):113–125, 2021 33174760 [Erratum Can J Psychiatry Aug 12: 7067437211035276, 2021 34382885]

Szymkowicz SM, Finnegan N, Dale RM: Failed response to repeat intravenous ketamine infusions in geriatric patients with major depressive disorder. J Clin Psychopharmacol 34(2):285–286, 2014 24525638

Tanaka M, Kusaga M, Nyamathi AM, et al: Effects of brief cognitive behavioral therapy for insomnia on improving depression among community-dwelling older adults: a randomized controlled comparative study. Worldviews Evid Based Nurs 16(1):78–86, 2019 30714310

Tannenbaum C, Paquette A, Hilmer S, et al: A systematic review of amnestic and non-amnestic mild cognitive impairment induced by anticholinergic, antihistamine, GABAergic and opioid drugs. Drugs Aging 29(8):639–658, 2012 22812538

Tapia-Munoz T, Mascayano F, Toso-Salman J: Collaborative care models to address late-life depression: lessons for low-and-middle-income countries. Front Psychiatry 6(64):1–4, 2015 25999866

Tay KW, Subramaniam P, Oei TP: Cognitive behavioural therapy can be effective in treating anxiety and depression in persons with dementia: a systematic review. Psychogeriatrics 19(3):264–275, 2019 30548731

Taylor WD: Clinical practice. Depression in the elderly. N Engl J Med 371(13):1228–1236, 2014 25251617

Thompson LW, Gallagher D, Breckenridge JS: Comparative effectiveness of psychotherapies for depressed elders. J Consult Clin Psychol 55(3):385–390, 1987 3597953

Thorp SR, Glassman LH, Wells SY, et al: A randomized controlled trial of prolonged exposure therapy versus relaxation training for older veterans with military-related PTSD. J Anxiety Disord 64:45–54, 2019 30978622

Trauer JM, Qian MY, Doyle JS, et al: Cognitive behavioral therapy for chronic insomnia: a systematic review and meta-analysis. Ann Intern Med 163(3):191–204, 2015 26054060

Trevizol AP, Goldberger KW, Mulsant BH, et al: Unilateral and bilateral repetitive transcranial magnetic stimulation for treatment-resistant late-life depression. Int J Geriatr Psychiatry 34(6):822–827, 2019 30854751

UK ECT Review Group: Efficacy and safety of electroconvulsive therapy in depressive disorders: a systematic review and meta-analysis. Lancet 361(9360):799–808, 2003 12642045

Unützer J, Park M: Older adults with severe, treatment-resistant depression. JAMA 308(9):909–918, 2012 22948701

Unützer J, Katon W, Callahan CM, et al: Collaborative care management of late-life depression in the primary care setting: a randomized controlled trial. JAMA 288(22):2836–2845, 2002 12472325

Unützer J, Tang L, Oishi S, et al: Reducing suicidal ideation in depressed older primary care patients. J Am Geriatr Soc 54(10):1550–1556, 2006 17038073

Uttley L, Stevenson M, Scope A, et al: The clinical and cost effectiveness of group art therapy for people with non-psychotic mental health disorders: a systematic review and cost-effectiveness analysis. BMC Psychiatry 15:151, 2015 26149275

van Schaik DJF, van Marwijk HWJ, Beekman ATF, et al: Interpersonal psychotherapy (IPT) for late-life depression in general practice: uptake and satisfaction by patients, therapists and physicians. BMC Fam Pract 8:52, 2007 17854480

van Schaik AM, Comijs HC, Sonnenberg CM, et al: Efficacy and safety of continuation and maintenance electroconvulsive therapy in depressed elderly patients: a systematic review. Am J Geriatr Psychiatry 20(1):5–17, 2012 22183009

Vasudev A, Chaudhari S, Sethi R, et al: A review of the pharmacological and clinical profile of newer atypical antipsychotics as treatments for bipolar disorder: considerations for use in older patients. Drugs Aging 35(10):887–895, 2018 30187288

Victoria LW, Gunning FM, Bress JN, et al: Reward learning impairment and avoidance and rumination responses at the end of Engage therapy of late-life depression. Int J Geriatr Psychiatry 33(7):948–955, 2018 29573471

Volkmann C, Bschor T, Köhler S: Lithium treatment over the lifespan in bipolar disorders. Front Psychiatry 11:377, 2020 32457664

Vozoris NT, Fischer HD, Wang X, et al: Benzodiazepine drug use and adverse respiratory outcomes among older adults with COPD. Eur Respir J 44(2):332–340, 2014 24743966

Wallace J, Paauw DS: Appropriate prescribing and important drug interactions in older adults. Med Clin North Am 99(2):295–310, 2015 25700585

Wetherell JL, Afari N, Ayers CR, et al: Acceptance and commitment therapy for generalized anxiety disorder in older adults: a preliminary report. Behav Ther 42(1):127–134, 2011a 21292059

Wetherell JL, Stoddard JA, White KS, et al: Augmenting antidepressant medication with modular CBT for geriatric generalized anxiety disorder: a pilot study. Int J Geriatr Psychiatry 26(8):869–875, 2011b 20872925

Wetherell JL, Petkus AJ, White KS, et al: Antidepressant medication augmented with cognitive-behavioral therapy for generalized anxiety disorder in older adults. Am J Psychiatry 170(7):782–789, 2013 23680817

Wijkstra J, Burger H, van den Broek WW, et al: Treatment of unipolar psychotic depression: a randomized, double-blind study comparing imipramine, venlafaxine, and venlafaxine plus quetiapine. Acta Psychiatr Scand 121(3):190–200, 2010 19694628

Wilkinson P, Izmeth Z: Continuation and maintenance treatments for depression in older people. Cochrane Database Syst Rev 9:CD006727, 2016 27609183

Wilkinson ST, Ballard ED, Bloch MH, et al: The effect of a single dose of intravenous ketamine on suicidal ideation: a systematic review and individual participant data meta-analysis. Am J Psychiatry 175(2):150–158, 2018 28969441

Williams JW Jr, Barrett J, Oxman T, et al: Treatment of dysthymia and minor depression in primary care: a randomized controlled trial in older adults. JAMA 284(12):1519–1526, 2000 11000645

Williams NR, Heifets BD, Blasey C, et al: Attenuation of antidepressant effects of ketamine by opioid receptor antagonism. Am J Psychiatry 175(12):1205–1215, 2018 30153752

Wuthrich VM, Rapee RM: Randomised controlled trial of group cognitive behavioural therapy for comorbid anxiety and depression in older adults. Behav Res Ther 51(12):779–786, 2013 24184427

Wuthrich VM, Rapee RM, Kangas M, et al: Randomized controlled trial of group cognitive behavioral therapy compared to a discussion group for co-morbid anxiety and depression in older adults. Psychol Med 46(4):785–795, 2016 26498268

Xie M, Jiang W, Yang H: Efficacy and safety of the Chinese herbal medicine shuganjieyu with and without adjunctive repetitive transcranial magnetic stimulation (rTMS) for geriatric depression: a randomized controlled trial. Shanghai Jingshen Yixue 27(2):103–110, 2015 26120260

Yatham LN, Kennedy SH, Parikh SV, et al: Canadian Network for Mood and Anxiety Treatments (CANMAT) and International Society for Bipolar Disorders (ISBD) 2018 guidelines for the management of patients with bipolar disorder. Bipolar Disord 20(2):97–170, 2018 29536616

Young RC, Mulsant BH, Sajatovic M, et al: GERI-BD: A randomized double-blind controlled trial of lithium and divalproex in the treatment of mania in older patients with bipolar disorder. Am J Psychiatry 174(11):1086–1093, 2017 29088928

Zhang JX, Liu XH, Xie XH, et al: Mindfulness-based stress reduction for chronic insomnia in adults older than 75 years: a randomized, controlled, single-blind clinical trial. Explore (NY) 11(3):180–185, 2015 25843539

Zhao K, Bai ZG, Bo A, et al: A systematic review and meta-analysis of music therapy for the older adults with depression. Int J Geriatr Psychiatry 31(11):1188–1198, 2016 27094452

Zhao X, Ma J, Wu S, et al: Light therapy for older patients with non-seasonal depression: a systematic review and meta-analysis. J Affect Disord 232:291–299, 2018 29500957

Zhong G, Wang Y, Zhang Y, et al: Association between benzodiazepine use and dementia: a meta-analysis. PLoS One 10(5):e0127836, 2015 26016483

Zullo AR, Gray SL, Holmes HM, et al: Screening for medication appropriateness in older adults. Clin Geriatr Med 34(1):39–54, 2018 29129216

CHAPTER 6

Comprehensive Cultural Assessment of the Older Adult With Depression and Anxiety

Eileen Ahearn, M.D., Ph.D.

PRÉCIS

In this chapter, we review important factors that can affect the evaluation and treatment of older adults with depression and anxiety. Because culture influences the presentation of psychological symptoms, we present information on how to conduct a culturally informed interview. In this chapter, we review special epidemiological and treatment con-

The author would like to express thanks to Lisa L. Boyle, M.D., M.P.H., for her contribution on social determinants of health in older adults with anxiety disorders.

siderations in minority groups, including ethnic minorities, LGBTQ+ individuals, and those with intellectual disabilities. Aging adults may receive treatment in different settings, and we need to understand the rate of mental illness and the unique challenges in those settings. Social determinants of health have important influences on risk for late-life depression and are reviewed. Meaning, purpose, and social connection can also affect psychological well-being. Finally, we discuss the issues of capacity for medical decision-making and elder abuse.

Cultural Assessment of the Older Adult

Culture is defined as the customs, beliefs, and values shared by a group of people and is manifested by the behavior and lifestyle of the group (Tseng 2003). Cultural psychiatry is the study of the impact of culture on the expressions of psychological symptoms and psychiatric illness (Tseng 2003). Understanding the impact of culture in the care of patients is critical to providing effective care. Studies have found that using a standard approach to culturally diverse populations, especially immigrants, can lead to misinterpretation, incorrect diagnoses, poor rapport, and suboptimal care (Kirmayer et al. 2003; Zandi et al. 2008). In one retrospective study of cultural consultations in Canada, nearly half of patients initially referred with a psychotic disorder were rediagnosed as not having psychosis after clinicians used a cultural interview (Adeponle et al. 2012). Initial misdiagnosis was significantly associated with recent arrival into Canada (odds ratio 6.05, 95% CI 1.56–23.46). Evidence of inadequate assessment and treatment has led to a focus on the development of cultural competence in psychiatry.

A focus on culture is important not only for patients from foreign countries but in all patients, even those who are in the majority in a given society. All patients are impacted by the influences of their culture, and so too are their responses to stress, behaviors, and psychological symptoms (Kirmayer 2006). In geriatrics, particular challenges for elders from any cultural group, such as menopause, retirement, grief and loss, and physical infirmity, may lead to psychological symptoms and conditions such as depression (Aggarwal 2010). A more robust assessment and fuller understanding of the impact of culture on the expression of symptoms can only improve understanding, enhance care, and help the individual build rapport with a given treatment provider.

An approach to cultural formulation in psychiatric care was first introduced formally in DSM-IV (American Psychiatric Association 1994) as the Outline for Cultural Formulation (OCF). Organized as a list of cultural topics for clinicians to consider in diagnosis and treatment, the OCF was cumbersome, unstructured, and time-consuming for clinicians (Kirmayer et al. 2008). The DSM-5 Cross-Cultural Issues Subgroup developed a semistructured interview to operationalize the OCF (Lewis-Fernández et al. 2014). The result was the Cultural Formulation Interview (CFI), a 16-question interview that focuses on cultural definitions of the presenting problem, including perceptions of cause, context, and support. The clinician inquires as to the patient's cultural identity and its role as well as cultural factors affecting coping and help-seeking behavior.

The CFI follows the basic conceptual constructs of the OCF: cultural identity, cultural explanations of illness, cultural factors related to psychosocial environment and functioning, and cultural elements of the relationship between the individual and the clinician. There is an informant version of the CFI (American Psychiatric Association 2013a) as well as supplementary modules (American Psychiatric Association 2013b). A summary of the CFI for older adults (from Supplementary Module 10) is displayed in Table 6–1.

Although testing of the CFI is ongoing and training protocols for residents and practicing psychiatrists alike are being developed (Mills et al. 2017), the CFI interview questions may be useful to incorporate into a standard geriatric interview. We illustrate the use of the CFI in the case example.

CASE EXAMPLE: "I DON'T WANT TO FEEL BETTER ABOUT DOING NOTHING"

Mr. Jones is a 68-year-old recently retired businessman who presents to his primary care doctor at the urging of his wife. During the course of his visit, he reports decreased enjoyment of life; loss of interest in doing things; lethargy; sleeping "too much"; and overeating, with a recent 10-pound weight gain. He denies suicidal ideation. He spends most of the day watching TV, reading the paper, and napping. He has mild hypertension that is being treated with hydrochlorothiazide, and otherwise he has been healthy. His wife reports that he has "lost his zest for life" and that the family can't seem to get him to do anything. His primary care physician does a physical examination and finds nothing unusual. The doctor orders laboratory work, including thyroid studies. The doctor suspects depression and offers an antidepressant, which Mr. Jones refuses. They schedule a 1-month follow-up visit.

During his subsequent visit, Mr. Jones reports no improvement in how he is feeling. His doctor shares that all of the lab tests came back as normal. He asks Mr. Jones what he thinks might be the issue, and Mr. Jones is unclear about why he is feeling the way he does: "I thought that maybe it was something physical." The doctor refers Mr. Jones to a psy-

---

Table 6–1.   Cultural Formulation Interview for older adults

Conceptions of aging and cultural identity

1. How would you describe a person of your age?

2. How does your experience of aging compare to that of your friends and relatives who are of a similar age?

3. Is there anything about being your age that helps you cope with your current life situation?

Conceptions of aging in relationship to illness attributions and coping

4. How does being older influence your [PROBLEM]? Would it have affected you differently when you were younger?

5. Are there ways that being older influences how you deal with your [PROBLEM]? Would you have dealt with it differently when you were younger?

Influence of comorbid medical problems and treatments on illness

6. Have you had health problems due to your age?

7. How have your health conditions or the treatments for your health conditions affected your [PROBLEM]?

8. Are there any ways that your health conditions or treatments influence how you deal with your [PROBLEM]?

9. Are there things that are important to you that you are unable to do because of your health or age?

Quality and nature of social supports and caregiving

10. Who do you rely on for help or support in your daily life in general? Has this changed now that you are going through [PROBLEM]?

11. How has [PROBLEM] affected your relationships with family and friends?

12. Are you receiving the amount and kind of support you expected?

13. Do the people you rely on share your view of your [PROBLEM]?

Additional age-related transitions

14. Are there other changes you are going through related to aging that are important for us to know about in order to help you with your [PROBLEM]?

Positive and negative attitudes towards aging and clinician-patient relationship

15. How has your age affected how health providers treat you?

16. Have any people, including health care providers, discriminated against you or treated you poorly because of your age? Can you tell me more about that? How has this experience affected your [PROBLEM] or how do you deal with it?

Table 6–1. Cultural Formulation Interview for older adults *(continued)*

17. Do you think that the difference in our ages will influence our work in any way? If so, how?[a]

Note. The goal of the Cultural Formulation Interview for Older Adults is to identify the role of cultural conceptions of aging and aging-related transition in the patient's presenting problem, referred to above as "[PROBLEM]." A clinician can incorporate these questions into their psychiatric diagnostic interview.

[a]Question 17 may be asked if there is a significant age difference between the clinician and the patient.

Source. Reprinted from American Psychiatric Association: Supplementary module 10. Older adults, in Supplementary Modules to the Core Formulation Interview (CFI). Arlington, VA, American Psychiatric Association, 2013b. Available at: www.psychiatry.org/ File%20Library/Psychiatrists/Practice/DSM/APA_DSM5_Cultural-Formulation-Interview-Supplementary-Modules.pdf. Accessed May 20, 2021. Copyright © 2013 American Psychiatric Association. Used with permission.

---

chologist to try to better understand what is causing his symptoms and so he can talk about options for treatment.

The psychologist uses the CFI for older adults. She discovers that Mr. Jones has negative views of aging in general and that this has made it harder for him to accept growing older. She also learns that he has been going through a difficult age-related transition, namely, his retirement: "When I was working, I felt valuable and I enjoyed going to work," he says. "I had a lot of friends at the office. I worked hard. I felt like I was accomplishing things." Mr. Jones adds, "I wanted to retire so I could enjoy other things, but now I feel lonely, isolated, and worthless. I feel like I am not contributing to society anymore, and I just don't know what to do with myself." When asked about the treatment offered so far, he says: "I don't want to take medication just so that I can feel better about doing nothing."

Most of Mr. Jones's friendships and outside supports were through his job, and when he retired, he lost those supports. He occasionally sees friends from the office, but they are younger and busy with their jobs and families. He also did not really plan for his retirement. Helping others, working hard, and feeling valued are important issues for him, and he feels feckless now. His general health is good, but his fitness level needs improvement.

Together, Mr. Jones and his new psychologist begin to plan a "better retirement" for him and address some of his fears of getting older. They focus on his goals of having friends, being productive, and using his skills as a businessman. He also wants to improve his fitness level.

Over the next 6 months, Mr. Jones makes some changes in his life. He looks into community opportunities to use his business skills and ends up advising the business club at the local high school. He enjoys this activity and discovers how much he likes mentoring young people. He joins the Silver Sneakers exercise group with his wife, and they both discover the fun of working out together and meeting other retirees. Mr. Jones offers to help advise minority small business startups through his community. He feels better and more purposeful and is happier. "I have met a lot of people that I might not otherwise know, and I feel like I am contributing to my community," he says. His struggles with retirement and depression abate; he feels less negative about getting older; and he eases into a new and fulfilling phase of his life, without an antidepressant. Taking the time to use a culturally formulated interview helped his treatment provider understand his views of aging and pinpoint his difficulty with his transition from work to retirement.

Ethnic and Racial Minority Elders

The number of adults in the United States older than age 64 years will increase from 17% in 2016 to 28% by 2060 (U.S. Census Bureau 2017). Importantly, the proportion of ethnic and racial minorities among those between ages 65 and 84 years will increase from 23% to 46% by 2060 (U.S. Census Bureau, Population Division 2017). Thus, ethnic minorities represent a rapidly increasing segment of the older adult population, further highlighting the need to consider how ethnicity and culture can influence the presentation of psychiatric illness.

There may be differences in the measured rates of psychiatric illness in different ethnic groups. In a study by Jimenez and colleagues (2010), researchers matched cultural background and language preferences of participants in a pooled sample of three epidemiological studies looking at lifetime and 12-month prevalence of psychiatric disorders in older adults. Latino and non-Latino whites had similar lifetime prevalence of depressive disorders (17% and 16.9%, respectively) and anxiety disorders (18.2% and 18.7%, respectively). In contrast, Asian Americans had much lower rates of these disorders (6.9% for depression and 9.4% for anxiety). Another study of Asian Americans also found a lower rate of mental illness overall (Alegria et al. 2004). There appears to be a cultural bias against reporting psychological symptoms or perhaps a different characterization or expression of psychological symptoms in Asian communities (Kleinman 1986). Research scales and instruments designed for Western culture also may not accurately identify symptoms.

In a study by Barry and colleagues (2014), 3,075 community-dwelling adults between ages 70 and 79 years were assessed at eight time periods over a decade. A greater percentage of Black enrollees were depressed (defined as scoring 8 or higher on the Center for Epidemiologic Studies Depression Scale [CES-D]) at almost every time point compared with white subjects. Even after adjusting for demographics, including education and socioeconomic status, as well as chronic conditions, the likelihood of depression remained higher (OR 1.22, 95% CI 1.03–1.43) in the African American group. A second study of 707 older adults found that

African American adults were also at higher risk for depression (Jang et al. 2005). However, a third study found lower rates of depression and anxiety disorders in older African Americans (Ford et al. 2007). Interestingly, the study by Barry and colleagues found that there may be a race-by-gender interaction in the United States: Black men may be at higher risk than white men of developing late-life depression, whereas Black and white women have roughly the same risk (Barry et al. 2014). In the United Kingdom, the prevalence of depressive symptoms is markedly higher in ethnic minority elders (specifically South Asian elders and Black Caribbean elders) than in white British elders (Mansour et al. 2020).

Immigrant versus U.S.-born status appears to be a significant variable for several different ethnic minority groups. Asian immigrants have significantly higher lifetime and 12-month prevalence of generalized anxiety disorder (GAD) than do U.S.-born Asians, and immigrant Latinos have higher rates of both GAD and dysthymia compared with U.S. born Latinos (Jimenez et al. 2010). Lower language proficiency is hypothesized to lead to isolation, anxiety, and depression (González et al. 2001; O'Donnell 1989).

Limited data exist to characterize the effectiveness of treatments in older racial and ethnic minorities (Fuentes and Aranda 2012; Miranda et al. 2003). Ethnic minority elders with depression report a higher disability burden (Williams et al. 2007), yet overall these groups have lower utilization of mental health services. In one study of older community-dwelling adults, 66% of those with major depressive disorder did not seek or receive care within the previous year (Garrido et al. 2011). Older adults with better physical health sought mental health care less often, as did those with higher cognitive functioning. Attitudes about seeking mental health treatment may be a factor. In addition, access to care may be different for some minority groups. In a study of minorities and depression treatment, all minority groups had significantly lower access to health care, and quality of care varied between groups (Alegría et al. 2008). There have also been reported disparities in both mental health diagnosis and treatment between different minority ethnic groups (Wu et al. 2018). Continued research is needed in this area to understand the differences in presentation, prevalence, and treatment of depression and anxiety in elder ethnic and racial minority groups.

LGBTQ+ Older Adults

An estimated 1.1 million adults in the United States older than age 65 identify as lesbian, gay, bisexual, transgender, or queer (LGBTQ+), and by 2060, that number is predicted to be at least 5 million (Fredriksen-Goldsen 2016). Anticipating the mental health needs of this important segment of our society is critical, yet a report from the Institute of Medicine (2011) highlighted the paucity of research and information regarding the health-related and aging needs of this group. Fortunately, there are active proposals for improving research, policy, and services for these aging adults (Fredriksen-Goldsen 2016).

Current older LGBTQ+ adults (>70 years old) grew up in a time when same-sex behaviors were criminalized and the American Psychiatric Association had declared homosexuality a psychiatric disorder. Often called the *Silent Generation*, this group reports high levels of identity concealment and internalized stigma (Fredriksen-Goldsen 2016). LGBTQ+ adults younger than 70 grew up in a time of activism and social change with regard to sexual orientation and identity and are often referred to as the *Pride Generation*. Same-sex behavior was decriminalized, and in 1973 homosexuality was removed as a psychiatric disorder in DSM. The rates of identity concealment are lower for the younger cohort of elders, but studies show a higher rate of overall victimization in this group (Fredriksen-Goldsen 2016).

In a study of health outcomes screened by gender and sexual orientation (Fredriksen-Goldsen et al. 2013), lesbian and gay elders reported poorer overall mental health and a greater risk of disability relative to heterosexual adults. This study also showed a higher rate of some physical illnesses, such as cardiovascular disease and obesity, in lesbian women compared with their heterosexual counterparts. In other studies, gay, bisexual, and transgender male cancer survivors had higher rates of depression (Kamen et al. 2014). In general, older transgender adults experience worse physical health, psychological distress, and disability compared with the lesbian, gay, and bisexual cohort (Fredriksen-Goldsen et al. 2013).

Several studies of mood and anxiety disorders in LGBTQ+ older adults have been conducted (Yarns et al. 2016). The Institute of Medicine (2011) study found a higher rate of depression in the older adult LGBT community compared with the general older population. A review by King and colleagues (2008) found a 1.5-fold increase in the lifetime risk for major depression in the lesbian, gay, and bisexual community. In an important survey report by Fredriksen-Goldsen and colleagues (2011), 31% of LGBT older adults self-reported clinically significant depressive symptoms. Transgender individuals reported a rate of depression of 48%, the highest among the subgroups. Thirty-nine percent of older LGBTQ+ adults have contemplated suicide, including 71% of older transgender adults (Fredriksen-Goldsen et al. 2011). Nearly 40%

of those who had contemplated suicide reported that their suicidal ideation was related to sexual orientation or gender identity. Compared with the non-LGBTQ+ community, older LGBTQ+ adults have a two- to threefold higher risk of depression. Aging transgender adults seem to be at particularly high risk of poorer physical and mental health than are nontransgender adults. Further research is needed to better understand, identify, and treat depression and anxiety in these groups.

The mental health professional can play a pivotal role in providing care and mitigating treatment outcomes. Specific recommendations and guidance include assessment of gender dysphoria, education about treatment options, collaboration with other health care team members, treatment of mental health conditions, and advocacy for the rights of transgender persons within the larger community (Johnson et al. 2018). In addition, the American Medical Association (2016) has recommendations for creating a welcoming and inclusive environment for LGBTQ+ adults: inclusive intake forms; staff training; and additions to the environment, such as LGBTQ+ health brochures and other visual reminders of inclusiveness and safety. For an example of inclusive signage, see Figure 6–1.

Spirituality in Older Adults

Spirituality is defined as "the search and connection with the sacred and the transcendent" (Lucchetti et al. 2018, p. 373) and may or may not take place in an organized religious context. Numerous studies in the adult population have demonstrated a connection between spirituality, religion, and better mental health (Lucchetti et al. 2018). A modest number of studies in the geriatric population demonstrate a mental health benefit from religious belief and religious participation. A study by Koenig and colleagues (1998) showed significantly faster remission from depression in medically ill older adults with higher levels of religiosity. A 4-year community study of older adults showed better depression recovery in those with strong religious beliefs and religious involvement (Sun et al. 2012). A study of adults whose mean age was 68 showed that those who attended religious services frequently were 35% less likely to remain depressed after 2 years, even after controlling for other demographic and health factors (Ronneberg et al. 2016).

Religiosity, including spirituality and/or participation in spiritual practices, may protect against depression, as demonstrated in multiple studies. In a Brazilian study of 1,500 older adults, there was a significantly lower prevalence of depression and anxiety disorder in those

> *This office appreciates the diversity of human beings and does not discriminate on the basis of race, age, religion, ability, marital status, sexual orientation, sex, or gender identity.*

Figure 6–1. Recommended nondiscrimination statement to display in your clinical environment.

Source. American Medical Association 2016; www.ama-assn.org/sites/ama-assn.org/files/corp/media-browser/public/glbt/nondiscrimination_0.pdf.

who regularly attended religious services (Corrêa et al. 2011). A 14-year study of older women in the United States showed that religious attendance (at least once a week) predicted a lower number of suicide deaths (VanderWeele et al. 2016). In a study of Korean Americans in New York City, self-reported spirituality was inversely related to depression (Park and Roh 2013). A study of 48,984 women found that those with frequent and recent attendance at religious services had a lower likelihood of depression (OR=0.71, 95% CI, 0.62–0.82) (Li et al. 2016). This connection may be related to such factors as meaning in life, purpose, optimism, and forgiveness (Koenig et al. 2012). Perhaps faith enhances positive emotions, diminishes negative emotions, and improves overall coping (Koenig et al. 2012).

Given the importance of spirituality and religiosity to so many of our patients, mental health professional ought to ask about and attend to these needs. In one study of 79 adults who were in psychiatric treatment, 79% rated spirituality as very important, most believed that it helped them to cope, and 82% thought that their provider should be aware of their spiritual needs (D'Souza 2002). Obtaining a spiritual history is now considered a standard of care at intake. A review of different clinical instruments for this purpose is provided by Lucchetti and colleagues (2013), and we describe the FICA Spiritual History Tool in Chapter 3, "Assessment of Late-Life Depression and Anxiety" (Borneman et al. 2010).

Depression and Anxiety in Older Adults With Intellectual Disability

Improvements in health care have increased the life expectancy of persons with intellectual disability (ID). (Note that the term *intellectual disability* has generally replaced *mental retardation*, so we use the former throughout this section.) Bittles and colleagues' (2002) study of survival probability of 8,724 Australian individuals with ID found median survival ages of 74.0, 67.6, and 58.6 years for those with mild, moderate, and severe intellectual impairment, respectively. Janicki and colleagues' (1999) study of 2,752 adults ages 40 and older with ID in the United States found the average life expectancy of adults to be 66.1 years for mild to moderate ID and 53.6 years for persons with severe ID.

Diagnosis of psychiatric disorders in individuals with ID has been stymied by both the lack of studies and a lack of rigor of the few studies that have been conducted. Most studies of dual diagnosis (ID plus another mental health disorder) were done with small numbers of patients and relied on administrative data (Szymanski 1994)—and there are no studies specifically of older adults. There have also been differences in the diagnostic instruments and interviews used, making comparison of studies difficult. There has been a historical bias against diagnosing other mental health disorders in individuals with ID because symptoms were thought to be part of ID rather than an additional treatable condition (Eaton and Menolascino 1982). Making the diagnosis of other mental health disorders in persons with ID can be clinically difficult. In some individuals, severe cognitive limitations and communication difficulties may necessitate an overreliance on caregiver observation (Borthwick-Duffy and Eyman 1990). Finally, psychiatrists and other mental health professionals typically have had very limited training in working with this population.

A variety of rating instruments have been developed for dual diagnosis conditions such as depression and anxiety in individuals with ID. Both the Hamilton Depression Rating Scale (HDRS) and the Zung Self-Rating Depression Scale (SDS) have a version for persons with ID (Helsel and Matson 1988; Sireling 1986). Two anxiety scales, the Zung Self-Rating

Anxiety Scale (SAS) and the Glasgow Anxiety Scale, have versions for individuals with ID (Lindsay and Michie 1988; Mindham and Espie 2003). In addition, the more general Psychopathology Inventory for Mentally Retarded Adults (PIMRA; Matson et al. 1984) and Diagnostic Assessment Scale for the Severely Handicapped (DASH; Matson et al. 1991) can help confirm different psychiatric diagnoses.

Mental health diagnoses are more common in the ID population relative to the general population, with rate estimates that are threefold to sixfold higher (Eaton and Menolascino 1982). Anxiety disorders are higher in the ID population, with one report noting a prevalence of 28% (Day 1983) and a second study of individuals at a day program reporting a 31% prevalence (Reiss 1990). Depression is thought to be underdiagnosed in this population (Reiss 1994). Presentation may be different than in the general population and can include such symptoms as psychomotor agitation, aggression, and self-injurious behaviors (Meins 1995). Causes of depression in this population include biological and genetic factors, but stressful events and a lack of social support may also contribute (Laman and Reiss 1987).

There are no specific studies of treatment of comorbid psychiatric disorders in older adults with ID. In general, a variety of environmental, behavioral, and psychopharmacological approaches have been used. As noted by Antochi et al (2003), evaluation of adults with ID who have had a behavioral change should include consideration of possible comorbid psychiatric disorders.

A comprehensive literature review of published treatment studies from 1975 to 2001 (Antochi et al. 2003) found a range of psychiatric medications used in people with ID, including antidepressants, antianxiety medications, anticonvulsants, antipsychotics, stimulants, β-blockers, and opioid antagonists. A summary of medications used to treat mental illness in people with ID is provided in Table 6–2. Antidepressants are used for a range of symptoms, including depression, obsessive-compulsive disorder, self-injury, and aggression. Limited data support a trial of a selective serotonin reuptake inhibitor (SSRI) for depression (Campbell and Duffy 1995; Hellings et al. 1996), and sertraline and paroxetine (Davanzo et al. 1998) were found to help with aggression and self-injurious behavior. Antianxiety agents such as buspirone provided improvement with self-injury and anxiety symptoms in several small studies (Ratey et al. 1991; Ricketts et al. 1994). There were no reports of antipsychotic treatment for depression or anxiety in the review by Antochi et al. (2003), nor were stimulants or mood stabilizers evaluated for these diagnoses. Stimulants were used mainly for ADHD, and mood stabilizers were used for aggression and bipolar disorder.

Table 6–2. Studies of treatment of persons with intellectual disabilities and additional psychiatric diagnoses

	Indication	Number of subjects	Medication	Response
Masi et al. 1997	MDD	7	Paroxetine 20–40 mg/day	4 of 7 showed clinical improvement
Sovner et al. 1993	MDD+SIB	2	Fluoxetine 20–40 mg/day	Reduction of symptoms
Bodfish and Madison 1993	OCD	10 with OCD, 6 control subjects	Fluoxetine 40–80 mg/day	7 of 10 with OCD responded
Davanzo et al. 1998	Aggression+ SIB	15	Paroxetine	Aggression reduced; no change in SIB
Lewis et al. 1996	SIB	8	Clomipramine	6 of 8 had >50% reduction in SIB
Posey et al. 2001	Aggression, SIB, anxiety, depression	26	Mirtazapine	9 of 26 showed improvement

Note. The subjects in the Masi and Sovner studies were adolescents; subjects in other studies were adults.
Abbreviations. MDD=major depressive disorder; OCD=obsessive-compulsive disorder; SIB=self-injurious behavior.
Source. Adapted from Antochi et al. 2003.

Despite the paucity of evidence supporting the use of psychotropic medications in adults with ID and comorbid mental illness, medications are commonly prescribed. A study of 4,069 adults with intellectual disabilities (mean age 49.6) showed an overall psychotropic medications use rate of 58% (Tsiouris et al. 2013). Rates of use for specific medication categories were as follows: antidepressants 23%, antipsychotics 43%, mood stabilizers 19%, and antianxiety agents 16%. Of the 58% of individuals who received medication, 49% were being treated for a psychiatric disorder only, 13% for behavioral issues, and 38% for both. Table 6–3 shows the odds ratio for use (vs. nonuse) of antipsychotics, antidepressants, and antianxiety medications for depression, anxiety, and aggression in this population. Prior to 2000, Molyneux et al. (1999) had found an antidepressant prevalence rate of only 8%–10%. It appears that over time, practitioners increasingly recognized and treated depression in this population.

Table 6–3.   Odds ratio for the use of psychotropic medication for given comorbid diagnoses in adults with intellectual disabilities

	Antipsychotic	Antidepressant	Mood stabilizer	Anxiolytic
Depression	1.15	7.89 ***	0.80	1.08
Anxiety	1.32**	1.49***	0.95	2.57***
Aggression	2.12***	1.76***	2.36***	2.17***

Note.   Data were derived from four logistic regressions on use of the for major classes of medications (use versus non-use).
**P <0.01, ***P <0.001.
Source.   Adapted from Tsiouris et al. 2013.

Special Considerations by Setting

Aging adults who face a variety of physical and mental health needs may be receiving treatment in different settings. The following is a discussion of specific settings and includes the demographics of those settings as well as the needs and challenges of individuals served in those environments.

LONG-TERM CARE FACILITIES

According to a national survey, roughly 4% of American adults ages 65 years and older are living in nursing homes (Jones et al. 2009). The average adult age 65 or older will need 3 years of long-term care during their lifetime (Kemper et al. 2005–2006). In a national survey of nursing homes in the United States, mental health disorders were the second most common primary diagnosis among nursing home residents, both at admission and at the time of the survey, with a prevalence of 16.4% and 21.9%, respectively (Jones et al. 2009). Dementia is the most frequent diagnosis for long-term care residents, with a prevalence of about 50% in these settings.

Depression is common in nursing home residents, with an estimated 6%–26% of this population meeting criteria for major depressive disorder. (See Chapter 1, "Introduction to Late-Life Depression," section "Epidemiology," for additional review of the epidemiology of depression in long-term care.) Prevalence of any depressive symptoms may be as high as 50% in nursing homes (Blazer 2003; Grabowski et al. 2010). Given that depression has adverse effects on health outcomes, treatment is important. One study of 76,735 residents in 921 nursing homes found that 48% had a depression diagnosis, and of those with depression, 74% were prescribed an antidepressant and only 0.5% received psychotherapy (Levin et al. 2007). Yet it is unclear how effective antidepressant treatment is in this population. A review by Boyce and colleagues (2012) of the effectiveness of antidepressant treatment in nursing homes was inconclusive. Most of the studies they reviewed did not include a control group, and approximately 50% of residents who were treated also had cognitive impairment, most often due to dementia. In two 8-week studies that did have control groups (Burrows et al. 2002; Magai et al. 2000), there was no statistical difference between SSRIs and placebo. SSRIs were better tolerated than tricyclic antidepressants. More research needs to be done to understand the efficacy and tolerability of antidepressants in the nursing home population.

Anxiety disorders appear to be common in long-term care facilities, as noted in Chapter 2, "Introduction to Late-Life Anxiety and Related Disorders," subsection "Residents of Skilled Nursing Facilities." A study of 180 older residents in nursing home facilities found that approximately 20% met DSM-5 criteria for an anxiety disorder (American Psychiatric Association 2013a; Creighton et al. 2018). GAD (11.1%) and specific phobias (6.1%) were the most common. The prevalence of GAD was higher than that reported in the general older adult population and may correlate with the higher rate of physical illness and functional impairment found in elders in nursing homes (Beekman et al. 1998). The majority of residents were receiving psychiatric medication to treat their symptoms. A high rate of benzodiazepine and antidepressant use was noted.

In an interesting study of nursing home residents with normal cognitive function or mild cognitive impairment, Creighton and colleagues (2019) found that the variables that correlated most highly with self-rated anxiety were depression, lower self-perceived health, cognitive impairment, lower perceived control of one's life, excessive dependence, and worry that support in their current relationships is insufficient for their current needs.

EMERGENCY DEPARTMENTS

In the United States, the number of emergency department (ED) visits is on the rise. The number of individuals using EDs increased from 34.2 million to 40 million between 1996 and 2005 (Xu et al. 2009). A disproportionate numbers of these patients were older adults. Further, an increasing number of older adults with mental health disorders visit the ED. Hakenewerth and colleagues (Centers for Disease Control and Prevention 2013) analyzed ED visits of those with mental health disorders, sorted by age group. Older adults accounted for 27% of all ED visits for mental health, a rate disproportionately higher than the incidence of mental health issues in this age group in the general population. The most common diagnoses treated were psychosis, depression, anxiety, and stress. The number of visits for these diagnoses far exceeded visits for dementia in this population. In general, behavioral health care is lacking for the geriatric community because of a variety of factors necessitating use of the ED for care (Jeste et al. 1999).

Among geriatric patients presenting to the ED, depression is common. In one study of 259 patients ages 65 years and older, 27% were found to be depressed on the basis of a self-rated depression scale (Meldon et al. 1997). In this study, patients who reported poor health were more likely to be depressed. The study noted that ED personnel appeared to underdiagnose depression. In general, ED providers are also less likely to screen for suicidal ideation in older adults (Betz et al. 2016). In addition to training ED clinicians, the use of depression rating instruments such as the Geriatric Depression Scale (GDS) or the Patient Health Questionnaire nine-item rating scale (PHQ-9) are important and have been validated for this older population. The Columbia Suicide Severity Rating Scale (C-SSRS) can also be implemented in EDs as a screening tool for suicidal ideation. We present an overview of suicide risk factors in older adults in Table 6–4; for a more extensive discussion, see Chapter 4, "Suicide Risk Reduction in Older Adults," especially Table 4–1.

Basic laboratory workup of older adults presenting to an ED with psychiatric symptoms includes a metabolic panel, complete blood count, vitamin B_{12} level, thyroid panel, and urine toxicology screen (Bessey et al. 2018). Other lab work and evaluations may be indicated; for more details, see Chapter 3 (especially Table 3–10). Collateral information from family may be helpful. Safety is paramount, and patients with suicidal ideation and a plan should be admitted to an inpatient psychiatric unit. Safety planning can be done with those who may be at high risk but who do not meet criteria for involuntary commitment. A written safety plan can be developed and should identify risk factors, supports, steps taken to lower risk, referral for further treatment, and emergency contact information for the patient and/or family to use should symptoms worsen (Bessey et al. 2018); see Chapter 4, subsection "Suicide Safety Planning."

Anxiety disorders are common in older adults, with GAD being the most common (Lenze and Wetherell 2011). Anxiety in the older adult may be secondary to medical issues, substance use, medications, or dementia; a standard medical evaluation should include an examination,

Table 6–4. Suicide risk factors in older adults, in brief

Nonmodifiable risk factors	Modifiable risk factors
Older age	Substance use disorder
Male	Mood disorder
White	Medical illness
Unmarried	Psychosis
Recent psychiatric hospitalization	Chronic pain
Previous suicide attempt	Social isolation
	Family history of suicide
	Access to lethal means
	Stressful life event

Note. For a comprehensive discussion of suicide risk factors and risk assessment, see Chapter 4, "Suicide Risk Reduction in Older Adults" (in particular, Tables 4–1 and 4–2).
Source. Adapted from Bessey et al. 2018.

electrocardiogram, and basic blood work (Bessey et al. 2018). A psychiatric history is key; it is also important to obtain a current assessment of the duration and character of anxiety symptoms along with collateral information. Anxiety often co-occurs as part of depression, so screening for depression is also important. Treatment with benzodiazepines should be avoided if possible, given the significant risks associated with their use, including falls, fractures, and memory impairment (Marra et al. 2015). Reassurance and an outpatient plan for follow-up in mental health are needed.

INPATIENT MEDICAL UNITS

A significant number of patients in hospital medical units have comorbid mental health diagnoses, including depression. In one study of the National Health System in the United Kingdom, the prevalence of mental health conditions in older adults on inpatient units was estimated to be 60%, with specific estimates of depression and anxiety disorders at 29% and 8%, respectively (Royal College of Psychiatrists 2005). Estimates of undetected mental health conditions in hospitalized patients are as high as 50% (Parsonage et al. 2012). One review showed a detection rate of depression in older hospitalized medical patients of only 10% (Cole and Bellavance 1997). In a second study, suboptimal treatment of depression was noted: the majority of older patients with depression were neither treated with antidepressants nor provided psychological interventions (Holmes and House 2000).

The significance of unrecognized mental health disorders should be emphasized because it is well known that comorbid mental health issues bode poorly for health outcomes and functional status (Moussavi et al. 2007; Yohannes et al. 2010). In one study, patients with heart failure were eight times more likely to die within 30 months if they also had comorbid depression (Jünger et al. 2005). Underrecognition and undertreatment of mental health disorders can lead to poorer outcomes, increased length of stay, and increased number of readmissions (Royal College of Psychiatrists 2005).

A consultation-liaison inpatient team can serve a critical function in addressing and treating comorbid mental health conditions. The consultation-liaison team can provide early identification, recommend medication treatment, and educate inpatient teams about care of psychiatric disorders. Participation in discharge planning to ensure ongoing mental health care is also a critical function of this team.

INCARCERATED OLDER ADULTS

Older adults are the fastest-growing segment of incarcerated adults in the United States. Between 1993 and 2013, there was a 400% increase in incarcerated adults in the state prison population who were at least 55 years old (Carson and Sobol 2016). A 2014 survey found that older inmates (65 years and older) represented more than 246,000 prisoners, or 16% of the entire prison population in the United States (Osborne Association 2014). By 2030, older inmates will account for one-third of incarcerated adults in the United States. Most older prisoners have "aged-in" during their prison time, a phenomenon that is secondary to sentencing practices such as mandatory minimum sentences, longer sentences, the increased use of life sentences, and a decrease in parole (Prost et al. 2021).

Not only do older incarcerated adults have high rates of chronic medical illness; they also have higher rates of mental health issues than do nonincarcerated older adults. A survey of 186 incarcerated older adults found a prevalence rate of depression of 14% using a cutoff of 10 on the PHQ-8 (Prost et al. 2021). This prevalence was higher than community rates for older adults. Another study of older inmates found a 1-month prevalence of major depression of 10.5% and a 1-month prevalence of anxiety disorders (excluding simple phobia) of 4.2% (Koenig et al. 1995). The prevalence rates were also higher than those of the surrounding community. The rate of chronic physical disability was also high, and there is a phenomenon of *accelerated aging* that has been described among adults in prison that leads to increased health issues, including mental health issues (Yarnell et al. 2017).

Only 4% of U.S. prisons provide specialized geriatric care (Thivierge-Rikard and Thompson 2007). Some possible solutions to the lack of adequate geriatric mental health care include increasing the geriatric training of forensic psychiatrists, promoting collaboration with geriatric psychiatrists, and training geriatric psychiatrists in the area of forensics. Other proposals have included early release from prison given the low rate of recidivism in older prisoners or compassionate release for those with severe conditions. The increased numbers of older incarcerated adults and their more complex health needs require attention for future planning of the prison health care system.

PATIENTS IN PALLIATIVE CARE AND HOSPICE

Depression and anxiety symptoms are common in patients receiving palliative care, with up to 15% meeting criteria for major depressive disorder (Hotopf et al. 2002; Mitchell et al. 2011). The existence of comorbid depression not only adds to the physical burden of a terminal illness, with such symptoms as increased pain and fatigue, but these same somatic symptoms may appear to be part of the medical condition itself, making depression more difficult to detect.

European guidelines on the management of depression in palliative cancer care suggest that clinicians should focus more on affective symptoms during evaluation because somatic symptoms may be less reliable (Rayner et al. 2011b). Specifically, affective symptoms such as loss of interest in activities, low mood, hopelessness, feeling worthless, and suicidal ideation are better indicators than physical symptoms in this population.

Psychotherapy can be used in patients with mild to moderate depression. A meta-analysis of psychotherapies for depression and anxiety in palliative care found the strongest evidence for cognitive-behavioral therapy, acceptance and commitment therapy, and mindfulness-based stress reduction, with improvement in depression, anxiety, and quality of life (Fulton et al. 2018).

Medications may also be helpful. A meta-analysis of antidepressant treatment of depression in palliative care found superior benefit for medications as early as 4–5 weeks and improved benefit at subsequent time points (6–8 weeks, 9–18 weeks) compared with placebo (Rayner et al. 2011a). The number needed to treat was 5 at the 9- to 18-week time point. A separate Cochrane review also had similar findings (Rayner et al. 2010). For moderate depression, medication and/or psychological therapy are recommended, and for severe depression, both interventions are suggested (Rayner et al. 2011b).

Social Determinants of Late-Life Depression and Anxiety

Social determinants of health are nonmedical factors that can affect health, such as economic issues, education, access to health care, and factors in the neighborhood or environment. For example, in a longitudinal study of 220 community-dwelling elders, risk factors for depression included being less educated and having a smaller social network (Smit et al. 2006). A study of 22,777 Europeans at least 50 years old found that lower educational level (below high school education) predicted a 15% higher rate of depression (Ladin et al. 2010).

Poverty is a risk factor for late-life depression. Lower socioeconomic status has consistently been shown to predict late-life depression across a wide variety of countries, including the United States, Mexico, Europe, Africa, India, and China (Brinda et al. 2016; Ladin et al. 2010). Other socioeconomic risk factors for late-life depression include food insecurity (i.e., lack of access to nutritious and affordable food), indebtedness, fewer years of formal education, previous employment in the informal sector (e.g., as a street vendor), not owning one's residence, and structural inequality (i.e., countries with more economic inequality have higher rates of late-life depression) (Brinda et al. 2016; Ruiz et al. 2019a). A study of 10,969 older adults in Japan found that those with debt were at significantly higher risk of mild to moderate depression (OR=1.3) and severe depression (OR=2.1), as measured by the CES-D (Kaji et al. 2010). Similarly, a study of rural elders in Japan found that those with the lowest personal income were 1.6 times more like to have depression, as measured by the CES-D (Fang et al. 2019). Poverty is a risk factor for food insecurity, which in turn has been associated with "feeling extremely anxious and/or depressed" in elders living in Canada (Pirrie et al. 2020).

Where an older adult lives, which is also closely linked with race, ethnicity, and socioeconomic status, influences the risk of depression. For example, low perceived social cohesion of one's neighborhood is a risk factor for late-life depression (Ruiz et al. 2019b). *Built environment* refers to features of a neighborhood such as walkability, building density, and economic disadvantage; an unfavorable built environment may be associated with late-life depression in men (Saarloos et al. 2011). Exposure to environmental pollution also increases the risk of late-life depression (Petkus et al. 2019).

Retirement status may have an effect on risk for depression. In the Japan Gerontological Evaluation Study of 62,438 community-dwelling adults, depression symptoms increased significantly following retirement, which was especially notable in older men (Shiba et al. 2017). The Health and Retirement Study of older Americans also found that retirement status is associated with an increased risk for depression (Zivin et al. 2013).

The relationship between marital status and late-life depression is covered in Chapter 1. We add here information on the link between widowhood and depression: Recent widowhood was also associated with increased risk for depression in late life. In a longitudinal study of 1,940 older adults in Amsterdam, the loss of a spouse doubled the risk for depression (OR 2.29, CI 1.77–2.99) (Schoevers et al. 2006). A longitudinal study of 2,827 older adults in Costa Rica also demonstrated increased risk for depression for recent widows (Gertner et al. 2017).

Social support and family support are, not surprisingly, protective factors against depression in late life. Participants in a cross-sectional study of 220 older individuals in India found a lower risk of depression in those with strong family support (Nakulan et al.2015). In a 10-year longitudinal study of 21,728 U.S. women, low social support was associated with a higher risk for depression in older women (Chang et al. 2016). A study of 2,047 older adults in Ireland found that adults who reported strong social support had a lower risk for late-life depression (OR=0.35, 95% CI, 0.22–0.54) (Cheong et al. 2017). High social support in a study of 200 older adult Korean immigrants in New York City was also correlated with lower levels of depression (Park and Roh 2013).

Caregivers are also at greater risk for depression. Chang and colleagues (2016) found a higher depression risk in older women with caregiver burdens. In a study of 1,801 older adults in the United States, those reporting any caregiving responsibilities over a 24-month period had, on average, 30 more days of depression over that period than those without this burden (Thompson et al. 2008).

Social determinants of health also contribute to anxiety in older adults. Stress in the environment in which a person was raised or currently lives increases vulnerability to anxiety disorders. Poverty and childhood trauma, such as parental loss or separation, low affective support during childhood, and parental mental illness, have been identified as risk factors for late-onset GAD (Zhang et al. 2015b). Trauma experienced during childhood, compared with during adulthood, is associated with more severe PTSD (Ogle et al. 2013). Childhood trauma and adverse life events can also increase the likelihood of panic disorder (Tibi et al. 2013). Interestingly, providing care for an older adult with cognitive impairment has been associated with anxiety later in life (Remes et al. 2016). In a longitudinal study conducted in Europe, extreme experiences of World War II were a risk factor for experiencing any anxiety disorder, GAD, phobic disorder, panic disorder, and obsessive-compulsive disorder in late life (Beekman et al. 1998). Similarly, fleeing life-threatening experiences as a refugee increases the risk of late-life anxiety (Remes et al. 2016). Lower income and experience of more recent stressful events were more likely in older adults with panic disorder than those without panic disorder (Chou 2010). Loneliness has been identified as a risk factor for late-life GAD in women (Boehlen et al. 2020).

We summarize these social determinants of health contributing to late-life depression and anxiety in Table 6–5.

Table 6–5.   Social determinants of health that can contribute to late-life depression and anxiety

Less than high school education

Low annual income

Financial debt

Food insecurity

Not owning one's home

Decreased social cohesion of one's neighborhood

Being retired

Lower social support and loneliness

Caregiver burden

Living in a country with greater economic disparities

Environmental pollution

Note.   See text for discussion.
Source.   Adapted from Vyas and Okereke 2020.

Capacity Assessment

Decisional capacity necessarily involves four critical elements: understanding, appreciation, reasoning, and the expression of a choice. In the context of consenting to medical treatment, capacity refers to a person's ability to understand his or her illness and the medical options for treatment. Patients must be able to understand the relative risks and benefits of treatment options and be able to demonstrate adequate reasoning regarding how they would make their decision. Finally, they must be able to clearly communicate a choice of treatment based on all treatment options.

Hindmarch and colleagues (2013) reviewed 10 studies of decision-making ability in patients who had major depression and were being referred either to a research study or for clinical treatment. They also included 7 additional ethical case analyses in their review. A number of studies they reviewed cited impairment of appreciation in individuals with depression. Because of their emotional state, these patients were sometimes found incapable of applying medical facts and treatment consequences to their own situation. Young and colleagues (1993) found that depressed patients could not understand the consequences of their medical choices, and Meynen (2011) noted an altered perception of future possibilities as a serious limitation, affecting the construct of appreciation. Elliott (1997) observed a minimal level of concern regarding one's welfare in depression as well as a lack of "decisional authenticity," which he defined as decisions that reflect the "true" self. He found some patients did not care about risk, a state-related phenomenon associated with depression.

Certainly, symptoms of depression such as hopelessness and anhedonia may make an individual feel that life may never get better and that it will not offer happiness or fulfillment (Sullivan and Youngner 1994). Owen and colleagues (2018) evaluated 12 patients with major depression. They noted two significant issues in people with depression: a "constricted experience of the future," defined as a negative view of the future and an inability to imagine recovery, and a failure of inductive reasoning based on this inflexible and pessimistic view of the future. Other studies have noted deficits in reasoning in depressed patients (Cohen et al. 2004; Vollmann et al. 2003).

A research instrument, the MacArthur Competence Assessment Tool (MacCAT-T), has been used in studies of depressed patients with varying rates of incapacity ranging from a few percent to 31% in one study (Owen et al. 2008). However, this instrument has an emphasis on cognition and may not be as useful in evaluations of capacity in depression (Grisso et al. 1997).

Suggestions for clinicians include treatment of depression, supported decision-making, and an ethically based approach when patients' decisions about their medical care appear unduly influenced by their depression. Future approaches and instruments need to be developed to better allow clinicians to confidently assess medical decision-making ability in individuals with depression.

Elder Abuse

Elder abuse is a public health issue affecting approximately one in six older adults worldwide (Yon et al. 2017). In the United States, three epidemiological studies estimated overall rates of elder abuse ranging from 7.6% to 10% (Acierno et al. 2010; Burnes et al. 2015; Laumann et al. 2008). All three studies were based on self-report and excluded elders with dementia, so they are likely underestimates of true prevalence because dementia is an independent risk factor for abuse (Dong et al. 2014). A consensus of types of elder abuse has emerged and includes physical abuse, psychological abuse or verbal abuse, sexual abuse, financial exploitation, and neglect (Laumann et al. 2008).

Risk factors for abuse include female sex, younger age, lower income, poor social support, and a shared living environment (Amstadter et al. 2011; Brozowski and Hall 2010; Burnes et al. 2015; Laumann et al. 2008). Older adults who are younger in age are likely to still be living with family, who are most often the perpetrators of abuse. Having dementia is a risk factor for abuse, as are poor physical health and functional impairment in general. As noted by Lachs and Pillemer (2015), perpetrators of abuse most often are adult children or spouses; are male; and have a history of current or past substance use, a history of legal issues, or mental health or physical problems. In addition, perpetrators of abuse often have financial problems and are unemployed. Elders who experience abuse are at higher risk for hospitalization, placement in a nursing home, and death (Dong and Simon 2013; Lachs et al. 1998, 2002; Schofield et al. 2013). They also have higher rates of depression and anxiety (Dong et al. 2013; Gibbs and Mosqueda 2010; Mouton et al. 2010).

Identification and screening are challenging, with potential for both false positives and false negatives. Assessment for elder abuse should be done without family present, but family caregivers should also be interviewed. Lachs and Pillemer (2015) provide a detailed list of manifestations of types of abuse and assessment. Positive findings should lead to comprehensive evaluation by adult protective services or a comparable social services agency. For more information on assessment for elder abuse, see Chapter 3, subsection "Screening for Elder Abuse."

Specific interventions vary depending on the type of abuse detected. Physical or sexual violence needs treatment but also referral to local law enforcement and completion of a safety plan for the victim. When financial exploitation is suspected, the clinician should consider referral to law enforcement or recommendation of financial guardianship. Verbal abuse may be managed by educating the caregiver, addressing caregiver burden, finding alternative caregivers, and treating the mental health needs of the patient. Finally, neglect can be addressed by alternative placement such as in a nursing home, by use of day programs or respite programs, by increasing services in the home, and/or by educating the caregiver about the inadequacy of current care he or she is providing. Interprofessional teams are suggested as a way of assisting victims of elder abuse. In addition to medical personnel, these teams might include law enforcement, community partners, and attorneys (Rizzo et al. 2015; Teaster et al. 2003).

Elder abuse can occur in long-term care facilities, and there are reports of both staff-to-resident abuse and resident-to-resident abuse. A telephone survey of 452 relatives of older adults in nursing homes found a 24.3% incidence of at least one episode of physical abuse by staff (Schiamberg et al. 2012). Griffore and colleagues (2009) found that the frequency of reported abuse of residents according to family members was higher than that reported to the National Ombudsman System—that is, formal mechanisms of reporting abuse were being underused. With respect to resident-to-resident abuse, a 10-year study of 747 nursing home residents identified 79 incidents and 42 residents involved in resident-to-resident mistreatment (as either victim or perpetrator) that necessitated calls to police (Lachs et al. 2007). Another study found that 97% of nursing aides reported seeing residents push, grab, or pinch each other in the previous 90 days (Castle 2012). The residents most vulnerable to resident-to-resident abuse are those with communication problems and cognitive impairment (Sifford-Snellgrove et al. 2012).

Meaning, Purpose, and Social Connection in Late Life

Meaning and purpose in life can have health benefits in older adults. In the U.S. Health and Retirement Study (HRS) of 8,419 older adults, life purpose was found to be protective against all-cause mortality (hazard ratio of 2.43, 95% CI 1.57–3.75) (Alimujiang et al. 2019; Wallace and Herzog 1995). A meta-analysis of studies of life purpose and mortality also found increased survival for older adults who had strong life purpose (Cohen et al. 2016).

Why might this be the case? Engagement in health behaviors and preventive care correlates with life purpose (Kim et al. 2014). In Kim and colleagues' study, data from 7,168 subjects enrolled in the HRS study demonstrated that higher life purpose was associated with increased likelihood of obtaining a cholesterol test, a colonoscopy, a mammogram, or a prostate exam. Individuals also spent 17% fewer nights in the hospital (RR=0.83, 95% CI=0.77–0.89) for each additional point on the 6-point life purpose scale. A smaller study suggested that individuals with a higher life purpose have lower cortisol levels and lower proinflammatory cytokines (Ryff et al. 2004).

In an interesting study of psychological well-being, Wood and Joseph (2010) included measures of purpose in life. In this study, 5,566 adults ages 51–56 years were surveyed initially, and then 10 years later, on an 18-item measure of psychological well-being and a depression rating scale. After adjusting for prior depression, physical health variables, and other covariates, people with low purpose in life at the initial measurement were at significantly higher risk for depression 10 years later (OR 1.85, 95% CI 1.33–2.57). Even those with impaired (not low) purpose had an increased risk of depression at 10 years (OR 1.69, 95% CI 1.23–2.31). Purpose in life is a significant factor in predicting depression, independent of physical health and other demographic and socioeconomic variables.

Finally, purpose in life has been found to protect against cognitive decline. In an analysis of data from the HRS study, purpose in life was associated with cognitive scores even after controlling for covariates. During the 6-year study period, there was evidence of slower cognitive decline (Kim et al. 2019).

Lack of social connection in later life is associated with health risks, including increased morbidity and mortality, as well as increased risk for depression (Brummett et al. 2001; Heikkinen and Kauppinen 2004). In an interesting study by Cornwell and Waite (2009) of 3,005 older individuals, social disconnectedness and the perception of being isolated each contributed independently to lower self-ratings of health. Specifically, both variables were found to be associated with poorer physical health. The authors concluded that it was not only the actual measure of social connectedness but also the person's perception of it that had a measurable impact on health and well-being. For mental health measures in this study, the findings were different. Older adults with lack of social connectedness had worse mental health ratings when they felt socially isolated. In this case, perception may have been the mediating variable linking lack of social connection and poorer mental health. Further work on social relationships, connection, and perception of relationships is needed.

Summary: Doing the Right Thing in the Care of Older Adults With Depression and Anxiety

Culture is defined as the customs, beliefs, and values shared by a group of people. Understanding cultural influences in our patients can help give us diagnostic clarity and improved rapport and can assist us in providing optimal care to patients. The 16-question Cultural Formulation Interview in DSM-5 Supplementary Module 10 can be incorporated into a standard psychiatric interview.

The percentage of older adults in the United States is increasing, as is the percentage of ethnic minorities. Although older Latino and non-Latino whites have a similar lifetime prevalence of depression and anxiety disorders, Asian Americans have a much lower rate of both. Older African Americans may be at higher risk for depression. In general, immigrant minorities have higher rates of both depression and anxiety compared with U.S.-born minorities.

An estimated 1.1 million adults in the United States identify as LGBTQ+. Understanding their needs is important, but unfortunately, little research has been done to date. In general, LGBTQ+ elders report poorer mental health. Transgender individuals seem to be particularly at risk for mental health issues.

Another important group is adults with intellectual disabilities who are living longer. Estimates suggest higher rates of comorbid mental health diagnoses in this group. Few studies have been conducted in this population, and there has been a historical bias diagnosing other mental health disorders in this population. Communication difficulties due to cognitive limitations and the lack of training of mental health professionals make diagnosis and treatment difficult. Limited data support a trial of SSRIs for depression.

Older adults with depression or anxiety may be treated in different settings, and it is important to understand the demographic risk data and challenges in those settings. In nursing homes, the prevalence of any depression symptoms may be as high as 50%. Treatment studies of this population often lack control groups and have included patients with dementia, limiting conclusive findings. In general, SSRI medications seem better tolerated than tricyclic antidepressants. Anxiety disorders may be as high as 20% in nursing homes, with generalized anxiety disorder being the most common. In the emergency department, a disproportionate number of visits are by older adults, and a considerable number are for mental health issues, including depression and anxiety. This phenomenon may also reflect the lack of community mental health care for the geriatric community. In prison, older inmates represent 16% of the entire prison population, a percentage that is predicted to increase. Studies have shown higher rates of depression and anxiety in correctional facilities relative to the community. Finally, in hospice and palliative care, patients have higher rates of depression, and both medication and psychotherapy have shown benefit.

Psychosocial risk factors have been identified in late-life depression. These risk factors include being female, having a low income, being recently widowed, being retired, being separated or divorced, having poor family/social support, and having a high caregiver burden. Meaning and purpose in life are protective and can lower the risk for depression in late life, independent of physical health and other socioeconomic variables. Lack of social connectedness as well as the perception of being isolated puts older individuals at risk for depression.

Finally, individuals with depression may lack capacity for medical decision-making, with possible impairment in both understanding and appreciation of their illness. Assessment of capacity should be considered in older adults with significant depression. Clinicians should also be alert to the possibility of elder abuse, which can affect approximately 10% of older adults in the United States. Assessment should be done without family present, but family caregivers should also be interviewed.

KEY POINTS

- Understanding the cultural influences of mental health presentation can improve diagnosis and treatment. Older adults from ethnic groups have different rates of depression and anxiety disorders. Understanding the needs of specific groups of individuals, such as older LGBTQ+ adults, is important.

- Older adults are treated in different settings, such as nursing homes, the emergency department, hospice care, and the prison system. Data regarding the incidence of depression and anxiety in those settings indicate a need to address treatment of mental health disorders of these elders.

- It is important to be cognizant of psychosocial risks for late-life depression when screening older adults for depression and anxiety. Social connectedness and purpose in life are protective against depression.

- Patients who are depressed may lack decision-making capacity if depression is severe. Clinicians need to bear this in mind and may need to evaluate for this capacity.

- Screening for possible elder abuse is important, particularly in older patients with certain risk factors.

Resources for Patients, Families, and Caregivers

National Research Center on LGBT Aging

www.lgbtagingcenter.org

- "[T]he country's first and only technical assistance resource center aimed at improving the quality of services and supports offered to lesbian, gay, bisexual and/or transgender older adults"

National Center on Elder Abuse

https://ncea.acl.gov

- "[P]rovides the latest information regarding research, training, best practices, news and resources on elder abuse, neglect and exploitation to professionals and the public"

National Institute of Mental Health
"Older Adults and Depression"

www.nimh.nih.gov/health/publications/older-adults-and-depression/index.shtml

- Lay language discussion of signs of depression, types of depression, risk factors, and treatment

National Center on Aging

www.ncoa.org/article/evidence-based-program-pearls-program-to-encourage-active-rewarding-lives

- List of behavioral health programs for older adults (e.g., Program to Encourage Active, Rewarding Lives for Seniors [PEARLS])

American Association of Geriatric Psychiatry

www.aagponline.org/index.php?src=gendocsandref=Consumer%2FPatient%20Informationandcategory=Foundation

- Information for older adults, family members, and caregivers

References

Acierno R, Hernandez MA, Amstadter AB, et al: Prevalence and correlates of emotional, physical, sexual, and financial abuse and potential neglect in the United States: the National Elder Mistreatment Study. Am J Public Health 100(2):292–297, 2010 20019303

Adeponle AB, Thombs BD, Groleau D, et al: Using the cultural formulation to resolve uncertainty in diagnoses of psychosis among ethnoculturally diverse patients. Psychiatr Serv 63(2):147–153, 2012 22302332

Aggarwal NK: Reassessing cultural evaluations in geriatrics: insights from cultural psychiatry. J Am Geriatr Soc 58(11):2191–2196, 2010 20977437

Alimujiang A, Wiensch A, Boss J, et al: Association between life purpose and mortality among US adults older than 50 years. JAMA Netw Open 2(5):e194270, 2019 31125099

Alegria M, Takeuchi D, Canino G, et al: Considering context, place and culture: the National Latino and Asian American Study. Int J Methods Psychiatr Res 13(4):208–220, 2004 15719529

Alegría M, Chatterji P, Wells K, et al: Disparity in depression treatment among racial and ethnic minority populations in the United States. Psychiatr Serv 59(11):1264–1272, 2008 18971402

American Medical Association: Creating an LGBTQ-friendly practice. Chicago, IL, American Medical Association, 2016. Available at: www.ama-assn.org/delivering-care/population-care/creating-lgbtq-friendly-practice. Accessed May 20, 2021.

American Psychiatric Association: Diagnostic and Statistical Manual of Mental Disorders, 4th Edition. Washington, DC, American Psychiatric Association, 1994

American Psychiatric Association: Diagnostic and Statistical Manual of Mental Disorders, 5th Edition. Arlington, American Psychiatric Association, 2013a

American Psychiatric Association: Supplementary module 10. Older adults, in Supplementary modules to the Core Formulation Interview (CFI). Arlington, VA, American Psychiatric Association, 2013b. Available at: www.psychiatry.org/File%20Library/Psychiatrists/Practice/DSM/APA_DSM5_Cultural-Formulation-Interview-Supplementary-Modules.pdf. Accessed May 20, 2021.

Amstadter AB, Cisler JM, McCauley JL, et al: Do incident and perpetrator characteristics of elder mistreatment differ by gender of the victim? Results from the National Elder Mistreatment Study. J Elder Abuse Negl 23(1):43–57, 2011 21253929

Antochi R, Stavrakaki C, Emery PC: Psychopharmacological treatments in persons with dual diagnosis of psychiatric disorders and developmental disabilities. Postgrad Med J 79(929):139–146, 2003 12697912

Barry LC, Thorpe RJ Jr, Penninx BW, et al: Race-related differences in depression onset and recovery in older persons over time: the health, aging, and body composition study. Am J Geriatr Psychiatry 22(7):682–691, 2014 24125816

Beekman ATF, Bremmer MA, Deeg DJH, et al: Anxiety disorders in later life: a report from the Longitudinal Aging Study Amsterdam. Int J Geriatr Psychiatry 13(10):717–726, 1998 9818308

Bessey LJ, Radue RM, Chapman EN, et al: Behavioral health needs of older adults in the emergency department. Clin Geriatr Med 34(3):469–489, 2018 30031428

Betz M, Arias S, Segal D, et al: Screening for suicidal thoughts and behaviors in older adults in the emergency department. J Am Geriatr Soc 65(10):e72–e77, 2016 27596110

Bittles AH, Petterson BA, Sullivan SG, et al: The influence of intellectual disability on life expectancy. J Gerontol A Biol Sci Med Sci 57(7):M470–M472, 2002 12084811

Blazer DG: Depression in late life: review and commentary. J Gerontol A Biol Sci Med Sci 58(3):249–265, 2003 12634292

Bodfish JW, Madison JT: Diagnosis and fluoxetine treatment of compulsive behavior disorder of adults with mental retardation. Am J Ment Retard 98(3):360–367, 1993 8292312

Boehlen FH, Herzog W, Schellberg D, et al: Gender-specific predictors of generalized anxiety disorder symptoms in older adults: results of a large population-based study. J Affect Disord 262:174–181, 2020 31668601

Borneman T, Ferrell B, Puchalski CM: Evaluation of the FICA tool for spiritual assessment. J Pain Symptom Manage 40(2):163–173, 2010 20619602

Boyce RD, Hanlon JT, Karp JF, et al: A review of the effectiveness of antidepressant medications for depressed nursing home residents. J Am Med Dir Assoc 13(4):326–331, 2012 22019084

Brinda EM, Rajkumar AP, Attermann J, et al: Health, social, and economic variables associated with depression among older people in low and middle income countries: World Health Organization Study on Global AGEing and Adult Health. Am J Geriatr Psychiatry 24(12):1196–1208, 2016 27743841

Borthwick-Duffy SA, Eyman RK: Who are the dually diagnosed? Am J Ment Retard 94(6):586–595, 1990 2340136

Brozowski K, Hall DR: Aging and risk: physical and sexual abuse of elders in Canada. J Interpers Violence 25(7):1183–1199, 2010 19717787

Brummett BH, Barefoot JC, Siegler IC, et al: Characteristics of socially isolated patients with coronary artery disease who are at elevated risk for mortality. Psychosom Med 63(2):267–272, 2001 11292274

Burnes D, Pillemer K, Caccamise PL, et al: Prevalence of and risk factors for elder abuse and neglect in the community: a population-based study. J Am Geriatr Soc 63(9):1906–1912, 2015 26312573

Burrows AB, Salzman C, Satlin A, et al: A randomized, placebo-controlled trial of paroxetine in nursing home residents with non-major depression. Depress Anxiety 15(3):102–110, 2002 12001178

Campbell JJ III, Duffy JD: Sertraline treatment of aggression in a developmentally disabled patient. J Clin Psychiatry 56(3):123–124, 1995 7883733

Carson EA, Sobol W: Aging of the State Prison Population, 1993–2013 (Rep No NCJ 248766). Washington, DC, Bureau of Justice Statistics, 2016

Castle NG: Nurse aides' reports of resident abuse in nursing homes. J Appl Gerontol 31(3):402–422, 2012

Centers for Disease Control and Prevention: Emergency department visits by patients with mental health disorders—North Carolina, 2008–2010. MMWR Morb Mortal Wkly Rep 62(23):469–472, 2013 23760188

Chang SC, Pan A, Kawachi I, et al: Risk factors for late-life depression: a prospective cohort study among older women. Prev Med 91:144–151, 2016 27514249

Cheong EV, Sinnott C, Dahly D, et al: Adverse childhood experiences (ACEs) and later-life depression: perceived social support as a potential protective factor. BMJ Open 7(9):e013228, 2017 28864684

Chou KL: Panic disorder in older adults: evidence from the national epidemiologic survey on alcohol and related conditions. Int J Geriatr Psychiatry 25(8):822–832, 2010 19946867

Cohen BJ, McGarvey EL, Pinkerton RC, et al: Willingness and competence of depressed and schizophrenic inpatients to consent to research. J Am Acad Psychiatry Law 32(2):134–143, 2004 15281414

Cohen R, Bavishi C, Rozanski A: Purpose in life and its relationship to all-cause mortality and cardiovascular events: a meta-analysis. Psychosom Med 78(2):122–133, 2016 26630073

Cole MG, Bellavance F: Depression in elderly medical inpatients: a meta-analysis of outcomes. CMAJ 157(8):1055–1060, 1997 9347776

Cornwell EY, Waite LJ: Social disconnectedness, perceived isolation, and health among older adults. J Health Soc Behav 50(1):31–48, 2009 19413133

Corrêa AA, Moreira-Almeida A, Menezes PR, et al: Investigating the role played by social support in the association between religiosity and mental health in low income older adults: results from the São Paulo Ageing and Health Study (SPAH). Br J Psychiatry 33(2):157–164, 2011 21829909

Creighton AS, Davison TE, Kissane DW: The prevalence, reporting, and treatment of anxiety among older adults in nursing homes and other residential aged care facilities. J Affect Disord 227:416–423, 2018 29154158

Creighton AS, Davison TE, Kissane DW: The factors associated with anxiety symptom severity in older adults living in nursing homes and other residential aged care facilities. J Aging Health 31(7):1235–1258, 2019 29683028

Davanzo PA, Belin RT, Widawski MH, King BH: Paroxetine treatment of aggression and self-injury in persons with mental retardation. Am J Ment Retard 102(5):427–437, 1998 9544340

Day K: A hospital-based psychiatric unit for mentally handicapped adults. Mental Handicap 11:137–140, 1983

Dong X, Simon MA: Elder abuse as a risk factor for hospitalization in older persons. JAMA Intern Med 173(10):911–917, 2013 23567991

Dong X, Chen R, Chang ES, et al: Elder abuse and psychological well-being: a systematic review and implications for research and policy—a mini review. Gerontology 59(2):132–142, 2013 22922225

Dong X, Chen R, Simon MA: Elder abuse and dementia: a review of the research and health policy. Health Aff (Millwood) 33(4):642–649, 2014 24711326

D'Souza R: Do patients expect psychiatrists to be interested in spiritual issues? Australas Psychiatry 10(1):44–47, 2002

Eaton LF, Menolascino FJ: Psychiatric disorders in the mentally retarded: types, problems, and challenges. Am J Psychiatry 139(10):1297–1303, 1982 7124983

Elliott C: Caring about risks. Are severely depressed patients competent to consent to research? Arch Gen Psychiatry 54(2):113–116, 1997 9040277

Fang M, Mirutse G, Guo L, Ma X: Role of socioeconomic status and housing conditions in geriatric depression in rural China: a cross-sectional study. BMJ Open 9(5):e024046, 2019 31110082

Ford B, Bullard K, Taylor R, et al: Lifetime and 12-month prevalence of the Diagnostic and Statistical Manual of Mental Disorders (fourth edition) among older African Americans: findings from the National Survey of American Life. Am J Geriatr Psychiatry 15(8):652–659, 2007 17504908

Fredriksen-Goldsen KI: The future of LGBT+ aging: a blueprint for action in services, policies, and research. Generations 40(2):6–15, 2016 28366980

Fredriksen-Goldsen KI, Kim H, Emlet CA, et al: The Aging and Health Report: Disparities and Resilience Among Lesbian, Gay, Bisexual, and Transgender Older Adults. Seattle, WA, Institute for Multigenerational Health, 2011

Fredriksen-Goldsen KI, Kim HJ, Barkan SE, et al: Health disparities among lesbian, gay, and bisexual older adults: results from a population-based study. Am J Public Health 103(10):1802–1809, 2013 23763391

Fredriksen-Goldsen KI, Cook-Daniels L, Kim HJ, et al: Physical and mental health of transgender older adults: an at-risk and underserved population. Gerontologist 54(3):488–500, 2014 23535500

Fuentes D, Aranda MP: Depression interventions among racial and ethnic minority older adults: a systematic review across 20 years. Am J Geriatr Psychiatry 20(11):915–931, 2012 22828202

Fulton JJ, Newins AR, Porter LS, et al: Psychotherapy targeting depression and anxiety for use in palliative care: a meta-analysis. J Palliat Med 21(7):1024–1037, 2018 29676960

Garrido MM, Kane RL, Kaas M, et al: Use of mental health care by community-dwelling older adults. J Am Geriatr Soc 59(1):50–56, 2011 21198461

Gertner AK, Domino ME, Dow WH: Risk factors for late-life depression and correlates of antidepressant use in Costa Rica: results from a nationally representative longitudinal survey of older adults. J Affect Disord 208:338–344, 2017 27810716

Gibbs L, Mosqueda L: Elder abuse: a medical perspective. Aging Health 6(1):739–747, 2010

González HM, Haan MN, Hinton L: Acculturation and the prevalence of depression in older Mexican Americans: baseline results of the Sacramento Area Latino Study on Aging. J Am Geriatr Soc 49(7):948–953, 2001 11527487

Grabowski DC, Aschbrenner KA, Rome VF, et al: Quality of mental health care for nursing home residents: a literature review. Med Care Res Rev 67(6):627–656, 2010 20223943

Griffore RJ, Barboza GE, Mastin T, et al: Family members' reports of abuse in Michigan nursing homes. J Elder Abuse Negl 21(2):105–114, 2009 19347713

Grisso T, Appelbaum PS, Hill-Fotouhi C: The MacCAT-T: a clinical tool to assess patients' capacities to make treatment decisions. Psychiatr Serv 48(11):1415–1419, 1997 9355168

Heikkinen RL, Kauppinen M: Depressive symptoms in late life: a 10-year follow-up. Arch Gerontol Geriatr 38(3):239–250, 2004 15066310

Hellings JA, Kelley LA, Gabrielli WF, et al: Sertraline response in adults with mental retardation and autistic disorder. J Clin Psychiatry 57(8):333–336, 1996 8778118

Helsel WJ, Matson JL: The relationship of depression to social skills and intellectual functioning in mentally retarded adults. J Ment Defic Res 32(Pt 5):411–418, 1988 3199434

Hindmarch T, Hotopf M, Owen GS: Depression and decision-making capacity for treatment or research: a systematic review. BMC Med Ethics 14:54, 2013 24330745

Holmes J, House A: Psychiatric illness predicts poor outcome after surgery for hip fracture: a prospective cohort study. Psychol Med 30(4):921–929, 2000 11037100

Hotopf M, Chidgey J, Addington-Hall J, et al: Depression in advanced disease: a systematic review part 1: prevalence and case finding. Palliat Med 16(2):81–97, 2002 11969152

Institute of Medicine: The Health of Lesbian, Gay, Bisexual, and Transgender People: Building a Foundation for Better Understanding. Washington, DC, Institute of Medicine of the National Academies, 2011

Janicki MP, Dalton AJ, Henderson CM, et al: Mortality and morbidity among older adults with intellectual disability: health services considerations. Disabil Rehabil 21(5–6):284–294, 1999 10381241

Jang Y, Borenstein AR, Chiriboga DA, et al: Depressive symptoms among African American and white older adults. J Gerontol B Psychol Sci Soc Sci 60(6):313–P319, 2005 16260705

Jeste DV, Alexopoulos GS, Bartels SJ, et al: Consensus statement on the upcoming crisis in geriatric mental health: research agenda for the next 2 decades. Arch Gen Psychiatry 56(9):848–853, 1999 12884891

Jimenez DE, Alegría M, Chen CN, et al: Prevalence of psychiatric illnesses in older ethnic minority adults. J Am Geriatr Soc 58(2):256–264, 2010 20374401

Johnson K, Yarns BC, Abrams JM, et al: Gay and Gray session: an interdisciplinary approach to transgender aging. Am J Geriatr Psychiatry 26(7):719–738, 2018 29699765

Jones AL, Dwyer LL, Bercovitz AR, et al: The National Nursing Home Survey: 2004 overview. Vital Health Stat 13 (167):1–155, 2009 19655659

Jünger J, Schellberg D, Müller-Tasch T, et al: Depression increasingly predicts mortality in the course of congestive heart failure. Eur J Heart Fail 7(2):261–267, 2005 15701476

Kaji T, Mishima K, Kitamura S, et al: Relationship between late-life depression and life stressors: large-scale cross-sectional study of a representative sample of the Japanese general population. Psychiatry Clin Neurosci 64(4):426–434, 2010 20492557

Kamen C, Palesh O, Gerry AA, et al: Disparities in health risk behavior and psychological distress among gay versus heterosexual male cancer survivors. LGBT Health 1(2):86–92, 2014 26789618

Kemper P, Komisar HL, Alecxih L: Long-term care over an uncertain future: what can current retirees expect? Inquiry 42(4):335–350, 2005–2006 16568927

Kim ES, Strecher VJ, Ryff CD: Purpose in life and use of preventative health care services. Proc Natl Acad Sci U S A 111(46):16331–16336, 2014 25368165

Kim G, Shin SH, Scicolone MA, et al: Purpose in life protects against cognitive decline among older adults. Am J Geriatr Psychiatry 27(6):593–601, 2019 30824327

King M, Semlyen J, Tai SS, et al: A systematic review of mental disorder, suicide, and deliberate self harm in lesbian, gay and bisexual people. BMC Psychiatry 8:70, 2008 18706118

Kirmayer LJ: Beyond the "new cross-cultural psychiatry": cultural biology, discursive psychology and the ironies of globalization. Transcult Psychiatry 43(1):126–144, 2006 16671396

Kirmayer LJ, Groleau D, Guzder J, et al: Cultural consultation: a model of mental health service for multicultural societies. Can J Psychiatry 48(3):145–153, 2003 12728738

Kirmayer LJ, Thombs BD, Jurcik T, et al: Use of an expanded version of the DSM-IV outline for cultural formulation on a cultural consultation service. Psychiatr Serv 59(6):683–686, 2008 18511590

Kleinman A: Social Origins of Distress and Disease: Neurasthenia, Depression, and Pain in Modern China. New Haven, CT, Yale University, 1986

Koenig HG, George LK, Peterson BL: Religiosity and remission of depression in medically ill older patients. Am J Psychiatry 155(4):536–542, 1998 9546001

Koenig HG, Johnson S, Bellard J, et al: Depression and anxiety disorder among older male inmates at a federal correctional facility. Psychiatr Serv 46(4):399–401, 1995 7788465

Koenig HG, King DE, Carson VB: Handbook of Religion and Health, 2nd Edition. New York, Oxford University Press, 2012

Lachs M, Bachman R, Williams CS, et al: Resident-to-resident elder mistreatment and police contact in nursing homes: findings from a population-based cohort. J Am Geriatr Soc 55(6):840–845, 2007 17537083

Lachs MS, Pillemer KA: Elder abuse. N Engl J Med 373(20):1947–1956, 2015 26559573

Lachs MS, Williams CS, O'Brien S, et al: The mortality of elder mistreatment. JAMA 280(5):428–432, 1998 9701077

Lachs MS, Williams CS, O'Brien S, et al: Adult protective service use and nursing home placement. Gerontologist 42(6):734–739, 2002 12451154

Ladin K, Daniels N, Kawachi I: Exploring the relationship between absolute and relative position and late-life depression: evidence from 10 European countries. Gerontologist 50(1):48–59, 2010 19515635

Laman DS, Reiss S: Social skill deficiencies associated with depressed mood of mentally retarded adults. Am J Ment Defic 92(2):224–229, 1987 3434593

Lenze EJ, Wetherell JL: A lifespan view of anxiety disorders. Dialogues Clin Neurosci 13(4):381–399, 2011 22275845

Laumann EO, Leitsch SA, Waite LJ: Elder mistreatment in the United States: prevalence estimates from a nationally representative study. J Gerontol B Psychol Sci Soc Sci 63(4):S248–S254, 2008 18689774

Levin CA, Wei W, Akincigil A, et al: Prevalence and treatment of diagnosed depression among elderly nursing home residents in Ohio. J Am Med Dir Assoc 8(9):585–594, 2007 17998115

Lewis MH, Bodfish JW, Powell SB, et al: Clomipramine treatment for self-injurious behavior of individuals with mental retardation: a double blind comparison with placebo. Am J Ment Retard 100(6):654–665, 1996 8735578

Lewis-Fernández R, Aggarwal NK, Bäärnhielm S, et al: Culture and psychiatric evaluation: operationalizing cultural formulation for DSM-5. Psychiatry 77(2):130–154, 2014 24865197

Li S, Okereke OI, Chang SC, et al: Religious service attendance and lower depression among women—a prospective cohort study. Ann Behav Med 50(6):876–884, 2016 27393076

Lindsay WR, Michie AM: Adaptation of the Zung self-rating anxiety scale for people with a mental handicap. J Ment Defic Res 32(Pt 6):485–490, 1988 3236373

Lucchetti A, Barcelos-Ferreira R, Blazer DG, et al: Spirituality in geriatric psychiatry. Curr Opin Psychiatry 31(4):373–377, 2018 29847345

Lucchetti G, Bassi RM, Lucchetti AL: Taking spiritual history in clinical practice: a systematic review of instruments. Explore (NY) 9(3):159–170, 2013 23643371

Magai C, Kennedy G, Cohen CI, et al: A controlled clinical trial of sertraline in the treatment of depression in nursing home patients with late-stage Alzheimer's disease. Am J Geriatr Psychiatry 8(1):66–74, 2000 10648297

Mansour R, Tsamakis K, Rizos E, et al: Late-life depression in people from ethnic minority backgrounds: differences in presentation and management. J Affect Disord 264:340–347, 2020 32056770

Marra EM, Mazer-Amirshahi M, Brooks G, et al: Benzodiazepine prescribing in older adults in U.S. ambulatory clinics and emergency departments. J Am Geriatr Soc 63(10):2074–2081, 2015 26415836

Masi G, Marchesci M, Planner P: Paroxetine in depressed adolescents with intellectual disability: an open label study. J Intellect Disabil Res 41(pt 3):268–272, 1997 9219077

Matson JL, Kazdin AE, Senatore V: Psychometric properties of the psychopathology instrument for mentally retarded adults. Appl Res Ment Retard 5(1):81–89, 1984 6721483

Matson JL, Gardner WI, Coe DA, et al: A scale for evaluating emotional disorders in severely and profoundly mentally retarded persons: development of the Diagnostic Assessment for the Severely Handicapped (DASH) scale. Br J Psychiatry 159:404–409, 1991 1958951

Meins W: Symptoms of major depression in mentally retarded adults. J Intellect Disabil Res 39(Pt 1):41–45, 1995 7719061

Meldon SW, Emerman CL, Schubert DS, et al: Depression in geriatric ED patients: prevalence and recognition. Ann Emerg Med 30(2):141–145, 1997 9250635

Meynen G: Depression, possibilities, and competence: a phenomenological perspective. Theor Med Bioeth 32(3):181–193, 2011 21207153

Mills S, Xiao AQ, Wolitzky-Taylor K, et al: Training on the DSM-5 Cultural Formulation Interview improves cultural competence in general psychiatry residents: a pilot study. Transcult Psychiatry 54(2):179–191, 2017 28358239

Mindham J, Espie CA: Glasgow Anxiety Scale for People ith an Intellectual Disability (GAS-ID): development and psychometric properties of a new measure for use with people with mild intellectual disability. J Intellect Disabil Res 47(Pt 1):22–30, 2003 12558692

Miranda J, Nakamura R, Bernal G: Including ethnic minorities in mental health intervention research: a practical approach to a long-standing problem. Cult Med Psychiatry 27(4):467–486, 2003 14727681

Mitchell AJ, Chan M, Bhatti H, et al: Prevalence of depression, anxiety, and adjustment disorder in oncological, haematological, and palliative-care settings: a meta-analysis of 94 interview-based studies. Lancet Oncol 12(2):160–174, 2011 21251875

Molyneux P, Emerson E, Caine A: Prescription of psychotropic medication to people with intellectual disabilities in primary health-care settings. J Appl Res Intellect Disabil 12:46–57, 1999

Moussavi S, Chatterji S, Verdes E, et al: Depression, chronic diseases, and decrements in health: results from the World Health Surveys. Lancet 370(9590):851–858, 2007 17826170

Mouton CP, Rodabough RJ, Rovi SL, et al: Psychosocial effects of physical and verbal abuse in postmenopausal women. Ann Fam Med 8(3):206–213, 2010 20458103

Nakulan A, Sumesh TP, Kumar S, et al: Prevalence and risk factors for depression among community resident older people in Kerala. Indian J Psychiatry 57(3):262–266, 2015 26600579

O'Donnell R: Functional disability of the Puerto Rican elderly. Journal of Aging and Health 1(2):244–246, 1989

Ogle CM, Rubin DC, Siegler IC: The impact of the developmental timing of trauma exposure on PTSD symptoms and psychosocial functioning among older adults. Dev Psychol 49(11):2191–2200, 2013 23458662

Osborne Association: The High Costs of Low Risk: The Crisis of America's Aging Prison Population. New York, Osborne Association, 2014. Available at: www.osborneny.org/assets/files/Osborne_HighCostsofLowRisk.pdf. Accessed September 12, 2021.

Owen GS, Richardson G, David AS, et al: Mental capacity to make decisions on treatment in people admitted to psychiatric hospitals: cross sectional study. BMJ 337:a448, 2008 18595931

Owen GS, Martin W, Gergel T: Misevaluating the future: affective disorder and decision-making capacity for treatment—a temporal understanding. Psychopathology 51(6):371–379, 2018 30485862

Park J, Roh S: Daily spiritual experiences, social support, and depression among elderly Korean immigrants. Aging Ment Health 17(1):102–108, 2013 22881195

Parsonage M, Fossey M, Tutty C: Liaison psychiatry in the modern NHS. London, Centre for Mental Health, 2012. Available at: www.centreformentalhealth.org.uk/sites/default/files/2018-09/Liaison_psychiatry_in_the_modern_NHS_2012_0.pdf. Accessed May 21, 2021.

Petkus AJ, Younan D, Wang X, et al: Particulate air pollutants and trajectories of depressive symptoms in older women. Am J Geriatr Psychiatry 27(10):1083–1096, 2019 31311712

Pirrie M, Harrison L, Angeles R, et al: Poverty and food insecurity of older adults living in social housing in Ontario: a cross-sectional study. BMC Public Health 20(1):1320, 2020 32867736

Posey DJ, Guerin KD, Kohn AE, et al: A naturalistic open-label study of mirtazapine in autistic and other pervasive developmental disabilities. J Child Adolesc Psychopharmacol 11(3):267–277, 2001 11642476

Prost SG, Archuleta AJ, Golder S: Older adults incarcerated in state prison: health and quality of life disparities between age cohorts. Aging Mental Health 25(2):260–268, 2021 31782313

Ratey J, Sovner R, Parks A, et al: Buspirone treatment of aggression and anxiety in mentally retarded patients: a multiple-baseline, placebo lead-in study. J Clin Psychiatry 52(4):159–162, 1991 2016248

Rayner L, Price A, Evans A, et al: Antidepressants for depression in physically ill people. Cochrane Database Syst Rev (3):CD007503, 2010 20238354

Rayner L, Price A, Evans A, et al: Antidepressants for the treatment of depression in palliative care: systematic review and meta-analysis. Palliat Med 25(1):36–51, 2011a 20935027

Rayner L, Price A, Hotopf M, et al: The development of evidence-based European guidelines on the management of depression in palliative cancer care. Eur J Cancer 47(5):702–712, 2011b 21211961

Reiss S: Prevalence of dual diagnosis in community-based day programs in the Chicago metropolitan area. Am J Ment Retard 94(6):578–585, 1990 2340135

Reiss S: Psychopathology in mental retardation, in Mental Health in Mental Retardation. Edited by Bouras N. Cambridge, UK, Cambridge University Press, 1994, pp 67–78

Remes O, Brayne C, van der Linde R, et al: A systematic review of reviews on the prevalence of anxiety disorders in adult populations. Brain Behav 6(7):e00497, 2016 27458547

Ricketts RW, Goza AB, Ellis CR, et al: Clinical effects of buspirone on intractable self-injury in adults with mental retardation. J Am Acad Child Adolesc Psychiatry 33(2):270–276, 1994 8150800

Rizzo VM, Burnes D, Chalfy A: A systematic evaluation of a multidisciplinary social work-lawyer elder mistreatment intervention model. J Elder Abuse Negl 27(1):1–18, 2015 24965802

Ronneberg CR, Miller EA, Dugan E, et al: The protective effects of religiosity on depression: a 2 year prospective study. Gerontologist 56(3):421–431, 2016 25063937

Royal College of Psychiatrists: Who Cares Wins: Improving the Outcome for Older People Admitted to the General Hospital. London, Royal College of Psychiatrists, 2005

Ruiz M, Hu Y, Martikainen P, et al: Life course socioeconomic position and incidence of mid-late life depression in China and England: a comparative analysis of CHARLS and ELSA. J Epidemiol Community Health 73(9):817–824, 2019a 31255999

Ruiz M, Malyutina S, Pajak A, et al: Congruent relations between perceived neighbourhood social cohesion and depressive symptoms among older European adults: an East-West analysis. Soc Sci Med 237:112454, 2019b 31376532

Ryff CD, Singer BH, Dienberg Love G: Positive health: connecting well-being with biology. Philos Trans R Soc Lond B Biol Sci 359(1449):1383–1394, 2004 15347530

Saarloos D, Alfonso H, Giles-Corti B, et al: The built environment and depression in later life: the health in men study. Am J Geriatr Psychiatry 19(5):461–470, 2011 20808136

Schiamberg LB, Oehmke J, Zhang Z, et al: Physical abuse of older adults in nursing homes: a random sample survey of adults with an elderly family member in a nursing home. J Elder Abuse Negl 24(1):65–83, 2012 22206513

Schoevers RA, Smit F, Deeg DJ, et al: Prevention of late-life depression in primary care: do we know where to begin? Am J Psychiatry 163(9):1611–1621, 2006 16946188

Schofield MJ, Powers JR, Loxton D: Mortality and disability outcomes of self-reported elder abuse: a 12-year prospective investigation. J Am Geriatr Soc 61(5):679–685, 2013 23590291

Shiba K, Kondo N, Kondo K, et al: Retirement and mental health: does social participation mitigate the association? A fixed-effects longitudinal analysis. BMC Public Health 17(1):526, 2017 28558670

Sifford-Snellgrove KS, Beck C, Green A, et al: Victim or initiator? Certified nursing assistants' perceptions of resident characteristics that contribute to resident-to-resident violence in nursing homes. Res Gerontol Nurs 5(1):55–63, 2012 21678883

Sireling L: Depression in mentally handicapped patients: diagnostic and neuro-endocrine evaluation. Br J Psychiatry 149:274–278, 1986 3779289

Smit F, Ederveen A, Cuijpers P, et al: Opportunities for cost-effective prevention of late-life depression: an epidemiological approach. Arch Gen Psychiatry 63(3):290–296, 2006 16520434

Sovner R, Fox CJ, Lowry MJ, et al: Fluoxetine treatment of depression and associated self-injury in two adults with mental retardation. J Intellect Disabil Res 37(pt 3):301–311, 1993 8334322

Sullivan MD, Youngner SJ: Depression, competence, and the right to refuse life-saving medical treatment. Am J Psychiatry 151(7):971–978, 1994 8010382

Sun F, Park NS, Roff LL, et al: Predicting the trajectories of depressive symptoms among southern community-dwelling older adults: the role of religiosity. Aging Ment Health 16(2):189–198, 2012 22032625

Szymanski L: Mental retardation and mental health: concepts, aetiology, and incidence, in Mental Health in Mental Retardation. Edited by Bouras N. Cambridge, UK, Cambridge University Press, 1994, pp 19–33

Teaster PB, Nerenberg L, Stansbury KL: A national look at elder abuse multidisciplinary teams. J Elder Abuse Negl 15(3–4):91–107, 2003

Thivierge-Rikard RV, Thompson MS: The association between aging inmate housing management models and non-geriatric health services in state correctional institutions. J Aging Soc Policy 19(4):39–56, 2007 18032207

Thompson A, Fan MY, Unützer J, et al: One extra month of depression: the effects of caregiving on depression outcomes in the IMPACT trial. Int J Geriatr Psychiatry 23(5):511–516, 2008 17944005

Tibi L, van Oppen P, Aderka IM, et al: Examining determinants of early and late age at onset in panic disorder: an admixture analysis. J Psychiatr Res 47(12):1870–1875, 2013 24084228

Tseng WS: Cultural Competence in Clinical Psychiatry. Boston, MA, Academic Press, 2003

Tsiouris JA, Kim SY, Brown WT, et al: Prevalence of psychotropic drug use in adults with intellectual disability: positive and negative findings from a large scale study. J Autism Dev Disord 43(3):719–731, 2013 22829245

U.S. Census Bureau: Table 2. Projected age groups and sex composition of the population: projections for the United States 2017–2060, in Projections for the United States: 2017–2060. Suitland, MD, U.S. Census Bureau, 2017. Available at: www2.census.gov/programs-surveys/popproj/tables/2017/2017-summary-tables/np2017-t2.xlsx. Accessed May 21, 2021.

U.S. Census Bureau, Population Division: Table 6. Race and Hispanic origin by age groups, in 2017 National Population Projections Tables: Main Series. Suitland, MD, U.S. Census Bureau, 2017. Available at: www.census.gov/data/tables/2017/demo/popproj/2017-summary-tables.html. Accessed May 21, 2021.

VanderWeele TJ, Li S, Tsai AC, et al: Association between religious service attendance and lower suicide rates among US women. JAMA Psychiatry 73(8):845–851, 2016 27367927

Vollmann J, Bauer A, Danker-Hopfe H, et al: Competence of mentally ill patients: a comparative empirical study. Psychol Med 41(1):119–128, 2003 14672255

Vyas CM, Okereke OI: Late-life depression: a narrative review on risk factors and prevention. Harv Rev Psychiatry 28(2):72–99, 2020 31977599

Wallace RB, Herzog AR: Overview of the health measures in the Health and Retirement Study. Journal of Human Resources 30:S84–S107, 1995

Williams DR, González HM, Neighbors H, et al: Prevalence and distribution of major depressive disorder in African Americans, Caribbean blacks, and non-Hispanic whites: results from the National Survey of American Life. Arch Gen Psychiatry 64(3):305–315, 2007 17339519

Wood AM, Joseph S: The absence of positive psychological (eudemonic) well-being as a risk factor for depression: a ten year cohort study. J Affect Disord 122(3):213–217, 2010 19706357

Wu C, Chiang M, Harrington A, et al: Racial disparity in mental disorder diagnosis and treatment between non-hispanic White and Asian American patients in a general hospital. Asian J Psychiatr 34:78–83, 2018 29674132

Xu KT, Nelson BK, Berk S: The changing profile of patients who used emergency department services in the United States: 1996 to 2005. Ann Emerg Med 54(6):805.e1-7–810.e1-7, 2009 19811852

Yarnell SC, Kirwin PD, Zonana HV: Geriatrics and the legal system. J Am Acad Psychiatry Law 45(2):208–217, 2017 28619861

Yarns BC, Abrams JM, Meeks TW, et al: The mental health of older LGBT adults. Curr Psychiatry Rep 18(6):60, 2016 27142205

Yohannes AM, Willgoss TG, Baldwin RC, et al: Depression and anxiety in chronic heart failure and chronic obstructive pulmonary disease: prevalence, relevance, clinical implications and management principles. Int J Geriatr Psychiatry 25(12):1209–1221, 2010 20033905

Yon Y, Mikton CR, Gassoumis ZD, et al: Elder abuse prevalence in community settings: a systematic review and meta-analysis. Lancet Glob Health 5(2):e147–e156, 2017 28104184

Young EW, Corby JC, Johnson R: Does depression invalidate competence? Consultants' ethical, psychiatric, and legal considerations. Camb Q Healthc Ethics 2(4):505–515, 1993 8149005

Zandi T, Havenaar JM, Limburg-Okken AG, et al: The need for culture sensitive diagnostic procedures: a study among psychotic patients in Morocco. Soc Psychiatry Psychiatr Epidemiol 43(3):244–250, 2008 18060339

Zhang X, Norton J, Carrière I, et al: Risk factors for late-onset generalized anxiety disorder: results from a 12-year prospective cohort (the ESPRIT study). Transl Psychiatry 5:e536, 2015b 25826111

Zivin K, Wharton T, Rostant O: The economic, public health, and caregiver burden of late-life depression. Psychiatr Clin North Am 36(4):631–649, 2013 24229661

INDEX

*Page numbers printed in **boldface** refer to tables and figures.*

Endocrine disease
    in assessment of anxiety or
        depression in older adults,
        113–114
    association with anxiety, **63**
End-stage renal disease, association
    with anxiety, **64**
Engage (adaptation of CBT), 227
Epidemiologic Catchment Area
    study, 40
Erikson, Erik, 228
Escitalopram, for treatment of late-life
    depression, **236**
Esketamine, for treatment of late-life
    depression and anxiety, 255–257
Estrogens, as factor in late-life
    depression and anxiety, **119**
Eszopiclone, for treatment of insomnia,
    39, **241**
Ethical considerations
    involuntary commitment, 203–204
    suicide at the end of life, 204–206
Ethnicity
    in assessment of late-life
        depression, 125–126
    rating scales and, 147
    suicide rates and, **180**
Ethnic minority elders, 3, 9, 90, 219,
    221–222, 230, **252**, 253, 308–309
    challenges faced by, 12
    depression and anxiety and, 11, 19,
        29, 124, **306–307**
    late-life anxiety and, 66
Executive dysfunction syndrome, 25,
    221
Exercise
    for management of late-life
        depression and anxiety, 228–
        229, 278
    resources for patients, families, and
        caregivers, 280

FAB. *See* Frontal Assessment Battery

Failure to thrive (FTT), as comorbidity
    of late-life depression, 40–41
Falls, 232, 233
Familismo, 11
Family
    anxiety and, 90–91
    communicating with, 156–157, 164
    impact of late-life depression on,
        32–33
    patient support and, 323
    psychoeducation of, 214–217, **215**
    resources for anxiety, 98
    resources for assessment of late-
        life depression and anxiety,
        164–165
    resources for cultural assessment
        of the older adult with
        depression and anxiety, 331
    resources for late-life depression,
        43
    resources for suicide, 208
Fear of falling, 76, **77,** 88–89
Filial piety, 11
Firearms, in suicide attempt, 179–180
Fish oil, 257, **258**
Fluoxetine, **315**
Folic acid, 257, **258**
Frailty, as comorbidity of late-life
    depression, 40–41
Friendship Line, 208
Frontal Assessment Battery (FAB), **139**
FTT. *See* Failure to thrive

GAD. *See* Generalized anxiety disorder
GAD-7. *See* Generalized Anxiety
    Disorder-7
GAI. *See* Geriatric Anxiety Inventory
GAI-SF. *See* Geriatric Anxiety
    Inventory-Short Form
GAS. *See* Geriatric Anxiety Scale
GDS. *See* Geriatric Depression Scale
Gender. *See also* LGBTQ+ older
    adults; Men; Women